Encyclopedia of Drug Discovery and Development: Advanced Research in Drug Discovery

Volume VII

Encyclopedia of Drug Discovery and Development: Advanced Research in Drug Discovery Volume VII

Edited by **Ned Burnett**

New Jersey

Published by Foster Academics,
61 Van Reypen Street,
Jersey City, NJ 07306, USA
www.fosteracademics.com

Encyclopedia of Drug Discovery and Development:
Advanced Research in Drug Discovery
Volume VII
Edited by Ned Burnett

International Standard Book Number: 978-1-63242-142-5 (Hardback)

Contents

Preface   VII

Chapter 1 **Data Analysis Approaches in High Throughput Screening**   1
           Asli N. Goktug, Sergio C. Chai and Taosheng Chen

Chapter 2 **Discovery of Selective and Potent Inhibitors of
           Palmitoylation**   27
           Sonia Lobo Planey

Chapter 3 **Air, Water and Soil: Resources for Drug Discovery**   65
           Luis Jesús Villarreal-Gómez, Irma Esthela Soria-Mercado, Ana Leticia
           Iglesias and Graciela Lizeth Perez-Gonzalez

Chapter 4 **Suppression of Pro-Inflammatory Cytokines via Targeting of
           STAT-Responsive Genes**   81
           Charles J. Malemud

Chapter 5 **The Antibacterial Drug Discovery**   120
           Jie Yanling, Liang Xin and Li Zhiyuan

Chapter 6 **Transition State Analogues of Enzymatic Reaction as
           Potential Drugs**   139
           Karolina Gluza and Pawel Kafarski

Chapter 7 **Colon Cancer: Current Treatments and Preclinical Models for
           the Discovery and Development of New Therapies**   187
           Samuel Constant, Song Huang, Ludovic Wiszniewski and
           Christophe Mas

Chapter 8 **Coupled Enzyme Activity and Thermal Shift Screening of the
           Maybridge Rule of 3 Fragment Library Against *Trypanosoma
           brucei* Choline Kinase; A Genetically Validated
           Drug Target**   212
           Louise L. Major, Helen Denton and Terry K. Smith

Chapter 9   **Applications of Snake Venom Proline-Rich Oligopeptides (Bj-PROs) in Disease Conditions Resulting from Deficient Nitric Oxide Production**   **231**
Claudiana Lameu and Henning Ulrich

Permissions

List of Contributions

Preface

Natural products are a consistent source of potentially effective compounds for the treatment of several disorders. It is believed that the tropical and Middle East regions have the most abundant supplies of natural products across the globe. Secondary metabolites obtained from plants have been employed by humans to treat health disorders, acute infections and chronic illness for a large number of years. Natural products have been greatly replaced by synthetic drugs in the past 100 years. Estimates of 200,000 natural products in plant species have been revised upward as mass spectrometry methodologies have advanced. For advancing countries the recognition and use of endogenous medicinal plants as cures for cancers have become appealing. This book covers important topics such as antibacterial drug discovery, resources for drug discovery, colon cancer: current treatments and preclinical models, etc.

This book is a comprehensive compilation of works of different researchers from varied parts of the world. It includes valuable experiences of the researchers with the sole objective of providing the readers (learners) with a proper knowledge of the concerned field. This book will be beneficial in evoking inspiration and enhancing the knowledge of the interested readers.

In the end, I would like to extend my heartiest thanks to the authors who worked with great determination on their chapters. I also appreciate the publisher's support in the course of the book. I would also like to deeply acknowledge my family who stood by me as a source of inspiration during the project.

Editor

Data Analysis Approaches in High Throughput Screening

Asli N. Goktug, Sergio C. Chai and Taosheng Chen

Additional information is available at the end of the chapter

1. Introduction

With the advances in biotechnology, identification of new therapeutic targets, and better understanding of human diseases, pharmaceutical companies and academic institutions have accelerated their efforts in drug discovery. The pipeline to obtain therapeutics often involves target identification and validation, lead discovery and optimization, pre-clinical animal studies, and eventually clinical trials to test the safety and effectiveness of the new drugs. In most cases, screening using genome-scale RNA interference (RNAi) technology or diverse compound libraries comprises the first step of the drug discovery initiatives. Small interfering RNA (siRNA, a class of double-stranded RNA molecules 20-25 nucleotides in length capable of interfering with the expression of specific genes with complementary nucleotide sequence) screen is an effective tool to identify upstream or downstream regulators of a specific target gene, which may also potentially serve as drug targets for a more efficient and successful treatment. On the other hand, screening of diverse small molecule libraries against a known target or disease-relevant pathway facilitates the discovery of chemical tools as candidates for further development.

Conducting either genome-wide RNAi or small molecule screens has become possible with the advances in high throughput (HT) technologies, which are indispensible to carry out massive screens in a timely manner (Macarron 2006; Martis et al. 2011; Pereira and Williams 2007). In screening campaigns, large quantities of data are collected in a considerably short period of time, making rapid data analysis and subsequent data mining a challenging task (Harper and Pickett 2006). Numerous automatic instruments and operational steps participate in an HT screening process, requiring appropriate data processing tools for data quality assessment and statistical analysis. In addition to quality control (QC) and "hit" selection strategies, pre- and post-processing of the screening data are essential steps in a comprehensive HT operation for subsequent interpretation and annotation of the large data sets. In this chapter, we review statistical data analysis methods developed to meet the needs for handling large datasets generated from HT campaigns. We first discuss the influence of proper assay design on statistical outcomes of the HT screening data. We then highlight similarities and differences among various methods for data normalization, quality assessment and "hit" selection. Information presented here provides guidance to researchers on the major aspects of high throughput screening data interpretation.

2. Role of statistics in HT screening design

2.1. HT screening process

A typical HT screening campaign can be divided into five major steps regardless of the assay type and the assay read-out (Fig. 1). Once target or pathway is identified, assay development is performed to explore the optimal assay conditions, and to miniaturize the assay to a microtiter plate format. Performance of an HT assay is usually quantified with statistical parameters such as signal window, signal variability and Z-factor (see definition in section 4). To achieve acceptable assay performances, one should carefully choose the appropriate reagents, experimental controls and numerous other assay variables such as cell density or protein/substrate concentrations.

The final distribution of the activities from a screening data set depends highly on the target and pathway (for siRNA) or the diversity of the compound libraries, and efforts have been continuously made to generate more diverse libraries (Entzeroth et al. 2009; Gillet 2008; Kummel and Parker 2011; Zhao et al. 2005). Furthermore, the quality and reliability of the screening data is affected by the stability and the purity of the test samples in the screening libraries, where storage conditions should be monitored and validated in a timely manner (Baillargeon et al. 2011; Waybright et al. 2009). For small molecules, certain compounds might interfere with the detection system by emitting fluorescence or by absorbing light, and they should be avoided whenever possible to obtain reliable screening results.

Assay development is often followed by a primary screen, which is carried out at a single concentration (small molecule) or single point measurements (siRNA). As the "hits" identified in the primary screen are followed-up in a subsequent confirmatory screen, it is crucial to optimize the assay to satisfactory standards. Sensitivity - the ability to identify an siRNA or compound as a "hit" when it is a true "hit", and specificity - the ability to classify an siRNA or compound as a "non-hit" when it is not a true "hit", are two critical aspects to identify as many candidates while minimizing false discovery rates. Specificity is commonly emphasized in the confirmatory screens which follow the primary screens. For instance, the confirmatory screen for small molecules often consists of multiple measurements of each compound's activity at various concentrations using different assay formats to assess the compound's potency and selectivity. The confirmatory stage of an RNAi screen using pooled siRNA may be performed in a deconvolution mode, where each well contains a single siRNA. Pooling strategy is also applicable to primary small molecule screens, where a keen pooling design is necessary (Kainkaryam and Woolf 2009). The confirmatory screens of compounds identified from small molecule libraries are followed by lead optimization efforts involving structure-activity relationship investigations and molecular scaffold clustering. Pathway and genetic clustering analysis, on the other hand, are widespread hit follow-up practices for RNAi screens. The processes encompassing hit identification from primary screens and lead optimization methods require powerful software tools with advanced statistical capabilities.

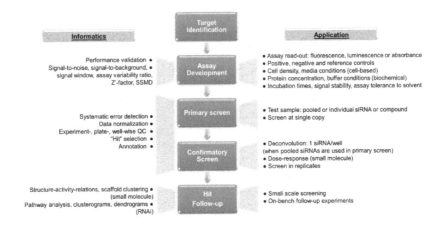

Figure 1. The HT screening process.

Accuracy and precision of an assay are also critical parameters to consider for a successful campaign. While accuracy is a measurement of how close a measured value is to its true value, precision is the proximity of the measured values to each other. Therefore, accuracy of an assay is highly dependent on the performance of the HT instruments in use. Precision, on the other hand, can be a function of sample size and control performances as well as instrument specifications, indicating that the experimental design has a significant impact on the statistical evaluation of the screening data.

2.2. Classical versus robust (resistant) statistics

One of the main assumptions when analyzing HT screening data is that the data is normally distributed, or it complies with the central limit theorem, where the mean of the distributed values converge to normal distribution unless there are systematic errors associated with the screen (Coma et al. 2009). Therefore, log transformations are often applied to the data in the pre-processing stage to achieve more symmetrically distributed data around the mean as in a normal distribution, to represent the relationship between variables in a more linear way especially for cell growth assays, and to make an efficient use of the assay quality assessment parameters (Sui and Wu 2007).

In HT screening practices, the presence of outliers - data points that do not fall within the range of the rest of the data - is generally experienced. Distortions to the normal distribution of the data caused by outliers impact the results negatively. Therefore, an HT data set with outliers needs to be analyzed carefully to avoid an unreliable and inefficient "hit" selection process. Although outliers in control wells can be easily identified, it should be clear that outliers in the test sample may be misinterpreted as real "hits" instead of random errors.

There are two approaches for statistical analysis of data sets with outliers: classical and robust. One can choose to replace or remove outliers based on the truncated mean or similar approaches, and continue the analysis process with classical methods. However, robust statistical approaches have gained popularity in HT screening data analysis in recent decades. In robust statistics, median and median absolute deviation (MAD) are utilized as statistical parameters as opposed to mean and standard deviation (std), respectively, to diminish the effect of outliers on the final analysis results. Although there are numerous approaches to detect and abolish/replace outliers with statistical methods (Hund et al. 2002; Iglewicz and Hoaglin 1993; Singh 1996), robust statistics is preferred for its insensitivity to outliers (Huber 1981). In statistics, while the robustness of an analysis technique can be determined by two main approaches, i.e. influence functions (Hampel et al. 1986) and breakdown point (Hampel 1971), the latter is a more intuitive technique in the concept of HT screening, where the breakdown point of a sample series is defined as the amount of outlier data points that can be tolerated by the statistical parameters before the parameters take on drastically different values that are not representing anymore distribution of the original dataset. In a demonstrated example on a five sample data set, robust parameters were shown to perform superior to the classical parameters after the data set was contaminated with outliers (Rousseeuw 1991). It was also emphasized that median and MAD have a breakdown point of 50%, while mean and std have 0%, indicating that sample sets with 50% outlier density can still be successfully handled with robust statistics.

2.3. False discovery rates

As mentioned previously, depending on the specificity and sensitivity of an HT assay, erroneous assessment of "hits" and "non-hits" is likely. Especially in genome-wide siRNA screens, false positive and negative results may mislead the scientists in the confirmatory studies. While the cause of false discovery results may be due to indirect biological regulations of the gene of interest through other pathways that are not in the scope of the experiment, it may also be due to random errors experienced in the screening process. Although the latter can be easily resolved in the follow-up screens, the former may require a better assay design (Stone et al. 2007). Lower false discovery rates can also be achieved by careful selection of assay reagents to avoid inconsistent measurements (outliers) during screening. The biological interference effects of the reagents in RNAi screens can be considered in two categories: sequence-dependent and sequence-independent (Echeverri et al. 2006; Mohr and Perrimon 2012). Therefore, off-target effects and low transfection efficiencies are the main challenges to be overcome in these screens. Moreover, selection of the appropriate controls for either small molecule or RNAi screens is very crucial for screen quality assessment as well as for "hit" selection, so that the false discovery rates can be inherently reduced. Positive controls are often chosen from small-molecule compounds or gene silencing agents that are known to have the desired effect on the target of interest; however, this may be a difficult task if very little is known about the biological process (Zhang et al. 2008a). On the other hand, selection of negative controls from non-targeting reagents is more challenging due to higher potential of biological off-target effects in RNAi screens compared to the negative controls used in small-molecule screens (Birmingham et al. 2009). Another factor that might interfere with the biological process in an HT screening assay is the bioactive contaminants that may be released from the consumables used in the screening campaign, such as plastic tips and microplates (McDonald et al. 2008; Watson et al. 2009). Unreliable and misleading screening results may be obtained from altered assay conditions caused by leached materials, and boosted false discovery rates may be unavoidable. Hence, the effects of laboratory consumables on the assay readout should be carefully examined during assay development.

The false discovery rates are also highly dependent on the analysis methods used for "hit" selection, and they can be statistically controlled. False discovery rate is defined as the ratio of false discoveries to the total number of discoveries. A t-test and the associated p value are often used for hypothesis testing in a single experiment and can be interpreted as the false positive discovery rate (Chen et al. 2010). However, the challenge arises when multiple hypothesis testing is needed or when the comparison of results across multiple experiments is required. For HT applications, a Bayesian approach was developed to enable plate-wise and experiment-wise comparison of results in a single process, while the false discovery rates can still be controlled (Zhang et al. 2008b). Another method utilizing the strictly standardized mean difference (SSMD) parameter was proven to control the false discovery and non-discovery rates in RNAi screens (Zhang 2007a; Zhang 2010 b; Zhang et al. 2010). By taking the data variability into account, SSMD method is capable of determining "hits" with higher assurance compared to the Z-score and t-test methods.

3. Normalization and systematic error corrections

3.1. Normalization for assay variability

Despite meticulous assay optimization efforts considering all the factors mentioned previously, it is expected to observe variances in the raw data across plates even within the same experiment. Here, we consider these variances as "random" assay variability, which is separate from the systematic errors that can be linked to a known reason, such as failure of an instrument. Uneven assay performances may unpredictably occur at any given time during screening. Hence, normalization of data within each plate is necessary to enable comparable results across plates or experiments allowing a single cut-off for the selection of "hits".

When normalizing the HT screening data, two main approaches can be followed: controls-based and non-controls-based. In controls-based approaches, the assay-specific in-plate positive and negative controls are used as the upper (100%) and lower (0%) bounds of the assay activity, and the activities of the test samples are calculated with respect to these values. Although, it is an intuitive and easily interpretable method, there are several concerns with the use of controls for normalization purposes. With controls-based methods, too high or too low variability in the control wells does not necessarily represent the variability in the sample wells, and the outliers and biases within the control wells might impair the upper and lower activity bounds (Brideau et al. 2003; Coma et al. 2009). Therefore, non-control-based normalizations are favored for better understanding of the overall activity distribution based on the sample activities per se. In this method, most of the samples are assumed to be inactive in order to serve as their own "negative controls". However, this approach may be misleading when the majority of the wells in a plate consist of true "hits" (such as screening a library of bioactive molecules) or siRNAs (e.g., focused library). Since the basal activity level would shift upwards under these conditions, non-controls-based method would result in erroneous decision making.

Plate-wise versus experiment-wise normalization and "hit" picking is another critical point to consider when choosing the best fitting analysis technique for a screen. Experiment-wise normalizations are advantageous in screens where active samples are clustered within certain plates. In this case, each plate is processed in the context of all plates in the experiment. On the other hand, plate-wise normalizations can effectively correct systematic errors occurring in a plate-specific manner without disrupting the results in other plates (Zhang et al. 2006). Therefore, the normalization method that fits best with one's experimental results should be carefully chosen to perform efficient "hit" selection with low false discovery rates.

The calculation used in the most common controls-based normalization methods are as follows:

- Percent of control (PC): Activity of the ith sample (S_i) is divided by the mean of either the positive or negative control wells (C).

$$PC= \frac{S_i}{mean(C)} \times 100 \qquad (1)$$

- Normalized percent inhibition (NPI): Activity of the ith sample is normalized to the activity of positive and negative controls. The sample activity is subtracted from the high control (C_{high}) which is then divided by the difference between mean of the low control (C_{low}) and the mean of the high control. This parameter may be termed normalized percent activity if the final result is subtracted from 100. Additionally, control means may be preferably substituted with the medians.

$$NPI= \frac{mean(C_{high})-S_i}{mean(C_{high})-mean(C_{low})} \times 100 \qquad (2)$$

The calculation used in the most common non-controls-based normalization methods are as follows.

- Percent of samples (PS): The mean of the control wells in the PC parameter (only when negative control is the control of interest) is replaced with the mean of all samples (S_{all}).

$$PS = \frac{S_i}{mean(S_{all})} \times 100 \qquad (3)$$

- Robust percent of samples (RPS): In order to desensitize the PS calculation to the outliers, robust statistics approach is preferred, where mean of S_{all} in PS calculation is replaced with the median of S_{all}.

$$RPS = \frac{S_i}{median(S_{all})} \times 100 \qquad (4)$$

Assay Variability Normalization				
Controls-based	Percent of control $PC = \frac{S_i}{mean(C)} \times 100$	**Non-controls-based**	Percent of samples $PS = \frac{S_i}{mean(S_{all})} \times 100$	Z-score Z-score$= \frac{S_i - mean(S_{all})}{std(S_{all})}$
	Normalized percent inhibition $NPI = \frac{mean(C_{high}) - S_i}{mean(C_{high}) - mean(C_{low})} \times 100$		Robust percent of samples $RPS = \frac{S_i}{median(S_{all})} \times 100$	Robust Z-score Robust Z-score$= \frac{S_i - median(S_{all})}{MAD(S_{all})}$ $MAD(S_{all}) = 1.4826 \times median(|S_i - median(S_{all})|)$
Systematic Error Corrections				
Non-controls-based	Median polish $r_{ijp} = S_{ijp} - \hat{\mu}_p - \hat{row}_i - \hat{col}_j$		BZ-score BZ-score$= \frac{r_{ijp} - mean((r_{ijp})_{all})}{std((r_{ijp})_{all})}$	Well-correction
	B-score B-score$= \frac{r_{ijp}}{MAD_p}$		Background correction $z_{ij} = \frac{1}{N} \sum_{p=1}^{N} S'_{ijp}$	Diffusion state model (can be controls-based too)

Table 1. Summary of HT screening data normalization methods.

- Z-score: Unlike the above parameters, this method accounts for the signal variability in the sample wells by dividing the difference of S_i and the mean of S_{all} by the std of S_{all}. Z-score is a widely used measure to successfully correct for additive and multiplicative offsets between plates in a plate-wise approach (Brideau et al. 2003).

$$Z\text{-score} = \frac{S_i - mean(S_{all})}{std(S_{all})} \qquad (5)$$

- Robust Z-score: Since Z-score calculation is highly affected by outliers, robust version of Z-score is available for calculations insensitive to outliers. In this parameter, the mean and std are replaced with median and MAD, respectively.

$$Robust\ Z\text{-score} = \frac{S_i - median(S_{all})}{MAD(S_{all})} \qquad (6)$$

$$MAD(S_{all})=1.4826 \times median(|S_i-median(S_{all})|) \qquad (7)$$

3.2. Normalization for systematic errors

Besides the data variability between plates due to random fluctuations in assay performance, systematic errors are one of the major concerns in HT screening. For instance plate-
wise spatial patterns play a crucial role in cell-based assay failures. As an example,
incubation conditions might be adjusted to the exact desired temperature and humidity set-
tings, but the perturbed air circulations inside the incubator unit might cause an uneven
temperature gradient, resulting in different cell-growth rates in each well due to evaporation issues. Therefore, depending on the positions of the plates inside the incubator, column-
wise, row-wise or bowl-shape edge effects may be observed within plates (Zhang 2008b;
Zhang 2011b). On the other hand, instrumental failures such as inaccurate dispensing of reagents from individual dispenser channels might cause evident temporal patterns in the final readout. Therefore, experiment-wise patterns should be carefully examined via proper
visual tools. Although some of these issues might be fixed at the validation stage such as
performing routine checks to test the instrument performances, there are numerous algorithms developed to diminish these patterns during data analysis, and the most common
ones are listed as follows and summarized in Table 1.

- Median polish: Tukey's two-way median polish (Tukey 1977) is utilized to calculate the
  row and column effects within plates using a non-controls-based approach. In this method, the row and column medians are iteratively subtracted from all wells until the maxi-
  mum tolerance value is reached for the row and column medians as wells as for the row
  and column effects. The residuals in p^{th} plate (r_{ijp}) are then calculated by subtracting the
  estimated plate average ($\hat{\mu}_p$), i^{th} row effect ($\hat{row}_i$) and j^{th} column effect ($\hat{col}_j$) from the true
  sample value (S_{ijp}). Since median parameter is used in the calculations, this method is rela-
  tively insensitive to outliers.

$$r_{ijp}=S_{ijp}-\hat{\mu}_p-\hat{row}_i-\hat{col}_j \qquad (8)$$

- B-score: This is a normalization parameter which involves the residual values calculated
  from median polish and the sample MAD to account for data variability. The details of
  median polish technique and an advanced B-score method, which accounts for plate-to-
  plate variances by smoothing are provided in (Brideau et al. 2003).

$$B\text{-score}=\frac{r_{ijp}}{MAD_p} \qquad (9)$$

$$MAD_p= 1.4826 \times median(|(r_{ijp})_{all}- median((r_{ijp})_{all})|) \qquad (10)$$

- BZ-score: This is a modified version of the B-score method, where the median polish is
  followed by Z-score calculations. While BZ-score is more advantageous to Z-score be-

cause of its capability to correct for row and column effects, it is less powerful than B-score and does not fit very well with the normal distribution model (Wu et al. 2008).

$$BZ\text{-score}=\frac{r_{ijp}- \text{mean}((r_{ijp})_{all})}{\text{std}((r_{ijp})_{all})} \tag{11}$$

- Background correction: In this correction method, the background signal corresponding to each well is calculated by averaging the activities within each well (S'_{ijp} representing the normalized signal of a well in i^{th} row and j^{th} column in p^{th} plate) across all plates. Then, a polynomial fitting is performed to generate an experiment-wise background surface for a single screening run. The offset of the background surface from a zero plane is considered to be the consequence of present systematic errors, and the correction is performed by subtracting the background surface from each plate data in the screen. The background correction performed on pre-normalized data was found to be more efficient, and exclusion of the control wells was recommended in the background surface calculations. The detailed description of the algorithm is found in (Kevorkov and Makarenkov 2005).

$$z_{ij}=\frac{1}{N}\sum_{p=1}^{N} S'_{ijp} \tag{12}$$

- Well-correction: This method follows an analogous strategy to the background correction method; however, a least-squares approximation or polynomial fitting is performed independently for each well across all plates. The fitted values are then subtracted from each data point to obtain the corrected data set. In a study comparing the systematic error correction methods discussed so far, well-correction method was found to be the most effective for successful "hit" selection (Makarenkov et al. 2007).

- Diffusion-state model: As mentioned previously, the majority of the spatial effects are caused by uneven temperature gradients across assay plates due to inefficient incubation conditions. To predict the amount of evaporation in each well in a time and space dependent manner, and its effect on the resulting data set, a diffusion-state model was developed by (Carralot et al. 2012). As opposed to the above mentioned correction methods, the diffusion model can be generated based on the data from a single control column instead of sample wells. The edge effect correction is then applied to each plate in the screening run based on the generated model.

Before automatically applying a systematic error correction algorithm on the raw data set, it should be carefully considered whether there is a real need for such data manipulation. To detect the presence of systematic errors, several statistical methods were developed (Coma et al. 2009; Root et al. 2003). In a demonstrated study, the assessment of row and column effects was performed based on a robust linear model, so called R score, and it was shown that performing a positional correction using R score on the data that has no or very small spatial effects results in lower specificity. However, correcting a data set with large spatial effects decreases the false discovery rates considerably (Wu et al. 2008). In the same study, receiver operating characteristics (ROC) curves were generated to compare the performance of several positional correction algorithms based on sensitivity and "1-specificity" values, and R-score was found to be the most superior. On the other hand, application of well-correction or diffusion model on data sets with no spatial effects was shown to have no adverse effect on the final "hit" selection (Carralot et al. 2012; Makarenkov et al. 2007). Additionally, reduction of thermal gradients and associated edge effects in cell-based assays was shown to be possible by easy adjustments to the assay workflow, such as incubating the plates at room temperature for 1 hour immediately after dispensing the cells into the wells (Lundholt et al. 2003).

4. QC methods

There are various environmental, instrumental and biological factors that contribute to assay performance in an HT setting. Therefore, one of the key steps in the analysis of HT screening data is the examination of the assay quality. To determine if the data collected from each plate meet the minimum quality requirements, and if any patterns exist before and after data normalization, the distribution of control and test sample data should be examined at experiment-, plate- and well-level. While there are numerous graphical methods and tools available for the visualization of the screening data in various formats (Gribbon et al. 2005; Gunter et al. 2003; Wu and Wu 2010), such as scatter plots, heat maps and frequency plots, there are also many statistical parameters for the quantitative assessment of assay quality. Same as for the normalization techniques, both controls-based and non-controls-based approaches exist for data QC methods. The most commonly-used QC parameters in HT screening are listed as follows and summarized in Table 2.

- Signal-to-background (S/B): This is a simple measure of the ratio of the positive control mean to the background signal mean (i.e. negative control).

$$S/B = \frac{mean(C_{pos})}{mean(C_{neg})} \tag{13}$$

- Signal-to-noise (S/N): This is a similar measure to S/B with the inclusion of signal variability in the formulation. Two alternative versions of S/N are presented below. Both S/B and S/N are considered week parameters to represent dynamic signal range for an HT screen and are rarely used.

$$S/N = \frac{mean\left(C_{pos}\right) - mean\left(C_{neg}\right)}{std\left(C_{neg}\right)} (a)$$

$$S/N = \frac{mean\left(C_{pos}\right) - mean\left(C_{neg}\right)}{\sqrt{std\left(C_{pos}\right)^2 + std\left(C_{neg}\right)^2}} (b) \tag{14}$$

- Signal window (SW): This is a more indicative measure of the data range in an HT assay than the above parameters. Two alternative versions of the SW are presented below, which only differ by denominator.

$$SW=\frac{\left|mean\left(C_{pos}\right)-mean\left(C_{neg}\right)\right|-3x\left(std\left(C_{pos}\right)+std\left(C_{neg}\right)\right)}{std\left(C_{pos}\right)}(a)$$

$$SW=\frac{\left|mean\left(C_{pos}\right)-mean\left(C_{neg}\right)\right|-3x\left(std\left(C_{pos}\right)+std\left(C_{neg}\right)\right)}{std\left(C_{neg}\right)}(b)$$

(15)

- Assay variability ratio (AVR): This parameter captures the data variability in both controls as opposed to SW, and can be defined as (1-Z'-factor) as presented below.

$$AVR=\frac{3 \times std(C_{pos}) - 3 \times std(C_{neg})}{\left|mean(C_{pos}) + mean(C_{neg})\right|}$$

(16)

- Z'-factor: Despite of the fact that AVR and Z'-factor has similar statistical properties, the latter is the most widely used QC criterion, where the separation between positive (C_{pos}) and negative (C_{neg}) controls is calculated as a measure of the signal range of a particular assay in a single plate. Z'-factor has its basis on normality assumption, and the use of 3 std's of the mean of the group comes from the 99.73% confidence limit (Zhang et al. 1999). While Z'-factor accounts for the variability in the control wells, positional effects or any other variability in the sample wells are not captured. Although Z'-factor is an intuitive method to determine the assay quality, several concerns were raised about the reliability of this parameter as an assay quality measure. Major issues associated with the Z'-factor method are that the magnitude of the Z'-factor does not necessarily correlate with the hit confirmation rates, and that Z'-factor is not an appropriate measure to compare the assay quality across different screens and assay types (Coma et al. 2009; Gribbon et al. 2005).

$$Z'\text{-factor}=1 - \frac{3 \times std(C_{pos}) - 3 \times std(C_{neg})}{\left|mean(C_{pos}) + mean(C_{neg})\right|}$$

(17)

- Z-factor: This is the modified version of the Z'-factor, where the mean and std of the negative control are substituted with the ones for the test samples. Although Z-factor is more advantageous than Z'-factor due to its ability to incorporate sample variability in the calculations, other issues associated with Z'-factor (as discussed above) still apply. Additionally, in a focused library in which many possible "hits" are clustered in certain plates, Z-factor would not be an appropriate QC parameter. While assays with Z'- or Z-factor values above 0.5 are considered to be excellent, one may want to include additional measures, such as visual inspection or more advanced formulations in the decision process, especially for cell-based assays with inherently high signal variability. The power of the above mentioned parameters were discussed in multiple studies (Gribbon et al. 2005; Iversen et al. 2006; Macarron and Hertzberg 2009; Stevens et al. 1998).

$$Z\text{-factor}=1 - \frac{3 \times std(C_{pos}) - 3 \times std(S_{all})}{\lceil mean(C_{pos}) + mean(S_{all}) \rceil} \tag{18}$$

- SSMD: It is an alternative quality metric to Z'- and Z-factor, which was recently developed to assess the assay quality in HT screens (Zhang 2007a; Zhang 2007b). Due to its basis on probabilistic and statistical theories, SSMD was shown to be a more meaningful parameter than previously mentioned methods for QC purposes. SSMD differs from Z'- and Z-factor by its ability to handle controls with different effects, which enables the selection of multiple QC criteria for assays (Zhang et al. 2008a). The application of SSMD-based QC criterion was demonstrated in multiple studies in comparison to other commonly-used methods (Zhang 2008b; Zhang 2011b; Zhang et al. 2008a). Although SSMD was developed primarily for RNAi screens, it can also be used for small molecule screens.

$$SSMD= \frac{mean(C_{pos}) - mean(C_{neg})}{\sqrt{std(C_{pos})^2 + std(C_{neg})^2}} \tag{19}$$

Signal-to-background (S/B)	$\frac{mean(C_{pos})}{mean(C_{neg})}$
Signal-to-noise (S/N)	$\frac{mean(C_{pos}) - mean(C_{neg})}{std(C_{neg})}$ or $\frac{mean(C_{pos}) - mean(C_{neg})}{\sqrt{std(C_{pos})^2 + std(C_{neg})^2}}$
Signal window (SW)	$\frac{\lvert mean(C_{pos}) - mean(C_{neg}) \rvert - 3 \times (std(C_{pos}) + std(C_{neg}))}{std(C_{pos})}$ or $\frac{\lvert mean(C_{pos}) - mean(C_{neg}) \rvert - 3 \times (std(C_{pos}) + std(C_{neg}))}{std(C_{neg})}$
Assay variability ratio (AVR)	$\frac{3 \times std(C_{pos}) - 3 \times std(C_{neg})}{\lvert mean(C_{pos}) + mean(C_{neg}) \rvert} = 1 - Z'\text{-factor}$
Z'-factor	$1 - \frac{3 \times std(C_{pos}) - 3 \times std(C_{neg})}{\lvert mean(C_{pos}) + mean(C_{neg}) \rvert}$
Z-factor	$1 - \frac{3 \times std(C_{pos}) - 3 \times std(S_{all})}{\lvert mean(C_{pos}) + mean(S_{all}) \rvert}$
SSMD	$\frac{mean(C_{pos}) - mean(C_{neg})}{\sqrt{std(C_{pos})^2 + std(C_{neg})^2}}$

Table 2. Summary of HT screening data QC methods.

5. "Hit" selection methods

The main purpose of HT screens is to obtain a list of compounds or siRNAs with desirable activity for further confirmation. Therefore, the ultimate goal of an HT screening campaign is to narrow down a big and comprehensive compound or siRNA library to a manageable number of "hits" with low false discovery rates. While the initial library of test samples undergoes multiple phases of elimination, the most critical factor is to select as many true "hits" as possible. After data normalization is applied as necessary, "hit" selection is performed on the plates that pass the QC criterion. As stated previously in Section 2.1, HT processes in primary and confirmatory screens differ in design. The "hit" selection process following a primary screen is similar for RNAi and small-molecule screens, where the screening run is often performed in single copy, and a single data point (obtained from either endpoint or kinetic reading) is collected for each sample. On the other hand, a confirmatory RNAi screen is typically performed in replicates using pooled or individual siRNA, while the confirmatory small-molecule screens are executed in dose-response mode. Here, we classify the "hit" selection methodologies in two major categories: primary and confirmatory screen analysis.

5.1. "Hit" selection in primary screen

Although RNAi and small molecule assays differ in many ways, a common aim is to classify the test samples with relatively higher or lower activities than the reference wells as "hits". Hence, it is required to select an activity cut-off, where test samples with values above or below the cut-off are identified as "hits". It is very crucial to select a sensible cut-off value with enough difference from the noise level in order to reduce false positive rates. Depending on the specific goals of the projects, the cut-off might need to be a reasonable value that leads to a manageable quantity of "hits" for follow-up studies. To guide scientists in the process, numerous "hit" selection methods have been developed for HT screens as presented below.

- Percent inhibition cut-off: The "hits" from HT screening data that is normalized for percent inhibition (NPI method in Section 3.1) can be selected based on a percent cut-off value that is arbitrarily assigned relative to an assay's signal window. As this method does not have much statistical basis to it, it is primarily preferred for small molecule screens with strong controls.

- Mean +/- k std: In this method, cut-off is set to the value that is k std's above or below the sample mean. While the cut-off can be applied to the normalized data, a k value of 3 is typically used, which is associated with the false positive error rate of 0.00135 (Zhang et al. 2006). As this cut-off calculation method is primarily based on normality assumption, it is also equivalent to a Z-score of 3. Since the use of mean and std make this method sensitive to outliers, a more robust version is presented next.

- Median +/- k MAD: To desensitize the "hit" selection to outliers, a cut-off that is k MADs above or below the sample median was developed, and a study comparing the std- and MAD-based "hit" selection methods showed lower false non-discovery rates with the latter (Chung et al. 2008).

- Quartile-based method: Similar to the previous approaches, the quartile-based "hit" selection method is based on the idea of treating the true "hits" as outliers and identifying them by setting upper and lower cut-off boundaries based on the quartiles and interquartiles of the data. The major advantage of the quartile-based method over median +/- k MAD is its more effective cut-off calculation formulation for non-symmetrical data, where upper and lower cut-offs can be determined independently. In the comparison of the three "hit" selection criteria presented so far, the quartile-based method outperformed the other two methods to detect true "hits" with moderate effects (Zhang et al. 2006).

- SSMD and Robust SSMD: This parameter has become a widely-used method for RNAi screening data analysis mainly due to its ability to quantify RNAi effects with a statistical basis, and its better control on false negative and false positive rates (Zhang 2007a; Zhang 2007b; Zhang 2009; Zhang 2010a; Zhang 2010 b; Zhang 2011b; Zhang et al. 2010). SSMD is a robust parameter to capture the magnitude of the RNAi effects with various sample sizes. This scoring method also provides comparison of values across screens. Mean and std in the standard SSMD formula is substituted with median and MAD in the robust version. The SSMD parameter used for the primary screens without replicates holds a linear relationship with the Z-score method.

- Bayesian method: This method is used to combine both plate-wise and experiment-wise information within single "hit" selection calculation based on Bayesian hypothesis testing (Zhang et al. 2008b). Bayesian statistics incorporates a prior data distribution and a likelihood function to generate a posterior distribution function. In HT screening data analysis using this method, the experiment- and plate-wise information is incorporated into the prior and likelihood functions, respectively. With the availability of various prior distribution models, the Bayesian method can be applied either with positive and negative controls or with test sample wells. As this method enables the control of false discovery rates, it is a more powerful "hit" selection measure than the median +/- k MAD when the sample data is used to generate the prior distribution.

5.2. "Hit" selection in confirmatory screen

Different strategies are pursued for the confirmation of "hits" from RNAi and small molecule primary screens. While dose response screens are very common to test the compound activities in a dose-dependent manner in small molecule screens, this is not applicable to RNAi screens. Here, we will present the "hit" selection methods for screens with replicates in two categories: dose-response analysis and others.

5.2.1. Dose-response analysis

After running a primary screen, in which a single concentration of compound is used, a subset of compounds is selected for a more quantitative assessment. These molecules are tested at various concentrations and plotted against the corresponding assay response. These types of curves are commonly referred to as "dose-response" or "concentration-response" curves, and they are generally defined by four parameters: top asymptote (maximal response), bottom asymptote (baseline response), slope (Hill slope or Hill coefficient), and the EC_{50} value.

A plot of signal as a function of concentration results in a rectangular hyperbola when the hill coefficient is 1 (Fig. 2A). Because the concentration range covers several orders of magnitude, the x-axis is normally displayed in the logarithm scale, resulting in a sigmoidal curve (Fig. 2B), which is generally fitted with the Hill equation:

$$signal=B+\frac{T-B}{1+\left(\frac{EC_{50}}{x}\right)^h} \tag{20}$$

The most accepted benchmark for drug potency is the EC_{50} value, which corresponds to the concentration of compound (x) that generates a signal midway between the top (T) and bottom (B) asymptotes (Fig. 2B). The steepness is indicated by the Hill slope (h), also known as the Hill coefficient or the slope factor (Fig. 2C).

It is preferable to apply the Hill equation to concentrations on a logarithmic scale, because the error associated with the EC_{50} (log form) follows a Gaussian distribution (Motulsky and Neubig 2010), as indicated in Eq. 21. The x values represent log[compound].

$$signal=B+\frac{T-B}{1+\left(\frac{10^{Log\ EC_{50}}}{10^x}\right)^h} \tag{21}$$

In biochemical experiments, a Hill coefficient of 1 is indicative of a 1:1 stoichiometry of enzyme-inhibitor or protein-ligand complexes. Under such condition, an increase from 10% to 90% response requires 81-fold change in compound concentration. Hill coefficient values that deviate from unity could reflect mechanistic implications (such as cooperativity or multiple binding sites) or non-ideal behavior of the compound (acting as protein denaturant or causing micelle formation) (Copeland 2005).

For symmetrical curves, the inflection point corresponds to the relative EC_{50} value, which lies halfway between the asymptotes. This relative EC_{50} may be different from the actual EC_{50} if the top and bottom plateaus do not accurately represent 0% and 100% response. For instance, in Fig. 2D, the midpoint in the black curve dictates a value of 60% based on the positive and negative controls. When using the relative EC_{50}, careful analysis of data fitting is necessary to avoid deceptive results, as exemplified by the green curve in Fig. 2D. Curve fitting would provide a relative EC_{50} value of 1 for both the green and black curves, but based on controls, the compound associated with the green curve would inhibit the assay only by 20%. Therefore, it is argued that the best approach is to use a two-parameter curve fit, where only two parameters are allowed to float (EC_{50} and Hill coefficient values), while fixing the top and bottom boundaries as presented in Fig. 2E. (Copeland 2005).

Although EC_{50} is normally the main criterion to categorize compounds for downstream analysis, the value is highly dependent on assay conditions, such as cell number and enzyme/substrate amount (Copeland 2003). For enzymatic assays, a more attractive approach is to consider relative affinities. Cheng and Prusoff formulated a way to convert EC_{50} values to dissociation constants, thus reducing the overload of performing multiple titrations associated with standard enzyme kinetics (Cheng and Prusoff 1973). Nevertheless, the caveat of using this convenient alternative is to recognize the inhibitory modality of the compounds (Copeland 2005): competitive (Eq. 22), non-competitive (Eq. 23) and uncompetitive (Eq. 24).

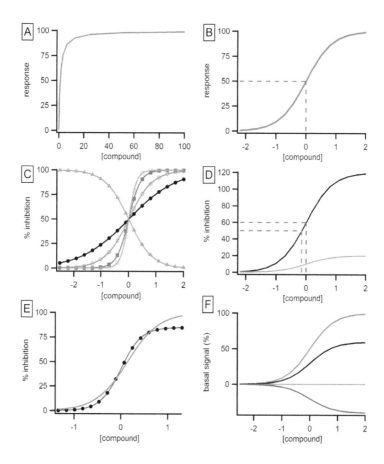

Figure 2. Dose-response curves. A) Response vs. compound concentration resulting in a rectangular hyperbola curve. B) Response vs. logarithm of compound concentration resulting in a sigmoidal curve. The dashed lines indicate the concentration corresponding to half-maximal signal. C) Curves at different Hill slopes: 0.5 (black, closed circles), 1 (red, open circles), 2 (blue, closed squares), 3 (green, open squares) and -1 (pink, closed triangles). D) Relative (blue dash lines) and actual (red dash lines) EC_{50} values for a curve with different top boundary from that of the control (black curve). The green and black curves have the same relative EC_{50}. E) The red curve fits the data points (black circles) allowing 2 parameters (EC_{50}, hill coefficient) to float, while the blue curve fits the data refining all 4 parameters (EC_{50}, hill coefficient, top and bottom asymptotes). F) Curves corresponding to a full agonist (red), partial agonist (black), antagonist (green) and inverse agonist (blue).

$$EC_{50} = K_i \left(1 + \frac{S}{K_M}\right) \tag{22}$$

$$EC_{50} = \frac{S + K_M}{\frac{K_M}{K_i} + \frac{S}{\alpha \times K_i}} \tag{23}$$

$$EC_{50} = \alpha \times K_i \left(1 + \frac{K_M}{S}\right) \tag{24}$$

The dissociation constant of a reversible compound (K_i) can be calculated based on a single substrate concentration (S) and the Michaelis constant (K_M). The constant α delineates the effect of inhibitor binding on the affinity of the substrate for the enzyme. It becomes evident that EC_{50} and K_i are roughly the same at much lower substrate concentration relative to K_M (Eq. 22) or when $\alpha = 1$ (Eq. 23).

Dose-response curves can follow various patterns, depending on the biological system to be investigated. For assays with certain basal level, increasing concentrations of a full agonist triggers a maximal response for the system (Fig. 2F, red curve). A partial agonist displays a reduced response (efficacy) relative to a full agonist (Fig. 2F, black curve), even though they both exhibit the same potency (i.e. same EC_{50} values). An antagonist might have certain affinity or potency, but it would not show any change in basal activity as the efficacy has a value of zero (Fig. 2F, green curve). However, an antagonist reverses the actions of an agonist. In pharmacological terms, the effects of a competitive antagonist can be overcome by augmenting the amount of agonist, but such agonist increment has no effect on the effects of non-competitive antagonists. Inverse agonists reduce the basal response of systems with constitutive activity (Fig. 2F, blue curve).

5.2.2. Other methods

In "hit" selection for confirmatory screens with single concentration of compound or siRNA, hypothesis testing is a commonly-used method to incorporate sample variability of each sample from its replicates. Therefore, confirmatory screens (or some primary screens) are chosen to be performed in replicates to statistically calculate the significance of the sample activity in relation to a negative reference group. Since previously listed Z- and robust Z-score methods assume that the variability of the test samples and the negative controls or references is equal, it is not a reliable measure for confirmatory screens with replicates, where the sample variability can be individually calculated. The most common methods to analyze screening data with replicates are listed below.

- *t*-test: For "hit" selection in confirmatory screens, *t* statistics and the associated *p* value is used to calculate if a sample compound or siRNA is behaving significantly different than the majority of the test samples or controls. A *t*-test determines whether the null hypothesis, which is the mean of a test sample being equal to the mean of the negative reference group, is accepted or not. Paired t-test (first pairing of the test sample and reference value within each plate, then calculating t statistic on the paired values) is often preferred to avoid the distortion of results due to inter-plate variability, whereas unpaired t-test is used for global comparison of the sample replicates with all reference values in the experiment (Zhang 2011a). The p value calculated from t statistic is then used to determine the significance of the sample activity compared to the reference. An alternative to standard t-test, namely randomized variance model (RVM) t-test (Wright and Simon 2003), was found to be more advantageous for screens with few replicates to detect relatively less strong "hits" (Malo et al. 2010).

- SSMD: While t-test is a useful method to calculate the significance of the sample activity by incorporating its variability across replicates, it lacks the ability to rank the samples by their effect sizes. As an alternative to t-test, SSMD-based "hit" selection method for replicates was proposed to enable the calculation of RNAi effects as previously illustrated in (Zhang 2011a). While SSMD-based method is more robust with small sample sizes as opposed to t-test (Zhang 2008a), at least 4 replicates is recommended in confirmatory screens to identify samples with moderate or higher effects (Zhang and Heyse 2009).

- Various other p value calculation methods (e.g., redundant siRNA activity, or RSA) (Konig et al. 2007) and rank products method (Breitling et al. 2004)) are available, which can be adapted to detect "hits" in RNAi screens (Birmingham et al. 2009).

6. Conclusion

HT screening is a comprehensive process to discover new drug targets using siRNA and drug candidates from small molecule libraries. Statistical evaluation of the assay performance is a very critical step in HT screening data analysis. A number of data analysis methods have been developed to correct for plate-to-plate assay variability and systematic errors, and assess assay quality. Statistical analysis is also pivotal in the "hit" selection process from primary screens and in the evaluation during confirmatory screens. While some of these methods may be intuitively applied using spreadsheet programs (e.g., Microsoft Excel), others may require the development of computer programs using more advanced programming environments (e.g., R, Perl, C++, Java, MATLAB). Besides commercially available comprehensive analysis tools, there are also numerous open-access software packages designed for HT screening data management and analysis for scientist with little or no programming knowledge. A short compilation of freely available analysis tools is listed in Table 3. The growing number of statistical methods will accelerate the discovery of drug candidates with higher confidence.

	Features	Programming Language
Screensaver	Web-based laboratory information management system for management of library and screen information (Tolopko et al. 2010)	Java
MScreen	Web-based compound library and siRNA plate management, QC and dose-response fitting tools (Jacob et al. 2012)	PHP, Oracle/MySQL
NEXT-RNAi	Library design and evaluation tools for RNAi screens (Horn et al. 2010)	Perl
K-Screen	Analysis, visualization, management and mining of HT screening data including dose-response curve fitting (Tai et al. 2011)	R, PHP, MySQL
HTS-Corrector	Statistical analysis, visualization and correction of systematic errors for all HT screens (Makarenkov et al. 2006)	C#
web cellHTS2	Web-based analysis toolbox for normalization, QC, "hit" selection and annotation for RNAi screens (Boutros et al. 2006; Pelz et al. 2010)	R/Bioconductor project
RNAither	Automated pipeline for normalization, QC, "hit" selection and pathway generation for RNAi screens (Rieber et al. 2009)	R/Bioconductor project
HTSanalyzeR	Gene set enrichment, network and gene set comparison analysis for post-processing of RNAi screening data (Wang et al. 2011)	R/Bioconductor project

Table 3. Examples of open-access software packages for library management and statistical analysis of HT screening data.

Acknowledgements

This work was supported by the American Lebanese Syrian Associated Charities (ALSAC), St. Jude Children's Research Hospital, and National Cancer Institute grant P30CA027165.

Author details

Asli N. Goktug, Sergio C. Chai and Taosheng Chen

High Throughput Screening Center, Department of Chemical Biology and Therapeutics, St. Jude Children's Research Hospital, USA

References

[1] Ang, K. L., Feroze, F., Ganji, G.,& Li, Y. (2004). Cell-based RNAi assay development for HTS. In: *Assay Guidance Manual*. Sittampalam, G. S., Gal-Edd, N., Arkin, M., Auld, D., Austin, C., Bejcek, B., Glicksman, M., Inglese, J., Lemmon, V., Li, Z., McGee, J., McManus, O., Minor, L., Napper, A., Riss, T., Trask, J., &Weidner J., pp. 1-20, Eli Lilly & Company, Retrieved from http://www.ncbi.nlm.nih.gov/books/NBK91998/

[2] Baillargeon, P., Scampavia, L., Einsteder, R., & Hodder, P. (2011). Monitoring of HTS compound library quality via a high-resolution image acquisition and processing instrument. *Journal of Laboratory Automation*, Vol. 16, No. 3, pp. 197-203.

[3] Birmingham, A., Selfors, L. M., Forster, T., Wrobel, D., Kennedy, C. J., Shanks, E., Santoyo-Lopez, J., Dunican, D. J., Long, A., Kelleher, D., Smith, Q., Beijersbergen, R. L., Ghazal, P., & Shamu, C. E. (2009). Statistical methods for analysis of high-throughput RNA interference screens. *Nature Methods*, Vol. 6, No. 8, pp. 569-75.

[4] Boutros, M., Bras, L. P., & Huber, W. (2006). Analysis of cell-based RNAi screens. *Genome Biology*, Vol. 7, No. 7, pp. R66.1-11.

[5] Breitling, R., Armengaud, P., Amtmann, A., & Herzyk, P. (2004). Rank products: a simple, yet powerful, new method to detect differentially regulated genes in replicated microarray experiments. *FEBS Letters*, Vol. 573, No. 1-3, pp. 83-92.

[6] Brideau, C., Gunter, B., Pikounis, B., & Liaw, A. (2003). Improved statistical methods for hit selection in high-throughput screening. *Journal of Biomolecular Screening*, Vol. 8, No. 6, pp. 634-47.

[7] Carralot, J. P., Ogier, A., Boese, A., Genovesio, A., Brodin, P., Sommer, P.,& Dorval, T. (2012). A novel specific edge effect correction method for RNA interference screenings. *Bioinformatics*,Vol. 28, No. 2, pp. 261-68.

[8] Chen, J. J., Roberson, P. K., & Schell, M. J. (2010). The false discovery rate: a key concept in large-scale genetic studies. *Cancer Control*, Vol. 17, No. 1, pp. 58-62.

[9] Cheng, Y., & Prusoff, W. H. (1973). Relationship between the inhibition constant (K1) and the concentration of inhibitor which causes 50 per cent inhibition (I50) of an enzymatic reaction. *Biochemical Pharmacology*, Vol. 22, No. 23, pp. 3099-108.

[10] Chung, N., Zhang, X. D., Kreamer, A., Locco, L., Kuan, P., Bartz, S., Linsley, P. S., Ferrer, M., & Strulovici, B. (2008). Median absolute deviation to improve hit selection

for genome-scale RNAi screens. *Journal of Biomolecular Screening*, Vol. 13, No. 2, pp. 149-58.

[11] Coma, I., Herranz, J., & Martin, J. (2009). Statistics and decision making in high-throughput screening. In: *High Throughput Screening, Methods in Molecular Biology, Methods and Protocols*, Janzen, W. P. & Bernasconi, P., pp. 69-106, Humana Press, ISBN 9781603272575, New York.

[12] Copeland, R. A. (2003). Mechanistic considerations in high-throughput screening. *Analytical Biochemistry*, Vol. 320, No. 1, pp. 1-12.

[13] Copeland, R. A. (2005). *Evaluation of Enzyme Inhibitors in Drug Discovery: A Guide for Medicinal Chemists and Pharmacologists*, John Wiley & Sons, ISBN 978-0-471-68696-5, Hoboken, New Jersey.

[14] Echeverri, C. J., Beachy, P. A., Baum, B., Boutros, M., Buchholz, F., Chanda, S. K., Downward, J., Ellenberg, J., Fraser, A. G., Hacohen, N., Hahn, W. C., Jackson, A. L.,Kiger, A., Linsley, P. S., Lum, L., Ma, Y., Mathey-Prevot, B., Root, D. E., Sabatini, D. M., Taipale, J., Perrimon, N.,& Bernards, R. (2006). Minimizing the risk of reporting false positives in large-scale RNAi screens. *Nature Methods*, Vol. 3, No. 10, pp. 777-79.

[15] Entzeroth, M., Flotow, H.,& Condron, P.(2009). Overview of high-throughput screening. In: *Current Protocols in Pharmacology*, pp. 9.4.1-27, John Wiley & Sons, Retrieved from http://onlinelibrary.wiley.com/doi/10.1002/0471141755.ph0904s44/abstract

[16] Gillet, V. J. (2008). New directions in library design and analysis. *Current Opinion in Chemical Biology*, Vol. 12, No. 3, pp. 372-78.

[17] Gribbon, P., Lyons, R., Laflin, P., Bradley, J., Chambers, C., Williams, B. S., Keighley, W., & Sewing, A. (2005). Evaluating real-life high-throughput screening data. *Journal of Biomolecular Screening*, Vol. 10, No. 2, pp. 99-107.

[18] Gunter, B., Brideau, C., Pikounis, B., &Liaw, A. (2003). Statistical and graphical methods for quality control determination of high-throughput screening data. *Journal of Biomolecular Screening*, Vol. 8, No. 6, pp. 624-33.

[19] Hampel, F. R. (1971). A General qualitative definition of robustness. *The Annals ofMathematical Statistics*, Vol. 42, No. 6, pp. 1887-96.

[20] Hampel, F. R., Ronchetti, E. M., Rousseeuw, P. J.,& Stahel, W. A. (1986). *Robust Statistics: The Approach Based on Influence Functions*. John Wiley & Sons, ISBN 9780471829218, New York.

[21] Harper, G., & Pickett, S. D. (2006). Methods for mining HTS data. *Drug Discovery Today*, Vol. 11, No. 16-16, pp. 694-99.

[22] Horn, T., Sandmann, T.,& Boutros, M. (2010). Design and evaluation of genome-wide libraries for RNA interference screens. *Genome Biology*, Vol. 11, No. 6, pp. R61.1-12.

[23] Huber, P. J. (1981). *Robust Statistics*. John Wiley& Sons, ISBN 9780471418054, New York.

[24] Hund, E., Massart, D. L., & Smeyers-Verbeke, J. (2002). Robust regression and outlier detection in the evaluation of robustness tests with different experimental designs. *AnalyticaChimica Acta*, Vol. 463, No. 1,pp. 53-73.

[25] Iglewicz, B., & Hoaglin, D. C. (1993). *How to detect and handle outliers.*ASQC Quality Press. ISBN 9780873892476, Wisconsin.

[26] Iversen, P. W., Eastwood, B. J., Sittampalam, G. S., &Cox, K. L. (2006). A comparison of assay performance measures in screening assays: Signal window, Z ' factor, andassay variability ratio. *Journal of Biomolecular Screening*, Vol. 11, No. 3, pp. 247-52.

[27] Jacob, R. T., Larsen, M. J., Scott, S. D., Kirchhoff, P. D., Sherman, D. H., & Neubig, R. R.(2012). MScreen: An Integrated Compound Management and High-Throughput Screening Data Storage and Analysis System. *Journal of Biomolecular Screening*, Vol. 20, No. 10, pp. 1-8.

[28] Kainkaryam, R. M.& Woolf, P. J. (2009). Pooling in high-throughput drug screening. Current Opinion in Drug Discovery &Development, Vo. 12, No. 3, pp. 339-50.

[29] Kevorkov, D. & Makarenkov, V. (2005). Statistical analysis of systematic errors in high-throughput screening. *Journal of Biomolecular Screening*, Vol. 10, No. 6, pp. 557-67.

[30] Konig, R., Chiang, C., Tu, B. P., Yan, S. F., DeJesus, P. D., Romero, A., Bergauer, T., Orth, A., Krueger, U., Zhou, Y., & Chanda, S. K. (2007). A probability-based approach for the analysis of large-scale RNAi screens. *Nature Methods*, Vol. 4, No. 10, pp. 847-49.

[31] Kummel, A., & Parker, C. N. (2011). The Interweaving of Cheminformatics and HTS. In: *Cheminformatics and Computational Chemical Biology, Methods in Molecular Biology*, Bajorath, J., pp. 435-457, Springer Science+Business Media, ISBN 9781607618393, New York.

[32] Lundholt, B. K., Scudder, K. M.,& Pagliaro, L. (2003). A simple techniquefor reducing edge effect in cell-based assays. *Journal of Biomolecular Screening*, Vol. 8, No. 5, pp. 566-70.

[33] Macarron, R. (2006). Critical review of the role of HTS in drug discovery. *Drug Discovery Today*, Vol. 11, No. 7-8, pp. 277-279.

[34] Macarron, R., &Hertzberg, R. P.(2009). Design and implementation of high throughput screening assays. In: *High Throughput Screening, Methods in Molecular Biology*, Janzen, W. P. & Bernasconi, P., pp. 1-32, Springer Science+Business Media, ISBN 9781603272582, New York.

[35] Makarenkov, V., Kevorkov, D., Zentilli, P., Gagarin, A., Malo, N., & Nadon, R. (2006). HTS-Corrector: software for the statistical analysis and correction of experimental high-throughput screening data. *Bioinformatics*, Vol. 22, No. 11, pp. 1408-09.

[36] Makarenkov, V., Zentilli, P., Kevorkov, D., Gagarin, A., Malo, N., &Nadon, R. (2007).An efficient method for the detection and elimination of systematic error in high-throughput screening. *Bioinformatics*, Vol. 23, No. 13, pp. 1648-57.

[37] Malo, N., Hanley, J. A., Carlile, G., Liu, J., Pelletier, J., Thomas, D. &Nadon, R. (2010). Experimental design and statistical methods for improved hit detection in high-throughput screening. *Journal of Biomolecular Screening*, Vol. 15, No. 8, pp. 990-1000.

[38] Martis, E. A., Radhakrishnan, R., & Badve, R. R. (2011). High-Throughput Screening: The Hits and Leads of Drug Discovery- An Overview. *Journal of Applied PharmaceuticalScience*, Vol. 1, No. 1, pp. 2-10.

[39] McDonald, G. R., Hudson, A. L., Dunn, S. M., You, H., Baker, G. B., Whittal, R. M., Martin, J. W., Jha, A., Edmondson, D. E., & Holt, A. (2008). Bioactive contaminants leach from disposable laboratory plasticware. *Science*, Vol. 322, No. 5903,pp. 917.

[40] Mohr, S., Bakal, C., & Perrimon, N. (2010). Genomic screening with RNAi: results and challenges. *Annual Review of Biochemistry*, Vol. 79, pp. 37-64.

[41] Mohr, S. E.,& Perrimon, N. (2012). RNAi screening: new approaches, understandings, and organisms. *Wiley Interdisciplinary Reviews*. RNA. Vol. 3, No. 2, pp. 145-158.

[42] Motulsky, H. J.,&Neubig, R. R. (2010). Analyzing binding data. In: *Currrent Protocols in Neuroscience*, pp. 7.5.1-65, John Wiley and Sons, Retrieved from http://onlinelibrary.wiley.com/doi/10.1002/0471142301.ns0705s52/full

[43] Pelz, O., Gilsdorf, M., & Boutros, M. (2010). web cellHTS2: a web-application for the analysis of high-throughput screening data. *BMC Bioinformatics*, Vol. 11, pp. 185-90.

[44] Pereira, D. A.,& Williams, J. A. (2007). Origin and evolution of high throughput screening. *British Journal of Pharmacology*, Vol. 152, No. 1, pp. 53-61.

[45] Rieber, N., Knapp, B., Eils, R.,& Kaderali, L. (2009). RNAither, an automated pipeline for the statistical analysis of high-throughput RNAi screens. *Bioinformatics*, Vol. 25, No. 5, pp. 678-679.

[46] Root, D. E., Kelley, B. P., & Stockwell, B. R. (2003). Detecting spatial patterns in biological array experiments. *Journal of Biomolecular Screening*, Vol. 8, No. 4, pp. 393-398.

[47] Rousseeuw, P. J. (1991). Tutorial to Robust Statistics. *Journal of Chemometrics*, Vol. 5, No. 1, pp. 1-20.

[48] Singh, A. (1996). Outliers and robust procedures in some chemometric applications. *Chemometrics and Intelligent Laboratory Systems*, Vol. 33, No. 2, pp. 75-100.

[49] Stevens, M. E., Bouchard. P. J., Kariv, I., Chung, T. D. Y., &Oldenburg, K. R. (1998). Comparison of automation equipment in high throughput screening. *Journal of Biomolecular Screening*, Vol. 3, No. 4, pp. 305-11.

[50] Stone, D. J., Marine, S., Majercak, J., Ray, W. J., Espeseth, A., Simon, A., & Ferrer, M. (2007). High-throughput screening by RNA interference: control of two distinct types of variance. *Cell Cycle*, Vol. 6, No. 8, pp. 898-901.

[51] Sui, Y., & Wu, Z. (2007). Alternative statistical parameter for high-throughput screening assay quality assessment. *Journal of Biomolecular Screening*, Vol. 12, No. 2, pp. 229-34.

[52] Tai, D., Chaguturu, R., & Fang, J. (2011). K-Screen: a free application for high throughput screening data analysis, visualization, and laboratory information management. *Combinatorial Chemistry & High Throughput Screening*, Vol. 14, No. 9, pp. 757-65.

[53] Tolopko, A. N., Sullivan, J. P., Erickson, S. D., Wrobel, D., Chiang, S. L., Rudnicki, K., Rudnicki, S., Nale, J., Selfors, L. M., Greenhouse, D., Muhlich, J. L., & Shamu, C. E. (2010). Screensaver: an open source lab information management system (LIMS) for high throughput screening facilities. *BMC Bioinformatics*, Vol. 11, pp. 260-73.

[54] Tukey, J. W. (1977). *Exploratory data analysis*. Addison-Wesley Publishing Company, ISBN 9780201076165, Massachusetts.

[55] Wang, X., Terfve, C., Rose, J. C., & Markowetz, F. (2011).HTSanalyzeR: an R/Bioconductor package for integrated network analysis of high-throughput screens. *Bioinformatics*, Vol. 27, No. 6, pp. 879-80.

[56] Watson, J., Greenough, E. B., Leet, J. E., Ford, M. J., Drexler. D. M., Belcastro, J. V., Herbst, J. J., Chatterjee, M., & Banks, M. (2009). Extraction, identification, and functional characterization of a bioactive substance from automated compound-handling plastic tips. *Journal of Biomolecular Screening*, Vol. 14, No. 5, pp. 566-72.

[57] Waybright, T. J., Britt, J. R., & McCloud, T. G. (2009). Overcoming problems of compound storage in DMSO: solvent and process alternatives. *Journal of Biomolecular Screening*, Vol. 14, No. 6, pp. 708-15.

[58] Wright, G. W.,& Simon, R. M. (2003). A random variance model for detection of differential gene expression in small microarray experiments. *Bioinformatics*, Vol. 19, No. 18, pp. 2448-55.

[59] Wu, Z., Liu, D.,&Sui, Y. (2008). Quantitative assessment of hit detection and confirmation in single and duplicate high-throughput screenings.*Journal of Biomolecular Screening*, Vol. 13, No. 2, pp. 159-167.

[60] Wu, Z., & Wu, Z., (2010). Exploration, visualization, and preprocessing of high-dimensional data. *Statistical Methods in Molecular Biology*, Vol. 620, pp. 267-84.

[61] Xin, H., Bernal, A., Amato, F. A., Pinhasov, A., Kauffman, J., Brenneman, D. E., Derian, C. K., Andrade-Gordon, P., Plata-Salaman, C. R., &Ilyin, S. E. (2004).High-

throughput siRNA-based functional target validation. *Journal of Biomolecular Screening*, Vol. 9, No. 4, pp. 286-93.

[62] Zhang, J., Chung, T. D. Y., & Oldenburg, K. R. (1999). A simple statistical parameter for use in evaluation and validation of high throughput screening assays. *Journal of Biomolecular Screening*, Vol. 4, No. 2, pp. 67-73.

[63] Zhang, X. D. (2007a). A new method with flexible and balanced control of false negatives and false positives for hit selection in RNA interference high-throughput screening assays. *Journal of Biomolecular Screening*, Vol. 12, No. 5, pp. 645-55.

[64] Zhang, X. D. (2007b). A pair of new statistical parameters for quality control in RNA interference high-throughput screening assays. *Genomics*, Vol. 89, No. 4, pp. 552-61.

[65] Zhang, X. D. (2008a). Genome-wide screens for effective siRNAs through assessing the size of siRNA effects. *BMC Research Notes*, Vol. 1, pp. 33-39.

[66] Zhang, X. D. (2008b). Novel analytic criteria and effective plate designs for quality control in genome-scale RNAi screens. *Journal of Biomolecular Screening*, Vol. 13, No. 5, pp. 363-77.

[67] Zhang, X. D. (2009). A method for effectively comparing gene effects in multiple conditions in RNAi and expression-profiling research. *Pharmacogenomics*, Vol. 10, No. 3, pp. 345-58.

[68] Zhang, X. D. (2010a). Assessing the size of gene or RNAi effects in multifactor high-throughput experiments. *Pharmacogenomics*, Vol. 11, No. 2, pp. 199-213.

[69] Zhang, X. D. (2010b). An effective method for controlling false discovery and false nondiscovery rates in genome-scale RNAi screens. *Journal of Biomolecular Screening*, Vol. 15, No. 9, pp. 1116-22.

[70] Zhang, X. D. (2011a). Illustration of SSMD, z score, SSMD*, z* score, and t statistic for hit selection in RNAi high-throughput screens. *Journal of Biomolecular Screening*, Vol. 16, No. 7, pp. 775-85.

[71] Zhang, X. D. (2011b). *Optimal high-throughput screening: practical experimental design and data analysis for genome-scale RNAi research*. Cambridge University Press, ISBN 9780521734448, New York.

[72] Zhang, X. D., Espeseth, Johnson. E. N., Chin, J., Gates, A., Mitnaul, L. J., Marine, S. D., Tian, J., Stec, E. M., Kunapuli, P., Holder, D. J., Heyse, J. F., Strulovici, B.,& Ferrer, M. (2008a). Integrating experimental and analytic approaches to improve data quality in genome-wide RNAi screens. *Journal of Biomolecular Screening*, Vol.13, No. 5, pp. 378-89.

[73] Zhang, X. D.,& Heyse, J. F. (2009). Determination of sample size in genome-scale RNAi screens. *Bioinformatics*, Vol. 25, No. 7, pp. 841-44.

[74] Zhang, X. D., Kuan, P. F., Ferrer, M., Shu, X., Liu, Y. C., Gates, A. T., Kunapuli, P., Stec, E. M., Xu, M., Marine, S. D., Holder, D. J., Strulovici, B., Heyse, J. F., & Espeseth,

A. S. (2008b). Hit selection with false discovery rate control in genome-scale RNAi screens. *Nucleic Acids Research*, Vol. 36, No. 14, pp. 4667-79.

[75] Zhang, X. D., Lacson, R., Yang, R., Marine, S. D., McCampbell, A., Toolan, D. M., Hare, T. R., Kajdas, J., Berger, J. P., Holder, D. J., Heyse, J. F., & Ferrer, M.(2010). The use of SSMD-based false discovery and false nondiscovery rates in genome-scale RNAi screens. *Journal of Biomolecular Screening*, Vol. 15, No. 9, pp. 1123-231.

[76] Zhang, X. D., Yang, X. C., Chung, N., Gates, A., Stec, E., Kunapuli, P., Holder, D. J., Ferrer, M., & Espeseth, A. S. (2006). Robust statistical methods for hit selection in RNA interference high-throughput screening experiments. *Pharmacogenomics*, Vol. 7, No. 3, pp. 299-309.

[77] Zhao, L., Li, T., Pan, Y., Ning, H., Liu, Z.,& Fan, D. (2005). Application of siRNA library in high-throughput genetic screens of mammalian cells. *Journal of Cancer Molecules*, Vol. 1, No. 1, pp. 19-25.

Chapter 2

Discovery of Selective and Potent Inhibitors of Palmitoylation

Sonia Lobo Planey

Additional information is available at the end of the chapter

1. Introduction

Palmitoylation is a reversible, post-translational modification of a protein through the addition of the 16-carbon fatty acid, palmitate, to a cysteine residue. There are two types of palmitoylation, one called thio- or S-palmitoylation in which palmitate is added to the thiol side chain of a cysteine residue via a labile thioester bond [1]. The other type, N-palmitoylation, is the addition of palmitate to an N-terminal cysteine via a stable amide bond [2]. The two forms of palmitoylation are regulated by different families of palmitoyl acyltransferases (PATs)—S-palmitoylation via a family of multi-pass transmembrane proteins called DHHC (Asp-His-His-Cys) proteins [3] and N-palmitoylation via a family of multi-pass transmembrane proteins termed membrane-bound O-acyltransferase [4]. S-palmitoylation, the focus of this chapter, is more common and because of the labile thioester bond, can dynamically regulate protein sorting and function.

Palmitoylation increases the lipophilicity of the modified protein often changing its subcellular distribution in both dramatic and subtle ways. The larger-scale changes occur when cytoplasmic proteins relocate from the cytoplasm to membrane and when integral membrane proteins move from one membrane system to another, such as from the endoplasmic reticulum (ER) to the plasma membrane (PM). The more subtle changes, in terms of distance, occur at the nanoscale level within a membrane. The increase in lipophilicity upon palmitoylation often results in an altered affinity for a particular lipid microenvironment within that membrane [5]. For example, lipid rafts are small islands in membranes with distinct lipid compositions that selectively attract or exclude both peripheral (often exclusively by virtue of palmitoylation) and integral membrane palmitoylated proteins. Palmitoylated proteins have affinity for lipid rafts that are rich in cholesterol, while prenylated proteins have little or no affinity for these rafts [5]. Such lipophilicity-driven changes in protein distribution may alter access of a palmitoylated protein to extracellular ligands (when the protein moves from the ER to the PM), protein-protein interactions, or the engagement of the palmitoyl-protein in multi-molecular signaling complexes. The role of palmitoylation as a versatile protein sorting signal, regulating intracellular protein trafficking and targeting to membrane microdomains has been reviewed recently [6]. Palmitate may be the most common lipid species to occupy cysteine residues, but it is not the only one. Marilyn Resh and colleagues identified the lipid moieties resident on the cysteine residue of the N-terminal tail of Src family kinases [7-9]. While for these proteins the cysteine residue near the N-terminus is most frequently palmitoylated, it is also modified by palmitoleate, stearate, or oleate with a frequency that is apparently related to the abundance of palmitate in cells [10]. The physiological differences that result from proteins being modified by these other lipids has not been explored extensively; however, given their different physical properties, it seems reasonable that their impact on a protein should be subtly different than palmitate.

Unlike other forms of lipidation such as myristoylation and prenylation, palmitoylation is reversible, by virtue of the labile thioester bond. This allows for dynamic regulation of the protein's lipophilicity [11-13]. By contrast, prenyl groups are attached to cysteines by a stable thioether bond and myristate to glycines by a stable amide bond. It is now apparent that many instances of palmitoylation are enzymatically mediated by a family of palmitoyl acyltransferases (PATs), whereas the mechanisms for depalmitoylation are poorly understood. Nevertheless, it is known that palmitate cycles on and off of many proteins at variable rates ranging from minutes to days. Such dynamic regulation makes palmitoylation unique among post-translational protein lipid modifications and places it in a category similar to phosphorylation. Discovering the molecular identity of PATs was a pivotal event that dramatically accelerated the pace of discovery in the field. Likewise, there has been increased interest in palmitoylation partly because many of the genes encoding PATs have been linked to human diseases like cancer. With a greater understanding of how palmitate is enzymatically attached to proteins, some of the most interesting questions include: What are the substrate(s) of each PAT?; how does a PAT recognize and palmitoylated a substrate?; how are PATs regulated?; and how is depalmitoylation regulated? The answers to these questions are beginning to unfold due to the recent discovery of pharmacological modulators of palmitoylation as well as the development of novel assays and refinement of existing assays. Our ability to understand palmitoylation and its importance to human health and disease is only as good as the methods we use to test our hypotheses. Thus, the discovery of potent and selective inhibitors of palmitoylation as well as the continued development of assays with increased sensitivity and selectivity is critical to this venture.

2. Palmitoylation and DHHC proteins

2.1. Molecular identity of palmitoyl acyltransferases (PATs)

It has been known for many years that palmitoylation is a critical regulator of diverse and complex signaling networks, but the mechanism responsible for palmitoylation of most proteins remained a mystery and somewhat controversial until only recently. The apparent absence of a consensus site for palmitoylation encoded by the sequence of amino acid residues surrounding palmitoyl cysteines, as well as the difficulty in purifying and identifying the enzymes capable of mediating the reaction, led many to believe that it was autocatalytic. Given these issues and the high reactivity of cysteines and palmitoyl-CoA, especially in *in vitro* protein palmitoylation assays, the possibility was not unreasonable [11, 14, 15]. Many of the arguments for and against autocatalytic palmitoylation have been reviewed recently [16].Yet, given the prevalence of palmitoylated proteins in parts of cells where signaling events are so highly concentrated, complex, and regulated, such as the neuronal synapse, it seemed somewhat unreasonable that all regulation of palmitoylation could be left to diffusion—a nagging reality that kept the search for an enzymatic mechanism alive despite the arguments to the contrary. Additionally, there was evidence over the years in support of the idea that these enzymes existed because PAT activity in detergent solubilized protein fractions had been measured using viral glycoproteins [17], p59*fyn* [18], and H-Ras [19] as substrates among others.

The experiments that conclusively provided the molecular identity of PATs were presented in a series of papers spanning almost a decade. The experimental model organism that ultimately provided the information was yeast. First, palmitoylation-dependent alleles of yeast *RAS2* were identified. A genetic screen designed to identify mutations that rendered cells non-viable if Ras2p was not palmitoylated was utilized to identify mutations in two genes- *ERF2* and *ERF4/SHR5* [20, 21]. These mutations resulted in diminished palmitoylation of Ras2p and mislocalization of GFP-Ras2p (respectively or it takes both mutations to cause both effects [20, 22]). However, it could not be decisively concluded if the mutations in *ERF2* and *ERF4* were affecting Ras2p palmitoylation directly or indirectly by altering Ras2p trafficking (which could have prevented an interaction between the palmitoyl acyltransferase and Ras2p).

In collaboration with Maurine Linder, Deschenes and colleagues used an *in vitro* palmitoylation assay to show that Erf2p and Erf4p together constituted a Ras2p PAT that used palmitoyl-CoA as a donor [23]. Erf2p is a ~42-kDa integral membrane protein that is expressed in the ER. The protein contains the DHHC-CRD (Asp-His-His-Cys-cysteine rich domain), also referred to as the NEW1 or zf-DHHC domain (PF01529), which is found in an extensive family of membrane proteins ranging from unicellular eukaryotes to humans [24, 25]. This domain is now recognized as the molecular signature for PATs that add palmitate to cysteines via a labile thioester bond.

At almost the same time that the Erf2p/Erf4p complex was identified as the Ras2p PAT, Akr1p was identified as a PAT with specificity for Yck2p [26]. An important clue leading to the relationship between these two proteins came from the fact that mutants in both Ras2p and Yck2P exhibited a reduced rate of pheromone receptor internalization [27, 28]. Akr1p contains a DHYC-CRD instead of a DHHC-CRD as well as ankyrin repeats not present in Erf2p. The DHYC motif present in three yeast proteins (Akr1p, Akr2p and Pfa5) does not appear to occur in the mammalian genome. Akr1p and Akr2p are most closely related to the mammalian HIP14 (DHHC17) and HIP14L (DHHC13) which contains the variant DQHC—the only observed mammalian deviation from DHHC [3].

2.2. The ZDHHC family of PATs

The mammalian genome contains at least 23 members of the *ZDHHC* PAT gene family identified by the presence of the signature DHHC-cysteine rich domain. Members of the family had been identified as being genes of interest (e.g., "REAM" in metastatic cancer [29]) prior to understanding their function. The genomic structure of *ZDHHC* genes varies widely, including the number and differential use of exons that are spliced together to generate the mRNA. EC gene analyses (http://genome.ewha.ac.kr/ECgene/) of the mRNAs that encode PATs suggest that all of the genes are alternatively spliced at various sites throughout the protein coding sequence as well as within untranslated regions. Many of the putative, alternatively-spliced exons are predicted to encode small peptides that change the structure of the protein in a way that may alter substrate specificity. Similarly, splicing may alter sites for other post-translational modifications, such as phosphorylation or glycosylation, all of which may regulate activity, substrate specificity, subcellular distribution, or interactions with non-substrate proteins. *ZDHHC7*, for example, alters the use of a 111 bp exon that is differentially and specifically expressed in tissues such as placenta, lung, liver, thymus, and small intestine [30]. This exon encodes a 37-residue peptide (EKSSDCRP-SACTVKTGLDPTLVGICGEGTESVQSLLL) within the intracellular loop between transmembrane domain 2 (TM2) and TM3 that contains a PKC phosphorylation site. It is conceivable that phosphorylation of this serine changes DHHC7 in such a way that substrate specificity or the rate of palmitate transfer activity is altered. In addition to alternative mRNA splicing, aberrant splicing induced by mutations or single nucleotide polymorphisms has been shown to occur in at least two ZDHHC genes. A splice-site mutation in highly conserved residues of *ZDHHC9*, a PAT that has been shown to palmitoylate H-Ras and N-Ras [31], has been described in families with X-linked mental retardation (XLMR) [32]. This mutation creates an additional, stronger splice-donor site 140 nt before (toward the 5' end) the normal donor site. Usage of the new site results in a mRNA that is frameshifted and that encodes a truncated protein. Single nucleotide polymorphisms that affect splicing of *ZDHHC8* have also been implicated in schizophrenia [33] (also see: [34-36]).

Hydropathy analyses predict that the PATs encoded by these genes all pass through a membrane multiple times (at least four) and are expressed predominantly in the ER and Golgi membranes [30, 37, 38]. Currently, there is little published data on the numbers of TM domains in any of the PATs with the exception of Akr1p in yeast [39]. Predictions using TopPred II 1.1 [40] as presented by Ohno and colleagues [30] show that most PATs have an even number of TM domains with the DHHC-CRD motif in the cytoplasm. However for DHHC13, -16, -11, and -22, the DHHC-CRD motif resides just C-terminal to the first or third TM domain. Assuming the N-terminus is cytoplasmic, this places the DHHC-CRD motif either in the lumen of the ER (the membrane compartment of residence reported for each by Ohno and colleagues 2006) or outside of the cell if expressed on the PM. Given that the environment in these two locations is oxidizing in nature [41, 42] and assuming this topological model is correct, it is possible that the cysteines of the DHHC-CRD motif could form inter- or intra-molecular disulfide bridges rather than being involved in the transfer of palmitate. However, while it is possible that PATs may assume duties in addition to palmitoylation, it seems somewhat unlikely they would do so in this arrangement as it represents a state in which it would be difficult to perform these functions. The highest-scoring predictions of the membrane topology using TMpred show that the human protein sequence of DHHC11 and -16 should contain four TM domains, DHHC13 eight TM domains, and DHHC22 either four or five TM domains, with each model placing the DHHC-CRD motif inside the cells. There is clear disparity among the predictions generated by the algorithms available and ultimately, any of these predictions of topology must be confirmed or disproved by experimental data. In any case, for a member of the PAT family to function as a PAT, the DHHC-CRD motif should probably reside in the cytoplasm (Figure 1A). The regions of the PAT proteins that contain the greatest diversity at the amino-acid level are the N- and C-terminal cytoplasmic tails (Figure 1B).

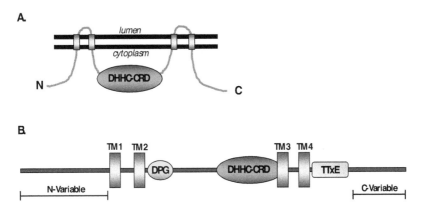

Figure 1. Predicted general structure of PATs. A) The predicted topology of PATs places the DHHC-CRD domain in the cytoplasm but such predictions must be confirmed experimentally. B) Each PAT is predicted to span the membrane four to six times; each is ~40 kDa with the greatest degree of sequence variability residing in the cytoplasmic N- and C-termini. The DHHC-CRD motif defines PATs. Palmitoylation of the cysteine in the DHHC portion is required for transfer of palmitate to a substrate. Most PATs also have a conserved DPG (aspartate-proline-glycine) motif and TTxE (threonine-threonine-asparagine-glutamate) motif, but their role in the function of PATs is not yet known.

In addition to the importance of PAT membrane topology, their membrane system of residence is likely to be an important aspect of their function. PATs have been localized to ER, Golgi, plasma membrane, endosomes, and the yeast vacuole [30, 43-48]; yet, little is known about how these proteins achieve their respective localizations. Immunolocalization of epitope-tagged DHHC proteins has been somewhat inconsistent among various cell types, between laboratories (e.g. DHHC2 [30, 37], and even in our own laboratory (unpublished observations SLP) in terms of within which membrane system a protein resides. Such inconsistencies suggest that the cell type, cell cycle, health of the cells, or even the location of the epitope tag may affect subcellular distribution. An interesting exception is DHHC2. DHHC2 has recently been shown to traffic between the PM and intracellular membranes via recycling endosomes [47]. Importantly, the C-terminal 68 amino acids of DHHC2 was shown to play an important role in defining its intracellular localization; however, a defined targeting signal present within this region of DHHC2 and in other DHHC proteins has yet to be defined.

2.3. PAT genes, palmitoylation and human disease

PATs have already been linked, in varying degrees, to human disease despite their recent discovery. At least 7 genes encoding PATs have been implicated in human disorders, including *ZDHHC8* with schizophrenia [33], *ZDHHC17* with Huntington's disease [49], *ZDHHC15* and *ZDHHC9* with X-linked mental retardation [32, 50], and *ZDHHC2*, *ZDHHC9*, *ZDHHC17*, and *ZDHHC11* with cancer [29, 51-53]; most of the demonstrated and putative connections are with cancer.

Overexpression of some PATs has also been shown to alter cancer-related signaling. DHHC17 (HIP14) is oncogenic. DHHC9 and DHHC11 display characteristics that strongly suggest they also are oncogenic. Overexpression of DHHC17 has the ability to induce colony formation and anchorage-independent growth in cell culture and tumors in mice [53]. It has been shown that these effects occur, at least in part, by DHHC17-mediated palmitoylation of H-, N-, and K2A- RAS proteins [53]. DHHC9 is strongly upregulated in some adenocarcinomas of the gastrointestinal tract at the transcript and protein levels [52] and has also been shown to palmitoylate H- and N- RAS proteins *in vitro* [31]. *ZDHHC11* has a high incidence of additional genomic copies in cases of non-small cell lung cancer and bladder cancer in which it is strongly linked to high-grade, advanced stage and disease progression [51].

Conversely to the behavior of the oncogenic PATs, a failure to express *ZDHHC2* results in an increase in metastasis in an *in vivo* model leading to the suggestion that *ZDHHC2* is a tumor/metastasis suppressor [29]. This absence of expression suggests that substrates of DHHC2 are no longer palmitoylated, and that whatever role palmitoylation had in signaling downstream from that event has been disrupted. Such is the case of DHHC2, where due to a lack of palmitoylation, one of its substrates, CKAP4, is no longer normally palmitoylated. One consequence of this is that CKAP4 no longer traffics efficiently (or at all) to the cell surface where it acts as a receptor for antiproliferative factor (APF) [37] [or presumably its other two known ligands, tissue plasminogen activator [54] and surfactant protein A [55]]. Without surface expression of CKAP4, APF is unable to initiate a wide range of downstream effects, including halting cellular proliferation and altering the expression of genes related to the progression of cancer [44].

CD9 and CD151, both tetraspanin proteins, have also been identified as substrates of DHHC2 [56]. CD9, which has been suggested to be a tumor suppressor [57, 58], is palmitoylated on multiple cysteines, but which of these are palmitoylated by DHHC2 is not known. Nonetheless, it is clear that suppression of DHHC2-mediated palmitoylation of CD9 in A431 cells affects cell behaviors that are consistent with it playing a role in tumor suppression. In particular, the cells undergo what appears to be epithelial-mesenchymal transition (EMT)— a process in which epithelial cells lose epithelial morphology and markers and gain a fibroblastic morphology during tumor progression [59-61]. It is not yet clear whether this change in cellular behavior was mediated solely by the reduction in CD9 palmitoylation or through reduced palmitoylation of this and other DHHC2 substrates such as CKAP4. It will be interesting to learn if a select subset of cysteines of CD9 is palmitoylated by DHHC2 and also how decreasing palmitoylation of specific cysteines results in the observed cellular behavior. Several other substrates of DHHC2 have been identified ranging from the neuronal adaptor/scaffold protein PSD95 [62], the SNARE proteins SNAP-23/25 [63], the non-receptor tyrosine kinase Lck [64], and the intracellular signaling proteins Gαi2 [65], GAP43 [62], R7BP [66], and eNOS [48]. Notably, there is no apparent structural similarity between the reported substrates of DHHC2, or even any sequence similarities surrounding the palmitoylated cysteine residues. Thus, DHHC2 can apparently palmitoylate cysteines located in the N-terminal regions (PSD-95, GAP-43, and Gα), internally in the protein sequence (SNAP-23/25), in the juxtamembrane region of transmembrane proteins (CD9, CD151, and CKAP4) and close to an N-terminal myristoylated glycine (Lck and eNOS).

From these examples, it is clear that upsetting the homeostatic balance of protein palmitoylation, in either direction, can have significant and deleterious effects on signaling networks. It is also clear that identification of PAT cognate substrates will provide important information concerning the molecular mechanisms underlying the oncogenic nature of the affiliated signaling systems as well as reveal important, novel targets for pharmacologic intervention. The development of specific DHHC protein inhibitors would provide vital reagents with which to study the physiological and pathophysiological importance of many palmitoylated proteins and may offer potential for therapeutic development.

2.4. PAT functions in addition to palmitoylation

It is not surprising that a disruption in the homeostatic balance of protein palmitoylation, in either direction, can have pathophysiological consequences. However, one must remain mindful that palmitoylation may not be the sole function of these proteins. Recently, two PATs—HIP14 (DHHC17) and HIP14L (DHHC13)—have been shown to mediate the transport of Mg^{2+} [67]. The first indication that these PATs were involved in Mg^{2+} regulation was that the abundance of their corresponding mRNAs was increased in cells grown in medium with reduced Mg^{2+} concentration. The authors then showed that Mg^{2+} (but not Ca^{2+}) transport was both electrogenic and voltage dependent, and that the transport required palmitoylation of the PAT. The authors concluded that these two PATs fall into a category of enzymes called "chanzymes" or ion channels that also have enzymatic activity; a type of protein previously represented only by the transient receptor potential melastatin (TRPM) family of transporters [68, 69]. The fact that GODZ (DHHC3) does not appear to mediate Mg^{2+} transport [70] but can mediate the transport of Ca^{2+} [71] suggests that this is not a general property of all PATs. The discovery that these PATs transport Mg^{2+} was astonishing especially in light of the fact that the DHHC-CRD motif appears, by sequence and predicted structure, to be a Zn^{2+}-binding protein; (a divalent cation with an atomic radius similar to Mg^{2+})—not Mg^{2+}. However, Goytain and colleagues also found that HIP14 and HIP14L transported Zn^{2+} with approximately half the efficiency as Mg^{2+}. The role of these and other PATs in binding to and/or transporting Zn^{2+} remains to be elucidated, but demonstrates the importance of not limiting ones view of PAT function (or many other proteins for that matter) only to palmitoylation.

2.5. Enzymatic mechanisms of palmitoylation

The physical and chemical mechanisms that result in enzymatic palmitoylation have yet to be defined clearly, but some progress has been made using purified proteins. It has been established that mutation of the cysteine in the DHHC motif of all PATs studied to date abolishes autoacylation of the PAT and palmitoylation of the substrate [23, 56, 62, 72]. This literature as well as discussion of potential physical mechanisms for the reaction have been reviewed recently [3, 73].

3. Palmitoyl-Cysteine prediction

Prior to the discovery of PATs, attempts were made to define stretches of amino acids that were preferred for palmitoylation. Palmitoylation near the N-terminus, following myristoylation, is among the predictable places for palmitoylation to occur provided there is one or more nearby cysteines. Navarro-Lérida et al (2002) fused a myristoylation motif (MGCTLS) to GFP with a short intervening sequence containing cysteines at various locations. These authors found a preference for cysteine palmitoylation at positions 3, 9, 15 and (to a much lesser degree) 21 residues away from the N-terminal methionine, but intervening residues were not evaluated. Commonalities in the composition of amino acid residues surrounding palmitoylated cysteines have been noted among members of the family of yeast amino acid permeases [74].

As more palmitoylated proteins and specific palmitoyl-cysteines are discovered, the task of predicting which adjacent amino acids provide a favorable environment for palmitoylation becomes easier. Algorithms trained with data from identified palmitoyl cysteines and adjacent amino acid residues are now able to provide predictions of the statistical likelihood that a cysteine of interest may be palmitoylated [75-78]. CSS-Palm 2.0, which was designed to predict potential palmitoylation sites, has been published [75]. The algorithm was trained to recognize potential palmitoyl-cysteines using a dataset of 263 experimentally determined palmitoylation sites from 109 distinct proteins. Interestingly, CSS-Palm 2.0 also successfully predicted most (~75%) of the same novel palmitoyl-cysteines in yeast proteins previously identified by Roth. et al [74] as well as palmitoyl-cysteines predicted by Roth et al., to be palmitoylated but not experimentally determined. This rate of success in both cases suggests that CSS-PALM 2.0 is more conservative at calling a site, potentially resulting in a greater rate of false negative results but is reasonably accurate nonetheless. This algorithm should prove useful when prioritizing which cysteine(s), often among multiple potential cysteines of a candidate palmitoyl protein, to analyze experimentally.

Patterns of amino acid residues surrounding palmitoyl-cysteines have emerged from these analyses. A diagram of favored residues generated by an early version of CSS-Palm 2.0 (NBA-Palm) [76] shows that leucines and additional cysteines are more commonly observed around palmitoyl-cysteines. The subsequent versions of NBA-palm used significantly improved predictive tests, but the rough sequence of preferred residues remains. An important aspect that cannot yet be considered when attempting to predict cysteine palmitoylation with these algorithms is the complexity of the PAT-substrate recognition that is encoded by residues outside of those that immediately surround the palmitoyl-cysteine; the higher order components of the recognition sites.

3.1. The physical properties of cysteines and thioester bonds

The unique physical and biochemical nature of the thioester bond that links palmitate to cysteine residues is the basis for the design of many recent assays for palmitoylation. The cysteine residue is among the most nucleophilic entities in a cell [79] and is the most common site of palmitoylation. Other residues can be modified by palmitate, but their occurrence is relatively rare and the bond chemistries are different [2, 80-83]. Palmitoylation can also occur in other ways, for example, on an amine of an N-terminal cysteine as is the case with Hedgehog [2, 83, 84], a secreted signaling protein. An example of palmitate modifying the weaker –OH nucleophile of threonine occurs on the carboxyl terminus of a spider toxin [81]. The ε-amino group of lysine can also be modified by palmitate linked by an amide bond. This occurs in several secreted proteins including a bacterial toxin [80].

The reactivity of the thiolate anion of cysteine residues makes it a key component in the structure and function of many proteins by stabilizing higher order structures via disulfide bridges and post-translational modifications like nitrosylation, prenylation, and acylation [85-87]. The high degree of reactivity has also provided a well-characterized, indispensable target for modification by synthetic, thiol-reactive ligands, allowing capture and characterization of proteins [88]. An exceptionally useful application of such thiol-specific chemistry is isotope-coded affinity tags (ICAT) for mass spectrometric determination of relative protein or peptide abundance among two or more samples [89-91]. With these probes, changes in abundance of identified proteins or peptides are determined by changes in the ratio of heavy to light-isotope-modified peptides from mixed samples. Combining ICAT technology with functional genomics methods like siRNA-mediated PAT-gene knockdown is one of several mechanisms that will allow us to identify substrates of PATs [37].

In healthy cells the cytoplasm is generally a reducing environment, meaning that solvent-exposed cysteine side chains are not typically disulfides and thus available to engage in reactions with other molecules [92]. The reactivity of a free cysteine depends on the pKa of the cysteine which is a function of the local environment surrounding the residue within the context of the whole protein. Unlike other residues with nucleophilic side chains (-OH or –NH₂), thiol side chains undergo conjugations, redox, and exchange reactions [85]. Conjugation reactions (in addition to fatty acylation) include nitric oxide (NO) or S-nitrosylation, reactive oxygen species (ROS), and reactive nitrogen species (RNS) forming bonds that are not susceptible to cleavage by hydroxylamine at neutral pH. Hydroxylamine is a reagent used to selectively remove thioester-linked palmitate [93]. Importantly, we know that hydroxylamine does not perturb disulfides [94], and that it efficiently cleaves thioesters in a quantitative manner [95].

In addition to the linkage of palmitate to cysteines, another thioester bond that occurs in cells is the transient association between ubiquitin and the E1, E2, and certain E3 ubiquitination enzymes [87, 96]. However, these thioester bonds are easily distinguished from the thioester bond that links palmitate to cysteines by their pKa; the pKa in the case of palmitoylation is near neutral pH (~7.4) whereas, for the thioester in the ubiquitin system it is pH 10.5 or greater. This wide differential allows for a high degree of selectivity when using hydroxylamine to cleave palmitate from proteins on the physical characteristics of ubiquitin-related cysteines. It is highly unlikely that they are ever in a position to be palmitoylated [97, 98].

Retinoic acid (RA) and RA-CoA have also been shown to be enzymatically attached to cysteines via a thioester bond that can be cleaved by hydroxylamine and reducing reagents such as βME at neutral pH. The reaction can be inhibited, but not fully, by myristate and palmitate suggesting that RA competes for the same cysteines as palmitate [99-107]. There is some debate in the RA field about how it binds to proteins, particularly the nuclear RA receptors, to carry out its signaling functions. RA binding to a hydrophobic cleft is the favored mechanism; however, there are many effects of RA (e.g. [108, 109]) that are independent of RA-receptor binding suggesting that cysteine modification may also have a place in the molecular mechanism of RA action.

3.2. Mass spectrometric identification of acyl groups that modify cysteines via a thioester bond

Lipid-modified thiols have been successfully identified using MALDI-TOF (matrix-assisted laser desorption ionization time-of-flight) mass spectrometry [110]. Using this method, direct information on the nature of the endogenous lipids on proteins or peptides (revealing interesting variability) can be obtained, whereas most other methods rely on surrogate markers for palmitate including thiol-reactive probes or radiolabeled palmitate. Using MALDI-TOF mass spectrometry, Marilyn Resh and colleagues found that the cysteine in the N-terminal Met-Gly-Cys of Src family kinases and two cysteines near the N-terminus of GAP43 are modified not only by palmitate but also (and to a lesser degree) by palmitoleate, stearate, or oleate [7, 8]. While palmitate appears to be the most common acyl group that forms a thioester bond to modify internal, cytoplasmic cysteines, it is clearly not the only one. The 16-carbon palmitate acyl group represents the longest chain synthesized by mammalian fatty acid synthase and is apparently the most abundant chain length present in some tissue types [111]. This relatively greater abundance may underlie the dominance of palmitate as the main acyl group to modify free thiols by S-acylation. The functional implications of incorporating lipids with shorter or longer acyl chains and especially those with different degrees of saturation may be that the proteins have different affinities for various lipid microdomains present in membranes. The specificity of PATs for chain-lengths different than 16 carbons has not been rigorously defined. However, it is known that acyl groups with differing carbon chain lengths and degrees of saturation can also be incorporated [7, 112].

3.3. PAT/Substrate recognition

Determining the nature of PAT/substrate recognition remains one of the more important tasks to be undertaken. This is especially true for PATs encoded by genes that have been linked to disease. There are two general approaches to defining PAT/substrate relationships:

1. identification of the PAT with specificity for a known palmitoyl protein and

2. identification of an unknown substrate of an individual PAT.

The first of these has been the most common. With this forward approach, each one of the 23 PATs is independently co-overexpressed with a known palmitoyl protein; the cells expressing the pair are metabolically labeled with ^{3}H-palmitate and the proteins analyzed by SDS-PAGE and fluorography. The incorporation of ^{3}H-palmitate onto the substrate protein in one or more of the co-overexpressions at a level significantly above background suggests that a particular PAT is responsible for palmitoylating that known substrate. Similarly, the presumptive PAT and substrate proteins can be purified and combined with ^{3}H-palmitoyl-CoA in a tube, allowed to react, and the incorporation of ^{3}H-palmitate measured as above. The current level of understanding of PAT/substrate recognition makes it unreasonable to assume that the more closely two PATs are related by sequence homology, the more likely they should palmitoylate a particular substrate. For this reason, assigning substrate status of a protein to a single PAT among a select group of tested, more closely-homologous PATs, to the exclusion of others because they are less homologous, may lead to erroneous exclusions. Similarly, we cannot yet assume that homology among residues surrounding palmitoyl cysteines of different proteins is an indication that they are palmitoylated by a particular PAT. The mechanism for molecular recognition is likely to be defined in part by the higher order structure (even quaternary as is the case with ERF2p and AKR1p) of the PATs and substrates. The reverse approach, defining unknown substrates of a single PAT can occur without these same biases as has been demonstrated in yeast and in human cells [37, 74].

4. Novel methods to discover and identify PAT/substrate specificity

The chemistry supporting novel assays to study palmitoylation and the reagents that are being incorporated into them have, for the most part, been known and available for years [88] . Most of the methods that are now being developed to study palmitoylation capitalize on many years of knowledge and development of cysteine-specific chemistries, developed mainly as methods to purify and/or specifically target proteins and peptides with various reagents. Many of the reagents that specifically label cysteines have been created as both affinity and fluorescent tags, the former for purification and structure determinations [88]and the latter as cellular reporters of protein abundance, subcellular distribution, protein conformation changes, the formation of the Golgi, and even the concentration of cellular analytes in specific subcellular domains. The following references provide a short list of some of the most clever uses of thiol chemistry [113-119]. Given the wealth of information on the unique chemistry of the palmitoyl thioester bond and the tools for capturing and characterizing cysteines in proteins, it is somewhat surprising that we are only now developing innovative assays to increase our understanding of palmitoylation. This recent increase is most likely tied to the dramatic increase in the utility of mass spectrometry as a proteomic tool. To provide a general frame of reference for the recent shift in the types of assays that are being developed, we will briefly discuss other assays that have been used successfully for a longer period of time. These assays are by no means outdated and some continue to be the most appropriate way to answer specific questions.

4.1. Chemistry and physical properties of palmitoyl cysteines: Reactions and probes

Working with palmitoylated proteins is inherently difficult due to the labile nature of the thioester bond and the increased hydrophobicity of the protein or peptide due to palmitate. On the other hand, the unique physical and chemical properties of thiols, palmitoylated thiols, and the thioester bond make them particularly amenable to modification by highly specific chemistry and a wide variety of thiol reactive probes.

Reactions of free thiols in the cytoplasm

Thiol modification occurs most commonly in cells by one of two routes: disulfide exchange or alkylation. Many of the reactive groups that undergo these two reactions are relatively stable in aqueous environments; the reactions are rapid and provide high yields of thioether and disulfide bonds [88]. Thiols will also react with many amine reactive reagents including isothiocyanates and succinimidyl esters but lack a high degree of specificity, resulting in unstable bonds that are much less useful for routine modification of thiols in proteins. Thiol-specific reagents and chemistry figure strongly into the design and development of novel assays for palmitoylation. Most investigators are limited somewhat to reagents that are available from a catalog but, fortunately, there are already many useful reagents available. Among the most useful are thio-reactive chemicals that are linked to another moiety (reactive or reporter) by a spacer arm of variable length and physical characteristics. Such hetero- and homo-bifunctional crosslinking reagents have provided much of the foundation for recent developments in palmitoylation assays and provide a fairly rich toolbox for future assay development.

Chemical moieties that react with palmitoyl-cysteines

Iodoacetamide conjugates are among the most commonly used tools for modifying cysteine thiols. These undergo nucleophilic substitution to form stable thioether bonds at physiological pH in aqueous environments. When using iodoacetamide and its conjugates, one should remember that depending on the pH of the solution, they can also react with histidine, lysine, and methionine (at pH >1.7) residues and N-terminal amines. However, when used at slightly alkaline pH in the dark and in the absence of reducing reagents, cysteine modification will be the exclusive reaction [88]. A good example of iodoacetamide-based probes are the isotope-coded affinity tags or ICAT [120]. These have proved particularly useful in determining the substrates of DHHC2 [37].

Maleimides are also common constituents of heterobifunctional crosslinking reagents and blocking reagents that target cysteines. They are ~1000 times more specific for cysteine sulfhydryls at pH 6.5-7.5, but at higher pH some cross reactivity can occur with amines. Maleimides form stable thioether bonds by adding the sulfhydryl across the double bond of the maleimide.

Phenylmercury derivatives react with thiols, including nitrosothiols, under conditions similar to iodoacetamides and maleimides to form stable mercury-thiol bonds that can be reversed in 0.1N HCl and reducing reagents like dithiothreitol (DTT) but apparently not by TCEP. Phenylmercury derivatives also react faster with thiols than do the commonly used thiol-reactive N-ethylmaleimide (NEM).

Compounds containing disulfide bonds are able to undergo disulfide exchange reactions with another thiol by the free thiol attacking the disulfide bond and subsequent formation of a new mixed thiol. Two examples of useful compounds in this category are Methylmethane-thiosulfonate (MMTS) and pyridyl disulfide derivitives like biotin HPDP ((N-(6-(Biotinami-do)hexyl)-3'-(2'-pyridyldithio)-propionamide). MMTS can be used in some cases to block free thiols more effectively than NEM, as it is uncharged and thus more likely to modify all free reactive cysteines. MMTS has been shown not to react with nitrosothiols or existing disulfides [121].

4.2. Metabolic labeling with radiolabeled palmitate

The most common method to identify palmitoyl proteins and to determine the residence half-life of palmitate on a specific protein or palmitate turnover (e.g. [122] for a particularly interesting example) is to metabolically label cells with radiolabled palmitate. ^{14}C-, ^{3}H- and ^{125}I-labeled palmitate have all been used, but ^{3}H-palmitate is most common because it is relatively inexpensive and widely available. However, using ^{125}I -labeled palmitate provides some advantages. In practical terms, the time required for detection is considerably shorter - hours instead of (often) weeks with ^{3}H-palmitate. The γ-irradiation from the ^{125}I is also compatible with phosphorimaging technology which is much more rapid and quantitative than densitometric measurements from films generated by autofluorography (as is used with tritium). The principle downside of using ^{125}I-labeled palmitate is that it is not commercially available, and the labeling must be done by the investigator. Reviews of the methods using radiolabeled palmitate and including technical details have been published recently [123-125].

4.3. Fluorescently-labeled peptide substrates for palmitoylation

Fluorescently-labeled peptides that mimic PAT substrates have been used to characterize PAT activity and for the discovery of inhibitors of palmitoylation [123, 126, 127]. The use of these peptides over the last several years was reviewed recently [123]. Peptide substrates for palmitoylation have also been genetically fused to fluorescent proteins and expressed in cells. This strategy has been used to determine how palmitoylation affects subcellular trafficking both between and within membranes [124]. Monomeric GFP-based reporters and fluorescence resonance energy transfer proved to be helpful in the identification of lipid rafts with an affinity for palmitate on the inner leaflet of the plasma membrane [5].

4.4. Acyl-biotin exchange: ABE

Most of the novel assays for palmitoylation utilize the same basic foundation first described for a palmitoyl protein by Schmidt and colleagues [128] and now most commonly known as acyl-exchange. First, free cysteines are blocked on proteins that have been extracted from live cells or tissue. Next, palmitates are removed from cysteines by cleavage of the thioester bond with hydroxylamine (typically 1.0M) at neutral pH. This creates a new set of free thiols unique in that they were all formerly palmitoylated; ideally, no others should exist. Finally, this new set of formerly-palmitoylated cysteines is modified by any one of the many thiol-specific reagents. The uniqueness of the individual assays that incorporate these steps lies primarily in the choice of thiol-specific reagents, and this choice depends on what questions the investigator wants to answer. There are also variations in the reagents used to block free cysteines in the first step. Both NEM and MMTS have been used in the assays described below but NEM is used most commonly.

Cysteines that are palmitoylated can also be modified by fatty acids other that palmitate [7] including stearate and oleate. The acyl-exhange method cannot yet distinguish between palmitate and the other fatty acids modifying cysteines by a thioester bond. Two additional points that relate to the specificity of this method for palmitoylation are: 1) that it will not report modification of cysteines by prenyl groups (geranylgeranyl or farnesyl) because they are attached by a thioether bond that is not susceptible to cleavage by hydroxylamine and 2) it will not report myristoylated proteins because this 14-carbon acyl group is linked to an N-terminal glutamate by an amide bond which is also insensitive to cleavage by hydroxylamine.

The recent development of novel assays using the three-step acyl exchange method to study palmitoylation in a broader sense was invigorated by two publications describing a new twist on the method that incorporated the use of radiolabeled NEM assay [129, 130]. Work described in these papers showed that labeling palmitoyl cysteines with radiolabeled NEM resulted in a remarkable 5- to 12-fold increase in sensitivity to detect several known palmitoyl proteins, including PSD-95 and SNAP-25, when compared to labeling with ^{3}H-palmitate. In addition, the authors demonstrated the utility of the biotinylated, heterobifunctional crosslinker, 4-[4'-(maleimidomethyl)cyclohexanecarboxamido] butane (Btn-BMCC), as an effective tool to capture and purify (using streptavidin-agarose) palmitoylated proteins. In doing so, they also demonstrated the general potential of using the wide variety of existing thiol-specific probes for the development of additional assays for palmitoylation that are beginning to materialize.

4.5. The palmitoyl proteome

The demonstration that one can effectively replace palmitate with a biotin group led to development of the first, large-scale, proteomic analysis of palmitoylation [74] in yeast, the model system in which the molecular identify of PATs was first determined [23, 26]. This method was dubbed "acyl biotin exchange" or ABE and used the same basic three-steps as described above. As the name implies, the proteins were labeled with a thiol-reactive, biotinylated heterobifunctional probe, [6-(Biotinamido)hexyl]-3'-(2'-pyridyldithio)propionamide (HPDP-biotin), with subsequent capture on streptavidin affinity matrix (for a detailed protocol see Wan et al. 2007 [131]). It is interesting to note the number of proteins that Roth and colleagues captured in the negative control samples (Figure 1a;[74]). The degree of overlap among proteins captured in the experimental and control samples suggests that the step in which free thiols were blocked with NEM was not quantitative and/or that the wash steps following binding of biotinylated proteins to the streptavidin matrix were not sufficiently stringent (steps 7 and 16 respectively from Wan et al, 2007 [131]) thereby resulting in the potential for a higher number of false-positive hits. However, issues of signal to noise and limits of sensitivity are by no means unique to this work (avidin-biotin affinity purification is notoriously difficult); rather they are unavoidable issues faced by all developers of novel strategies and users of nascent technologies. Incremental improvements in important assays like this always follow.

One of the key features of all proteomic methods is the system used for detection of specifically-isolated proteins or peptides. Work by Roth et al. [74] identified proteins by multi-dimensional protein identification technology (MudPIT), a high-throughput, tandem mass spectrometry (MS/MS)-based proteomic technology [132] [see also [131, 133]]. Compared to other mass spectrometric methods, MudPIT has the potential to identify less abundant proteins with a higher degree of confidence, because multiple peptides of a single protein can be used to identify a protein of interest. One downside with MudPIT in this case is that the palmitoyl cysteine(s) cannot be pinpointed, as there may be many candidates among the individual peptides of a whole protein suspected as being a palmitoyl protein. After demonstrating the usefulness of this large-scale method for purification and identification of palmitoylated proteins, the authors used mutant strains of yeast lacking one or more of the seven yeast PAT proteins to identify substrates of individual PATs. Comparison of the degree of palmitoylation of individual proteins between wild type yeast (a full set of normally palmitoylated proteins) and those not expressing one or more of the yeast PATs (each with a specific set of hypo/depalmitoylated proteins) provided the identity of the substrates of individual PATs. Together, this work represents a very significant contribution to the identification and understanding of the yeast palmitoyl proteome and provided many important clues about potential homologous PAT-substrate pairs in other systems.

The complexity of palmitoylation is greater in a vertebrate system. With at least 23 genes encoding PATs identified in humans, the diversity at the most basic level is at least three-fold greater than in yeast. When one considers the additional variants encoded by alternative splicing of PAT mRNAs, the potential diversity increases even more. The greater number of PATs suggests (but does not prove) that there are also more palmitoylated proteins in mammals. The ability to genetically manipulate mammalian cells is improving but lags behind yeast. Nevertheless, defining the palmitoyl proteome or palmitoylosome and how it is regulated in mammals (humans in particular) is a task of significant importance and interest. Now that the enzymes capable of mediating palmitoylation have been identified, one of the most important questions that we face is which substrates are palmitoylated by each PAT— a question brought sharply into focus when one considers the known connections between mutations or deletions in PAT genes and human disease, in particular cancer. DHHC2 is deleted in many types of cancer (see above). Its absence is strongly correlated with an increase in the metastatic potential of cancer cells. The simplest inverse corollary in this case is that palmitoylated substrates of DHHC2 are responsible for keeping cells from metastasizing. Identification of these substrates and their associated signaling networks using novel assays for palmitoylation has begun to provide supporting evidence for known mechanisms of cancer progression [56] as well as a novel signaling pathway for the regulation of cellular proliferation and metastasis [37].

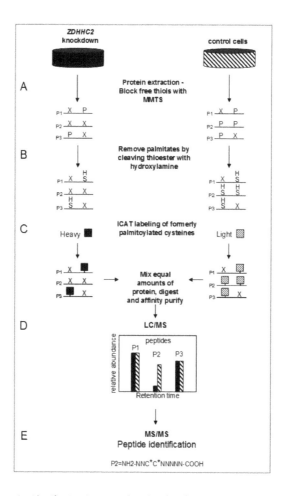

Figure 2. Palmitoyl-cysteine Identification Capture and Analysis (PICA): Determining PAT-substrate specificity by differential labeling of palmitoylated proteins with Isotope-coded Affinity Tags (ICAT) (A) In one set of cultures, *ZDHHC2* expression is knocked down by transfecting HeLa cells with *ZDHHC2*-specific siRNA (Dharmacon). Proteins are extracted from experimental and control cells and treated with the thiol-specific blocking reagent MMTS. This step chemically modifies or protects all thiols ("X" on the proteins P1-P3) that are free at physiological pH and leaves the palmitoylated cysteines (P) undisturbed as depicted on P1-P3. (B) Following the protection or blocking of free thiols, palmitates are removed by selective cleavage of the thioester bond with hydroxylamine at pH 7.4, which generates a distinctive set of free, formerly-palmitoylated, reactive thiols (C) that can be selectively labeled with ICAT reagents. Iodoacetamide at one end of the ICAT reagent binds to the thiol sidechain of cysteines; on the other end, biotin pro-

vides a mechanism for affinity purification of thiol-captured peptides on an avidin column. (D) Proteins from knockdown and control conditions are mixed in equal amounts and digested in-gel with trypsin. ICAT labeled peptides are enriched by avidin affinity and analyzed by LC/MS. A pair of ICAT-labeled peptides is chemically identical and is easily visualized, because they essentially coelute and there is a 9 Da mass difference measured in a scanning mass spectrometer. Even if equal amounts of a single protein exist in two different samples, the quantity of protein that is captured depends directly on its degree of palmitoylation; if all of a single protein is palmitoylated under one condition, then all of it will be captured; if only half of this protein is palmitoylated under another condition then the capture rate of that protein will be half as much, relative to control, making it appear half as abundant. Proteins for which there has been no change in palmitoylation (ie, equal capture rates) will yield a heavy:light (H/L) ratio of 1. The degree to which palmitoylation is diminished will register as a decrease in the H/L ratio (ie, 50% reduction in palmitoylation will correspond to a H/L ratio of 0.5). A change in the capture rate that results in a change in the post-purification abundance is measured in the LC/MS phase. (E) Finally, the peptides are further fragmented into their constituent amino acids by MS/MS, enabling identification of the proteins corresponding to the captured peptides.

4.6. Palmitoyl-cysteine Identification Capture and Analysis (PICA): Identification of PAT substrates and palmitoyl proteins in vertebrates

With the aim of defining PAT-substrate specificity in a living vertebrate system, we developed a method to identify substrates of specific PATs in mammalian cells and tissues called Palmitoyl cysteine Isolation Capture and Analysis or PICA [37]. We used this method to identify CKAP4/p63, a known palmitoyl protein [134] as one substrate of DHHC2 in HeLa cells [37]. This method is similar to ABE as described by Roth et al (2006) but was inspired [135] in part by the work of Drisdel and Green (2004) and incorporated several novel features that will be discussed below.

The ability of PICA to identify PAT substrates is based on the principle that it quantifies the differential frequency of palmitoylation of individual proteins or peptides in control conditions versus conditions in which the function of a single PAT is reduced by siRNA-mediated gene knockdown. The process to identify substrates of DHHC2 consisted of four basic steps outlined in Figure 2. In the first part we generated two distinct pools of palmitoylated proteins, one from control HeLa cells and the other from HeLa cells in which the activity of one PAT (DHHC2) was reduced. These two distinct pools of palmitoylated proteins were then captured and compared directly to identify differences in the degree of palmitoylation of individual proteins between the two pools. To do this, we reduced the expression of ZDDHC2 mRNA (and consequently the abundance of the encoded enzyme, DHHC2) in HeLa cells using siRNA-mediated gene knockdown which resulted in a reduced level of palmitoylation of DHHC2 substrates. Total protein from knockdown and control cells was prepared by first blocking free thiols with MMTS in the presence of SDS. This was followed by selective exposure of all palmitoyl cysteines by cleavage of the palmitoyl-cysteine thioester bond with 1.0M hydroxylamine at neutral pH, thereby generating a unique population of formerly palmitoylated cysteines. Second, we selectively and differentially labeled the exposed, formerly-palmitoylated cysteines from knockdown and control cells with biotinylated, thiol-reactive heavy (H) and light (L) ICAT reagents, respectively. Third, we combined equal quantities of the ICAT-labeled protein from ZDHHC2 knockdown and control cells and digested the mixture with trypsin. The resulting H and L ICAT-labeled tryptic peptides were captured and purified on an avidin affinity column. Finally, ICAT-labeled, putative, formerly-palmitoylated peptides were analyzed by mass spectrometry. Peptides with a reduced

H/L ratio over four independent runs were analyzed further to confirm that the identified cysteine was indeed palmitoylated by DHHC2 under physiological conditions. Details of the protocol and reagents used and outlined in Figure 2 can be found in [37].

There are several unique aspects in the PICA method. First, we used MMTS to block the free thiols in the first step. NEM is used most commonly at this step, but MMTS is more reactive and smaller than NEM or iodoacetamide, enhancing its ability to modify all free reactive cysteines. Inefficient blocking of free thiols in the first step is one factor that could easily contribute to false-positive capture of proteins in the purification step. Qualitative evaluation (silver-stained SDS-PAGE) of protein capture in experimental and control (no-hydroxylamine) conditions [Figure 2, [37]] suggests that it may be more efficient than NEM (for comparison see Figure 1A [74]). However, it may also be that we captured very few proteins under control conditions because of a more stringent wash protocol than described by Roth et al [74]. The use of ICAT reagents in PICA allowed us to combine formerly-palmitoylated peptides purified from control and experimental cells in the same pool, and subsequently, a direct, simultaneous analysis of palmitoylation in the two pools in a single analytical sample. We defined a substrate of DHHC2 as one that had a consistently reduced H/L ratio over four independent PICA runs. This approach provided us with many (the vast majority), convenient internal control peptides which are peptides that were not substrates of DHHC2 that had unchanged H/L ratios. This approach significantly reduces the potential for identification of false-positive hits because, if a protein can be falsely labeled by an ICAT, it should do so with equal efficiency in both the control and experimental cells yielding a peptide with an H/L ratio of ~1. The greater risk with this approach is the failure to identify substrates that exist in low abundance. Using tandem mass spectrometry, we analyzed a sample of significantly reduced complexity including only ICAT-tagged peptides. As is inherent in such analyses, the most abundant peptides dominate the report. However, one advantage of this approach is that when a peptide is identified, whether it is a substrate of a single PAT or not, the palmitoyl cysteine(s) is also identified. In the case of CKAP4/p63 (and the majority of other peptides) there was only a single cysteine, and it was already known to be a site for palmitoylation [134]. Spectral counting has the potential to positively identify palmitoyl proteins of lower abundance because more than a single peptide from any given protein is factored into to the identification. There is greater overall coverage (identified peptide fragments of a protein) using this method thereby increasing the confidence level of identification. However, the disadvantage inherent in analyzing a complex mixture, including nonpalmitoylated peptides by spectral counting, is that identification of the palmitoyl cysteine (in the cases where there are multiple candidate cysteines) must await subsequent and tedious analyses. The tradeoff between these two complementary approaches in mass spectrometric analysis is sensitivity versus specificity. Combining these analyses will provide a much greater depth of coverage.

4.7. Forward and reverse approaches to assigning PAT-substrate pairs

The first reports that identified PAT-substrate pairings took the reverse approach: start with a known palmitoylated protein then use metabolic labeling with radiolabeled palmitate and co-overexpression of one PAT and the substrate (for a review see: [72]). Using this method, an increase in the incorporation of radiolabeled palmitate on the overexpressed substrate in the presence of an overexpressed PAT is used to claim specificity. This method is an important tool for increasing our understanding of palmitoylation-related phenomena including confirmation of putative PAT-substrate pairs identified by other methods. Likewise, when starting with a known palmitoyl protein and the intention of identifying the PAT responsible for its palmitoylation, it remains a useful method. However, we should remember that just because overexpression of a PAT can increase the incorporation of palmitate onto a specific protein does not necessarily mean that it does so in a live cell. Again, problems like this are not unique to this method and simply reflect our lack of knowledge about where and when PATs and their substrates are expressed, the degree of promiscuity among PATs and, how PAT function is regulated.

The potential for specific cysteines to be modified by both palmitate and RA via a thioester bond is an issue that deserves attention from those of us interested primarily in palmitoylation for at least two reasons. One is the potential that an exchange between the two modifications is a physiologically relevant means of regulating signaling and second, the possibility that proteins identified as being palmitoylated in assays utilizing some form of ABE chemistry are RA-modified instead.

4.8. Labeling palmitoyl proteins with bioorthogonal probes

This particularly interesting approach labels cysteines with isosteric, azido-derivitives of fatty acids that are able to substitute for fatty acids that occur naturally in cells (Figure 3) [112, 136]. Once bound to cysteines, the azido group on the fatty acid is reacted, with a high degree of selectivity, via the Staudinger reaction [137] with (triaryl)phosphines that are themselves derivatized with Myc, biotin, a fluorophore, or others. Using this method Hang and colleagues [112] found that ω-azido fatty acids with 12 and 15 carbons can be efficiently metabolized by mammalian cells and accurately report myristoylation and thio-palmitoylation, respectively.

Work by Kostiuk and colleagues identified palmitoyl proteins from mitochondria using azido-palmitate [136]. To accomplish this they purified proteins from cellular mitochondrial fractions, first by differential centrifugation, then by further purification based first on charge and subsequently by size using chromatographic separation. Labeling of proteins in this study was outside of a living system presumably leaving only the possibility of autocatalytic/non-enzymatic palmitoylation. Mass spectrometric analysis of selected bands identified 21 palmitoylated proteins, 19 of which were novel. The majority of the proteins labeled were metabolic-type proteins unique to the mitochondrion. This raises the interesting possibility that the principle mechanism of palmitoylation in this organelle is autocatalytic rather than enzymatic, and that, as suggested by the authors, the key role of palmitoylation in the mitochondrion is to inhibit enzymes by palmitoylation of cysteines in the vicinity of the active site.

These so called bio-orthogonal probes have been reported to be nontoxic and very stable under physiological conditions. Importantly, this two-step reaction is rapid and more sensitive than labeling with ^{125}I-palmitoyl-CoA. These features, especially their ability to effectively substitute for endogenous fatty acids, make them ideal for labeling palmitoyl proteins in live cells, providing a significantly more direct measure of protein palmitoylation than can be achieved in any other assay format. It is easy to imagine that use of such probes will come to dominate in experimental systems for studying palmitoylation.

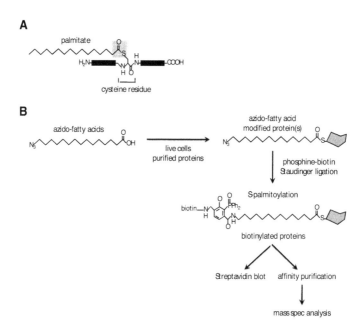

Figure 3. Using Click chemistry and bio-orthogonal probes to label palmitoyl cysteines. A) A palmitoylated protein; the shaded box indicates the thioester bond. B) Azido-palmitate is transferred to a protein forming a thioester bond with a cysteine residue. The azide moiety of the azido-palmitate reacts, via the Staudinger reaction, with the tagged (in this case biotin) phosphine, forming an amide bond. The biotin-tagged proteins can then be affinity purified and analyzed in various ways including mass spectrometry. Tags and reporters other than biotin can be added to the phosphine providing a wide array of potential methods for subsequent analyses.

5. Pharmacological modulation of Palmitoylation

5.1. Developing compounds that selectively target individual PATs

Existing chemicals used to inhibit palmitoylation are neither selective nor potent. The compounds used most commonly are 2-bromopalmitate (2BP), tunicamycin, and cerulenin. Each of these is a lipid-based molecule (Figure 4). 2BP has been used most frequently at a concentration of ~100 μM to block palmitoylation in spite of the fact that at least two studies have shown that the IC50 of 2-BP is ~10 μM [138, 139]. 2BP is not tolerated well by cultured cells and causes death even after a brief exposure to 100 µM. 2BP inhibits several enzymes involved in lipid metabolism, including carnitine palmitoyltransferase 1, fatty acid CoA ligase, glycerol-3-phosphate acyltransferase, and enzymes in the synthesis of triacylglycerol biosynthesis [140, 141]. This high degree of promiscuity as well as the toxicity of 2BP renders it nearly useless as a tool to determine anything specific about palmitoylation related signaling issues that equally plague cerulenin and tunicamycin. The uses and effects of these three inhibitors was reviewed recently [142].

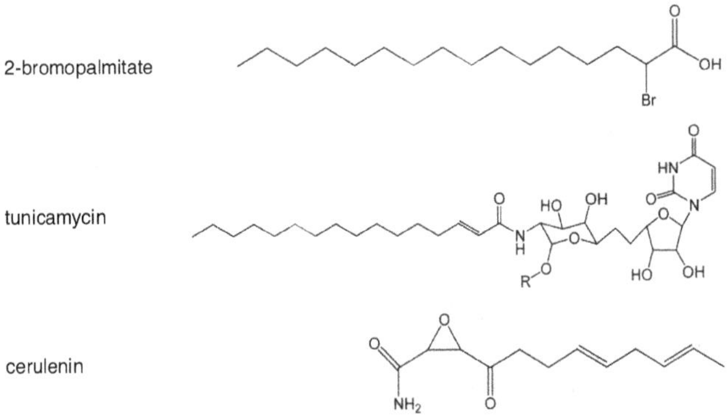

Figure 4. Lipid-based inhibitors of palmitoylation.

Smith and colleagues [126] recently screened a compound library in an attempt to identify more selective and potent inhibitors of palmitoylation, in particular inhibitors of PATs. This screen identified single compounds from five chemical classes (Compounds I-V) that inhibited cellular processes associated with palmitoylation. The assays used in the screens included: measuring the *in vivo* and *in vitro* growth rate of an NIH/3T3 cell line that overexpressed DHHC17, displacement from the plasma membrane of myristoylated or farnesylated GFP, and *in vitro* palmitoylation of small, non-complex, myristoylated or farnesylated, synthetic, fluorescent peptides intended to mimic known palmitoylation substrates [123, 126, 127]. These assays could not discriminate a direct effect of any compound on any PAT. They could only report the activity of compounds that acted at some point (not excluding direct PAT inhibition) in any pathway that leads to or affects palmitoylation; compounds like 2BP, cerulenin, and tunicamycin. This assertion was borne out in follow-up studies on the same compounds [138] (see below). Perhaps the most intriguing finding in this report was that compounds I-IV were able to suppress the oncogenic behavior of human cells that overexpressed DHHC17. However, there is no direct evidence to indicate that compounds I-IV exert these actions via inhibition of DHHC17 or through the palmitoylation of Ras proteins by DHHC17 as was speculated [53, 126]. Nevertheless, since these compounds reduced the *in vivo* growth of tumors from cells overexpressing DHHC17 [126], it would be worth determining their exact mechanism of action.

Subsequent studies by Linder, Deschenes and colleagues [138] tested four of the five compounds identified by Smith and colleagues and found that they were not selective for DHHC proteins. This report also included a wealth of information defining the mechanisms by which 2BP inhibits palmitoylation. Briefly, only one of the four compounds re-tested, compound V and 2BP, inhibited the activity of any of the four DHHC proteins tested. Neither compound V nor 2BP was selective for any of the PATs tested, and 2BP was more potent. Both compound V and 2BP blocked autoacylation of the PATs; compound V was reversible, 2BP was not. Even though compound V was able to inhibit the activity of the four PATs tested and in the same manner as 2BP, these experiments could not determine whether compound V also blocks palmitoylation indiscriminately at steps prior to the actual palmitoylation event, as is the case with 2BP, cerulenin, and tunicamycin.

There would be no compelling reason to begin a drug discovery program to identify inhibitors of just any PAT. Rather one would choose to begin with a PAT that is linked to a disease state—a situation where misregulated expression or function of that PAT was clearly linked to a pathological state. As discussed earlier, links between PAT expression (but not yet altered function) have been demonstrated for both neurological disorders and cancer; thus, candidate PATs that would be appropriate targets for drug development exist. Both overexpression and absence of PAT expression have been implicated in the development of cancer. Dampening the activity of an existing PAT is a conceptually and mechanistically simpler task than accurately restoring the specific activity of a PAT that is not expressed or absent. This review is concerned with PAT assays and PAT inhibitors, so we will address the case of PAT overexpression in ideal terms as well as the technical issues that surround the development and implementation of the assays designed to discover PAT inhibitors.

5.2. Considerations for development of high-throughput screens to discover PAT inhibitors

The DHHC motif in PATs defines the active site and is highly conserved in all mammalian PATs [3]. The regions of highest diversity are primarily in the N- and C-termini of the PAT. Mutation of the cysteine in the DHHC motif abolishes PAT autoacylation and palmitoylation of the substrate, a property of all DHHC proteins studied so far. This high degree of homology in the active site sequence among PATs could give the impression that developing highly specific, active-site inhibitors for palmitoylation will be impossible. However, this same issue exists with kinases [143, 144], and yet the development of selective and potent active-site, ATP-competitive inhibitors has been successful (eg, [145]).

The specificity of palmitoylation must be derived in part from the unique physical interactions of individual PATs with their substrates. The sequence of amino acids surrounding a substrate cysteine partially defines the potential for that cysteine to be palmitoylated. However, the physical determinants for substrate recognition will likely extend throughout the accessible portions of the PAT and substrate as was elegantly demonstrated for DHHC17 [146]. Other factors that are likely to regulate palmitoylation are the temporal and spatial aspects of PAT and substrate expression.

There are many more palmitoylated proteins than there are PATs; therefore, modulating the activity of a single PAT, even with complete compound selectivity, will likely yield a change in the palmitoylation of multiple substrates. This conundrum is common to the development of highly selective and potent pharmacological modulators of all enzymes that mediate post-translational protein modifications, again kinases being a classic example.

Another challenge is that each PAT traverses the plasma membrane multiple times. A conservative guess would suggest that the membrane environment is important for determining PAT structure and substrate recognition. However, Jennings et al.,[138] demonstrated that at least four PATs can be purified from a membrane environment and remain enzymatically active. These findings are both remarkable and encouraging evidence that enzyme activity-based and drug-binding screens for selective PAT inhibitors can be accomplished with purified proteins.

5.3. Primary screen for PAT inhibitors

The discovery and refinement of drugs to modulate PAT activity will require the use of multiple assay types. The initial success of each can only be a matter of speculation at the beginning of the project, and the success of the primary screen will influence the choice of follow up assays. However, one unique aspect of palmitoylation suggests a logical starting point. The most dramatic visible change that can occur when a protein is palmitoylated is when it moves from the cytoplasm to the plasma (or other) membrane. The technology to measure such a translocation in living cells using high-throughput microscopy has been demonstrated [139, 147] and along with many other such morphometric analyses, has become well established in drug discovery programs and the basic life sciences [148-150]. This technology is often referred to as high-content screening (HCS). To develop an assay to identify inhibitors of a single PAT using HCS, it would be ideal to have identified the most clinically relevant, cytosolic substrate of the PAT of interest and to have determined that this substrate is palmitoylated exclusively by this one PAT or, alternatively, by no other PAT expressed in the cell type that will be used for the screen. However, biological systems rarely offer ideal situations, and accommodations will inevitably need to be made. The ideal substrate would then be fused to a monomeric fluorescent protein (FP) [5, 151] to generate a fluorescent reporter of palmitoylation that localizes primarily or exclusively to the PM. Cells stably expressing this reporter would then be grown in multi-well imaging plates and exposed to a chemical compound library, and the subcellular distribution of the FP-tagged palmitoylation substrate evaluated by HCS. Compounds that cause redistribution of the fluorescent reporter from the PM to the cytoplasm are candidates (or hits) for follow up analyses that will determine if they blocked palmitoylation of the reporter by directly inhibiting the PAT of interest or indirectly by some other mechanism. Typically, compounds in a large library (tens to hundreds of thousands of compounds) are tested at a single concentration and replicated, often three times, to increase the confidence of selecting biologically active compounds. But, the relationship of replicates is solely statistical, not pharmacological. An alternative screening method for identifying hits is "titration-based screening" called qHTS [152]. This method, which has been used successfully by Jim Inglese, Doug Auld and Colleagues at the NIH Chemical Genomics Center, measures the assay system response to multiple (up to seven), different concentrations of a single compound. The increased density and accuracy of the data produced by this method can provide many benefits over screening at a single concentration (for a full description of the merits of qHTS see [152]). Among the most important benefits of screening at multiple concentrations is that it alleviates the problems of false-negatives and false-positives that plague screens run at a single concentration. The nominal, additional effort required at the front end of the process is generously compensated by a subsequent reduction in the effort required to choose which hits to pursue in follow-up assays.

Displacement or translocation of the fluorescent palmitoylation reporter from the PM to the cytoplasm in response to a compound cannot provide evidence that the compound has this effect by direct inhibition of a PAT. Secondary screens designed to determine which of the hits works by direct inhibition of PAT activity will be required. One option would be to determine the effects of each hit on the enzymatic activity of the PAT of interest. Jennings et al have demonstrated that a PAT can be purified from a membrane environment and retain its enzymatic function i.e., transfer of palmitate to a substrate. The metabolically active form of palmitate in a living system is palmitoyl-CoA. Transfer of palmitate to a substrate results in the liberation of CoA from palmitate, a chemical species that can be measured with accuracy and sensitivity in a high throughput manner (Figure 5) [153].

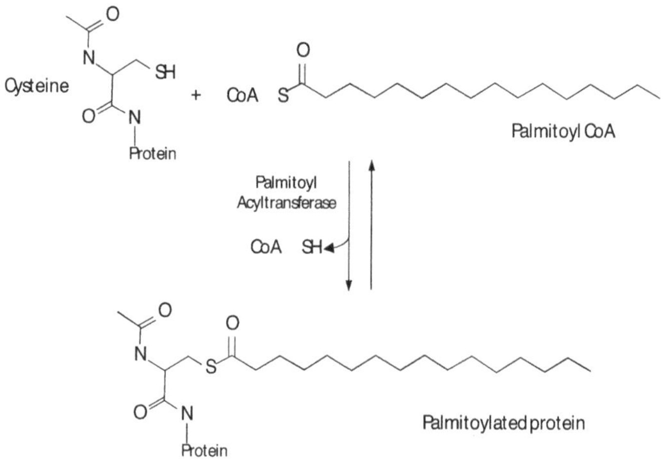

Figure 5.

Retesting hits from the primary screen in this secondary, enzymatic assay would determine if the compounds directly inhibited palmitoylation of the substrate in the reaction. It would also identify compounds that inhibit palmitoylation by competing with palmitoyl-CoA for access to the PAT active site, as well as allosteric inhibitors. Structural analysis of the compounds would provide information about how they inhibit palmitoylation. A binding assay in which compounds are tested for their ability to compete directly with palmitoyl-CoA for binding to the PAT would more conclusively determine the mechanism by which the compounds were inhibiting substrate palmitoylation.

It is likely that the inhibitors identified will represent multiple classes of compounds distinguished by their chemical structures. However, the chemicals identified in these screens are unlikely to represent the most potent or selective compounds that exist. Further refinement by probing and refining the chemical space of each compound in a medicinal chemistry effort will be required to achieve both objectives. Generating higher affinity analogs of the hit compounds for the PAT of interest will improve the selectivity and potency of the compounds for an individual PAT. However, the question of how selective any of these compounds is for a single PAT must be answered by determining their ability to inhibit other PATs—counterscreening. Since the family of PATs is relatively small (23 genes), it would not be unreasonable to measure the effects of the compounds on each of the other PATs in the enzymatic assay described above.

The assay development pathway proposed above is outlined only in very general and ideal terms, glossing over inevitable technical challenges that must be overcome for the project to be successful. However, even as brief as this description is, it exceeds by far the complexity of any published attempt to identify selective PAT inhibitors to date. A valuable, practical guide to choosing, developing, and validating assays including those proposed above is available at: http://ncgc.nih.gov/guidance/manual_toc.html.

6. Conclusion

The discovery of the molecular identity of PATs was a pivotal event that has fostered substantial progress in the field of lipidation, having a profoundly positive effect on many fields of biology. Many long-standing questions have been greeted with answers as well as a clearer direction in which new inquiries should proceed. While sometimes criticized as being stamp collecting, defining the palmitoyl proteome of specific cells and tissues would provide new and unforeseen insight into many cellular processes. The methods described here provide the technical foundation for defining the palmitoyl proteome. Defining the intrinsic and extrinsic mechanisms and factors that regulate PAT activity will also be crucial and challenging. Future assays to investigate such details will certainly benefit from the demonstrated usefulness of bioorthagonal probes that appear to be treated by cells as if they were palmitate. These probes may provide a more direct measure of palmitoylation than the exchange of cysteine-reactive probes for palmitate on purified proteins.

The number of signaling networks in which palmitoylation plays a pivotal role is large and growing. The relationship between PAT gene expression and cancer is perhaps the most evident as the fraction of PAT genes implicated in metastasis and tumorigenesis is notably high. There is also a remarkable confluence between our increasing understanding of palmitoylation and our increasing awareness of the importance of lipid rafts, one of the primary residences of palmitoylated proteins in cancer [154, 155]. In instances where there is a relationship between aberrant expression of PATs and cancer, the critical questions relate to the substrates of these PATs and their associated signaling networks. Identification of these signaling networks will potentially provide new therapeutic targets for the prevention or reversal of cancer progression. Given the preponderance of palmitoylated proteins resident in the neuronal synapse (which is itself a lipid raft of sorts), it is clearly another area of research that deserves (and has already received) a great deal of attention.

While there has been some progress made in identifying pharmacological modulators of palmitoylation [125, 126, 138], there is nothing yet known about how to specifically target individual PATs. From a practical standpoint, inhibiting specific PATs may be a simpler process than developing specific PAT agonists. The advent of assays with the ability to measure changes in the activity of a single PAT along with the identification of PAT-substrate associations should enable further development of new assays to identify specific pharmacological modulators of individual PATs as well as providing important information on the signaling networks associated with specific PATs.

Our ability to understand palmitoylation and its importance to human health and disease is only as good as the technological methods we use to make accurate and valid measurements. Our ability to investigate the basic mechanisms of how PATs work, of PAT/substrate relationships, and how palmitoylation affects signaling processes related to disease would be improved significantly by the development of selective and potent pharmacological tools. Until such tools are available, we should be mindful that using compounds such as 2-BP, cerulenin, and tunicamycin may lead to erroneous conclusions. Developing non-lipid, selective inhibitors that target the PAT active site is feasible. The challenges that exist are conceptually similar in some aspects to those faced during the development of selective, small-molecule inhibitors of kinases that do not resemble ATP. Based on current knowledge, the most logical PATs to target first are those for which overexpression is oncogenic. However, the motivation to initiate drug discovery programs on a large scale will probably remain below the required threshold until more conclusive data are available from more sophisticated, whole-animal experiments that link PATs to oncogenesis.

Author details

Sonia Lobo Planey

Address all correspondence to: splaney@tcmedc.org

The Commonwealth Medical College, Scranton, PA, USA

References

[1] Linder, M. E., & Deschenes, R. J. (2007). Palmitoylation: policing protein stability and traffic. *Nat Rev Mol Cell Biol. Jan*, 8(1), 74-84.

[2] Buglino, J. A., & Resh, M. D. Hhat is a palmitoylacyltransferase with specificity for N-palmitoylation of Sonic Hedgehog. *J Biol Chem*, 283(32), 22076-88.

[3] Mitchell, D. A., Vasudevan, A., Linder, M. E., & Deschenes, R. J. Protein palmitoylation by a family of DHHC protein S-acyltransferases. *J Lipid Res*, 47(6), 1118-27.

[4] Hofmann, K. A superfamily of membrane-bound O-acyltransferases with implications for wnt signaling. *Trends Biochem Sci*, 25(3), 111-2.

[5] Zacharias, D. A., Violin, J. D., Newton, A. C., & Tsien, R. Y. Partitioning of lipid-modified monomeric GFPs into membrane microdomains of live cells. *Science*, 296(5569), 913-6.

[6] Greaves, J., Prescott, G. R., Gorleku, O. A., & Chamberlain, L. H. The fat controller: roles of palmitoylation in intracellular protein trafficking and targeting to membrane microdomains (Review). *Mol Membr Biol*, 26(1), 67-79.

[7] Liang, X., Lu, Y., Neubert, T. A., & Resh, M. D. Mass spectrometric analysis of GAP-43/neuromodulin reveals the presence of a variety of fatty acylated species. *J Biol Chem*, 277(36), 33032-40.

[8] Liang, X., Lu, Y., Wilkes, M., Neubert, T. A., & Resh, M. D. The N-terminal SH4 region of the Src family kinase Fyn is modified by methylation and heterogeneous fatty acylation: role in membrane targeting, cell adhesion, and spreading. *J Biol Chem*, 279(9), 8133-9.

[9] Liang, X., Nazarian, A., Erdjument-Bromage, H., Bornmann, W., Tempst, P., & Resh, M. D. Heterogeneous fatty acylation of Src family kinases with polyunsaturated fatty acids regulates raft localization and signal transduction. *J Biol Chem*, 276(33), 30987-94.

[10] Jones, T. L., Degtyarev, M. Y., & Backlund, P. S. Jr. The stoichiometry of G alpha(s) palmitoylation in its basal and activated states. *Biochemistry*, 36(23), 7185-91.

[11] Bizzozero, O. A., Mc Garry, J. F., & Lees, M. B. Autoacylation of myelin proteolipid protein with acyl coenzyme A. *J Biol Chem*, 262(28), 13550-7.

[12] Morello, J. P., & Bouvier, M. (1996). Palmitoylation: a post-translational modification that regulates signalling from G-protein coupled receptors. *Biochem Cell Biol*, 74(4), 449-57.

[13] Wedegaertner, P. B., & Bourne, H. R. Activation and depalmitoylation of Gs alpha. *Cell*, 77(7), 1063-70.

[14] Bano, M. C., Jackson, C. S., & Magee, A. I. (1998). Pseudo-enzymatic S-acylation of a myristoylated yes protein tyrosine kinase peptide in vitro may reflect non-enzymatic S-acylation in vivo. Biochem J. Mar 1 , 330(Pt 2), 723-31.

[15] Duncan, J. A., & Gilman, A. G. (1996). Autoacylation of G protein alpha subunits. J Biol Chem. Sep 20; , 271(38), 23594-600.

[16] Dietrich, L. E., & Ungermann, C. (2004). On the mechanism of protein palmitoylation. EMBO Rep. Nov; , 5(11), 1053-7.

[17] Berger, M., & Schmidt, M. F. Cell-free fatty acid acylation of Semliki Forest viral polypeptides with microsomal membranes from eukaryotic cells. *J Biol Chem*, 259(11), 7245-52.

[18] Berthiaume, L., & Resh, M.D. Biochemical characterization of a palmitoyl acyltransferase activity that palmitoylates myristoylated proteins. *J Biol Chem*, 270(38), 22399-405.

[19] Liu, L., Dudler, T., & Gelb, M. H. Purification of a protein palmitoyltransferase that acts on H-Ras protein and on a C-terminal N-Ras peptide. *J Biol Chem*, 271(38), 23269-76.

[20] Bartels, D. J., Mitchell, D. A., Dong, X., & Deschenes, R. J. Erf2, a novel gene product that affects the localization and palmitoylation of Ras2 in Saccharomyces cerevisiae. *Mol Cell Biol*, 19(10), 6775-87.

[21] Mitchell, D. A., Farh, L., Marshall, T. K., & Deschenes, R. J. A polybasic domain allows nonprenylated Ras proteins to function in Saccharomyces cerevisiae. *J Biol Chem*, 269(34), 21540-6.

[22] Jung, V., Chen, L., Hofmann, S. L., Wigler, M., & Powers, S. Mutations in the SHR5 gene of Saccharomyces cerevisiae suppress Ras function and block membrane attachment and palmitoylation of Ras proteins. *Mol Cell Biol*, 15(3), 1333-42.

[23] Lobo, S., Greentree, W. K., Linder, M. E., & Deschenes, R. J. Identification of a Ras palmitoyltransferase in Saccharomyces cerevisiae. *J Biol Chem*, 277(43), 41268-73.

[24] Putilina, T., Wong, P., & Gentleman, S. (1999). The DHHC domain: a new highly conserved cysteine-rich motif. Mol Cell Biochem May; , 195(1-2), 219 -26 .

[25] Mesilaty-Gross, S., Reich, A., Motro, B., & Wides, R. The Drosophila STAM gene homolog is in a tight gene cluster, and its expression correlates to that of the adjacent gene ial. *Gene*, 231(1-2), 173-86.

[26] Roth, A. F., Feng, Y., Chen, L., & Davis, N. G. The yeast DHHC cysteine-rich domain protein Akr1p is a palmitoyl transferase. *J Cell Biol*, 159(1), 23-8.

[27] Feng, Y., & Davis, N. G. Akr1p and the type I casein kinases act prior to the ubiquitination step of yeast endocytosis: Akr1p is required for kinase localization to the plasma membrane. *Mol Cell Biol*, 20(14), 5350-9.

[28] Givan, S. A., & Sprague, G. F. Jr. The ankyrin repeat-containing protein Akr1p is required for the endocytosis of yeast pheromone receptors. *Mol Biol Cell*, 8(7), 1317-27.

[29] Oyama, T., Miyoshi, Y., Koyama, K., Nakagawa, H., Yamori, T., Ito, T., et al. Isolation of a novel gene on 8p21.3-22 whose expression is reduced significantly in human colorectal cancers with liver metastasis. *Genes Chromosomes Cancer*, 29(1), 9-15.

[30] Ohno, Y., Kihara, A., Sano, T., & Igarashi, Y. Intracellular localization and tissue-specific distribution of human and yeast DHHC cysteine-rich domain-containing proteins. *Biochim Biophys Acta*, 1761(4), 474-83.

[31] Swarthout, J. T., Lobo, S., Farh, L., Croke, M. R., Greentree, W. K., Deschenes, R. J., et al. DHHC9 and GCP16 constitute a human protein fatty acyltransferase with specificity for H- and N-Ras. *J Biol Chem*, 280(35), 31141-8.

[32] Raymond, F. L., Tarpey, P. S., Edkins, S., Tofts, C., O'Meara, S., Teague, J., et al. Mutations in ZDHHC9, which encodes a palmitoyltransferase of NRAS and HRAS, cause X-linked mental retardation associated with a marfanoid habitus. *Am J Hum Genet*, 80(5), 982-7.

[33] Mukai, J., Liu, H., Burt, R. A., Swor, D. E., Lai, W. S., Karayiorgou, M., et al. Evidence that the gene encoding ZDHHC8 contributes to the risk of schizophrenia. *Nat Genet*, 36(7), 725-31.

[34] Demily, C., Legallic, S., Bou, J., Houy-Durand, E., Van Amelsvoort, T., Zinkstok, J., et al. ZDHHC8 single nucleotide polymorphism rs175174 is not associated with psychiatric features of the 22q11 deletion syndrome or schizophrenia. *Psychiatr Genet*, 17(5), 311-2.

[35] Glaser, B., Schumacher, J., Williams, H. J., Jamra, R. A., Ianakiev, N., Milev, R., et al. No association between the putative functional ZDHHC8 single nucleotide polymorphism rs175174 and schizophrenia in large European samples. *Biol Psychiatry*, 58(1), 78-80.

[36] Saito, S., Ikeda, M., Iwata, N., Suzuki, T., Kitajima, T., Yamanouchi, Y., et al. No association was found between a functional SNP in ZDHHC8 and schizophrenia in a Japanese case-control population. *Neurosci Lett*, 374(1), 21-4.

[37] Zhang, J., Planey, S. L., Ceballos, C., Stevens, S. M. Jr, Keay, S. K., & Zacharias, D. A. Identification of CKAP4/63as a major substrate of the palmitoyl acyltransferase DHHC2, a putative tumor suppressor, using a novel proteomics method. *Mol Cell Proteomics*, 7(7), 1378-88.

[38] Rocks, O., Gerauer, M., Vartak, N., Koch, S., Huang, Z. P., Pechlivanis, M., et al. The palmitoylation machinery is a spatially organizing system for peripheral membrane proteins. *Cell*, 141(3), 458-71.

[39] Politis, E. G., Roth, A. F., & Davis, N. G. Transmembrane topology of the protein palmitoyl transferase Akr1. *J Biol Chem*, 280(11), 10156-63.

[40] Claros, M. G., & von, Heijne. G. TopPred II: an improved software for membrane protein structure predictions. *Comput Appl Biosci*, 10(6), 685-6.

[41] Freedman, R. B., Dunn, A. D., & Ruddock, L. W. Protein folding: a missing redox link in the endoplasmic reticulum. *Curr Biol*, 8(13), R 468-70.

[42] Huppa, J. B., & Ploegh, H. L. The eS-Sence of-SH in the ER. *Cell*, 92(2), 145-8.

[43] Hou, H., Subramanian, K., La Grassa, T. J., Markgraf, D., Dietrich, L. E., Urban, J., et al. The DHHC protein Pfa3 affects vacuole-associated palmitoylation of the fusion factor Vac8. *Proc Natl Acad Sci U S A*, 102(48), 17366-71.

[44] Planey, S. L., Keay, S. K., Zhang, C. O., & Zacharias, D. A. Palmitoylation of cytoskeleton associated protein 4 by DHHC2 regulates antiproliferative factor-mediated signaling. *Mol Biol Cell*, 20(5), 1454-63.

[45] Smotrys, J. E., & Linder, M. E. (2004). Palmitoylation of intracellular signaling proteins: regulation and function. *Annu Rev Biochem*, 73, 559-87.

[46] Lam, K. K., Davey, M., Sun, B., Roth, A. F., Davis, N. G., & Conibear, E. Palmitoylation by the DHHC protein Pfa4 regulates the ER exit of Chs3. *J Cell Biol*, 174(1), 19-25.

[47] Greaves, J., Carmichae, J. A., & Chamberlain, L. H. The palmitoyl transferase DHHC2 targets a dynamic membrane cycling pathway: regulation by a C-terminal domain. *Mol Biol Cell*, 22(11), 1887-95.

[48] Fernandez-Hernando, C., Fukata, M., Bernatchez, P. N., Fukata, Y., Lin, M. I., Bredt, D. S., et al. Identification of Golgi-localized acyl transferases that palmitoylate and regulate endothelial nitric oxide synthase. *J Cell Biol*, 174(3), 369-77.

[49] Yanai, A., Huang, K., Kang, R., Singaraja, R. R., Arstikaitis, P., Gan, L., et al. Palmitoylation of huntingtin by HIP14 is essential for its trafficking and function. *Nat Neurosci*, 9(6), 824-31.

[50] Mansouri, M. R., Marklund, L., Gustavsson, P., Davey, E., Carlsson, B., Larsson, C., et al. Loss of 5p15.33 ZDHHC15 expression in a woman with a balanced translocation t(X;15)(q13.3;cen) and severe mental retardation. *Eur J Hum Genet*, 13(8), 970-7.

[51] Yamamoto, Y., Chochi, Y., Matsuyama, H., Eguchi, S., Kawauchi, S., Furuya, T., et al. (2007). Gain of is associated with progression of bladder cancer. *Oncology*, 72(1-2), 132-8.

[52] Mansilla, F., Birkenkamp-Demtroder, K., Kruhoffer, M., Sorensen, F. B., Andersen, C. L., Laiho, P., et al. Differential expression of DHHC9 in microsatellite stable and instable human colorectal cancer subgroups. *Br J Cancer*, 96(12), 1896-903.

[53] Ducker, C. E., Stettler, E. M., French, K. J., Upson, J. J., & Smith, C. D. Huntingtin interacting protein 14 is an oncogenic human protein: palmitoyl acyltransferase. *Oncogene*, 23(57), 9230-7.

[54] Razzaq, T. M., Bass, R., Vines, D. J., Werner, F., Whawell, S. A., & Ellis, V. Functional regulation of tissue plasminogen activator on the surface of vascular smooth muscle

cells by the type-II transmembrane protein p63(CKAP4). *J Biol Chem*, 278(43), 42679-85.

[55] Gupta, N., Manevich, Y., Kazi, Tao. J. Q., Fisher, A. B., & Bates, S. R. Identification and characterization of p63 (CKAP4/ERGIC-63/CLIMP-63), a surfactant protein A binding protein, on type II pneumocytes. *Am J Physiol Lung Cell Mol Physiol*, 291(3), L 436-46.

[56] Sharma, C., Yang, X. H., & Hemler, M. E. DHHC2 Affects Palmitoylation, Stability, and Functions of Tetraspanins CD9 and CD151. *Mol Biol Cell*.

[57] Ikeyama, S., Koyama, M., Yamaoko, M., Sasada, R., & Miyake, M. Suppression of cell motility and metastasis by transfection with human motility-related protein (MRP-1/CD9) DNA. *J Exp Med*, 177(5), 1231-7.

[58] Miyake, M., Inufusa, H., Adachi, M., Ishida, H., Hashida, H., Tokuhara, T., et al. Suppression of pulmonary metastasis using adenovirally motility related protein-1 (MRP-1/CD9) gene delivery. *Oncogene*, 19(46), 5221-6.

[59] Zavadil, J., Bitzer, M., Liang, D., Yang, Y. C., Massimi, A., Kneitz, S., et al. Genetic programs of epithelial cell plasticity directed by transforming growth factor-beta. *Proc Natl Acad Sci U S A*, 98(12), 6686-91.

[60] Janda, E., Lehmann, K., Killisch, I., Jechlinger, M., Herzig, M., Downward, J., et al. Ras and TGF[beta] cooperatively regulate epithelial cell plasticity and metastasis: dissection of Ras signaling pathways. *J Cell Biol*, 156(2), 299-313.

[61] Thiery, J. P. Epithelial-mesenchymal transitions in tumour progression. *Nat Rev Cancer*, 2(6), 442-54.

[62] Fukata, M., Fukata, Y., Adesnik, H., Nicoll, R. A., & Bredt, . Identification of PSD-95 palmitoylating enzymes. *Neuron*, 44(6), 987-96.

[63] Greaves, J., Gorleku, O. A., Salaun, C., & Chamberlain, L. H. Palmitoylation of the SNAP25 protein family: specificity and regulation by DHHC palmitoyl transferases. *J Biol Chem*, 285(32), 24629-38.

[64] Zeidman, R., Buckland, G., Cebecauer, M., Eissmann, P., Davis, D. M., & Magee, A. I. DHHC2 is a protein S-acyltransferase for Lck. *Mol Membr Biol*, 28(7-8), 473-86.

[65] Tsutsumi, R., Fukata, Y., Noritake, J., Iwanaga, T., Perez, F., & Fukata, M. Identification of G protein alpha subunit-palmitoylating enzyme. *Mol Cell Biol*, 29(2), 435-47.

[66] Jia, L., Linder, M. E., & Blumer, K. J. Gi/o signaling and the palmitoyltransferase DHHC2 regulate palmitate cycling and shuttling of RGS7 family-binding protein. *J Biol Chem*, 286(15), 13695-703.

[67] Goytain, A., Hines, R. M., & Quamme, G. A. Huntingtin-interacting proteins, HIP14 and HIP14L, mediate dual functions, palmitoyl acyltransferase and Mg2+ transport. J. *Biol Chem*, 283(48), 33365-74.

[68] Schlingmann, K. P., & Gudermann, T. A critical role of TRPM channel-kinase for hu-
       man magnesium transport. *J Physiol*, 566(Pt 2), 301 -8 .

[69] Schlingmann, K. P., Waldegger, S., Konrad, M., Chubanov, V., & Gudermann, T.
       TRPM6 and TRPM7--Gatekeepers of human magnesium metabolism. *Biochim Biophys
       Acta*, 1772(8), 813-21.

[70] Goytain, A., Hines, R. M., & Quamme, G. A. Huntingtin-interacting proteins, HIP14
       and HIP14L, mediate dual functions:Palmitoyl acytransferase and Mg2+ transport. *J
       Biol Chem*.

[71] Hines, R. M., Kang, R., Goytain, A., & Quamme, G. A. Golgi-specific DHHC zinc fin-
       ger protein GODZ mediates membrane Ca2+ transport. *J Biol Chem*, 285(7), 4621-8.

[72] Fukata, Y., Iwanaga, T., & Fukata, M. Systematic screening for palmitoyl transferase
       activity of the DHHC protein family in mammalian cells. *Methods*, 40(2), 177-82.

[73] Nadolski, M. J., & Linder, M. E. Protein lipidation. *FEBS J*, 274(20), 5202-10.

[74] Roth, A. F., Wan, J., Bailey, A. O., Sun, B., Kuchar, J. A., Green, W. N., et al. Global
       analysis of protein palmitoylation in yeast. *Cell*, 125(5), 1003-13.

[75] Ren, J., Wen, L., Gao, X., Jin, C., Xue, Y., & Yao, X. CSS-Palm 2.0: an updated software
       for palmitoylation sites prediction. *Protein Eng Des Sel*.

[76] Xue, Y., Chen, H., Jin, C., Sun, Z., & Yao, X. (2006). NBA-Palm: prediction of palmi-
       toylation site implemented in Naive Bayes algorithm. *BMC Bioinformatics*, 7, 458 .

[77] Zhou, F., Xue, Y., Yao, X., & Xu, Y. (2006). A general user interface for prediction
       servers of proteins' post-translational modification sites. *Nat Protoc*, 1(3), 1318-21.

[78] Zhou, F., Xue, Y., Yao, X., & Xu, Y. CSS-Palm: palmitoylation site prediction with a
       clustering and scoring strategy (CSS). *Bioinformatics*, 22(7), 894-6.

[79] Bernstein, L. S., Linder, M. E., & Hepler, J. R. (2004). Analysis of RGS protein palmi-
       toylation. *Methods Mol Biol*, 237, 195-204.

[80] Basar, T., Havlicek, V., Bezouskova, S., Halada, P., Hackett, M., & Sebo, P. The con-
       served lysine 860 in the additional fatty-acylation site of Bordetella pertussis adeny-
       late cyclase is crucial for toxin function independently of its acylation status. *J Biol
       Chem*, 274(16), 10777-83.

[81] Branton, W. D., Rudnick, M. S., Zhou, Y., Eccleston, E. D., Fields, G. B., & Bowers, L.
       D. Fatty acylated toxin structure. *Nature*, 365(6446), 496-7.

[82] Kleuss, C., & Krause, E. Galpha(s) is palmitoylated at the N-terminal glycine. *Embo J*,
       22(4), 826-32.

[83] Pepinsky, R. B., Zeng, C., Wen, D., Rayhorn, P., Baker, D. P., Williams, K. P., et al.
       Identification of a palmitic acid-modified form of human Sonic hedgehog. *J Biol
       Chem*, 273(22), 14037-45.

[84] Bijlsma, M. F., Spek, C. A., & Peppelenbosch, M. P. Hedgehog: an unusual signal transducer. *Bioessays*, 26(4), 387-94.

[85] Di Simplicio, P., Franconi, F., Frosali, S., & Di Giuseppe, D. Thiolation and nitrosation of cysteines in biological fluids and cells. *Amino Acids*, 25(3-4), 323 -39 .

[86] Lipton, S. A., Choi, Y. B., Takahashi, H., Zhang, D., Li, W., Godzik, A., et al. Cysteine regulation of protein function--as exemplified by NMDA-receptor modulation. *Trends Neurosci*, 25(9), 474-80.

[87] Hershko, A., & Ciechanover, A. (1998). The ubiquitin system. *Annu Rev Biochem*, 67, 425-79.

[88] Hermanson, G. T. (1996). Bioconjugate Techniques. 1st ed. *San Diego: Academic Press*.

[89] Gygi, S. P., Rist, B., Gerber, S. A., Turecek, F., Gelb, M. H., & Aebersold, R. Quantitative analysis of complex protein mixtures using isotope-coded affinity tags. *Nat Biotechnol*, 17(10), 994-9.

[90] Schrimpf, S. P., Meskenaite, V., Brunner, E., Rutishauser, D., Walther, P., Eng, J., et al. Proteomic analysis of synaptosomes using isotope-coded affinity tags and mass spectrometry. *Proteomics*, 5(10), 2531-41.

[91] Gygi, S. P., Rist, B., Griffin, T. J., Eng, J., & Aebersold, R. Proteome analysis of low-abundance proteins using multidimensional chromatography and isotope-coded affinity tags. *J Proteome Res*, 1(1), 47-54.

[92] Sitia, R., & Molteni, S. N. Stress, protein (mis)folding, and signaling: the redox connection. *Sci STKE* [239], pe27.

[93] Munro, A. P., & Williams, D. L. H. (1999). Reactivity of nitrogen nucleophiles towards S-nitrosopenicillamine. *Journal of the Chemical Society, Perkin Transactions*, 2, 1989-93.

[94] Fenton, S. S., & Fahey, R. C. Analysis of biological thiols: determination of thiol components of disulfides and thioesters. *Anal Biochem*, 154(1), 34-42.

[95] Bizzozero, O. A., & Good, L. K. Rapid metabolism of fatty acids covalently bound to myelin proteolipid protein. *J Biol Chem*, 266(26), 17092-8.

[96] Passmore, L. A., & Barford, D. Getting into position: the catalytic mechanisms of protein ubiquitylation. *Biochem J*, 379(Pt3), 513-25.

[97] Bizzozero, O. A. (1995). Chemical analysis of acylation sites and species. *Methods Enzymol*, 250, 361-79.

[98] Tolbert, B. S., Tajc, S. G., Webb, H., Snyder, J., Nielsen, J. E., Miller, B. L., et al. The active site cysteine of ubiquitin-conjugating enzymes has a significantly elevated pKa: functional implications. *Biochemistry*, 44(50), 16385-91.

[99] Cione, E., Pingitore, A., Perri, M., & Genchi, G. Influence of all-trans-retinoic acid on oxoglutarate carrier via retinoylation reaction. *Biochim Biophys Acta*, 1791(1), 3-7.

[100] Cione, E., Tucci, P., Chimento, A., Pezzi, V., & Genchi, G. Retinoylation reaction of proteins in Leydig (TM-3) cells. *J Bioenerg Biomembr*, 37(1), 43-8.

[101] Cione, E., Tucci, P., Senatore, V., Ioele, G., & Genchi, G. (2005). Binding of all-trans-retinoic acid to MLTC-1 proteins. Mol Cell Biochem Aug; , 276(1-2), 55 -60 .

[102] Kubo, Y., Wada, M., Ohba, T., & Takahashi, N. Formation of retinoylated proteins from retinoyl-CoA in rat tissues. *J Biochem*, 138(4), 493-500.

[103] Takahashi, N., & Breitman, T. R. Retinoic acid acylation (retinoylation) of a nuclear protein in the human acute myeloid leukemia cell line HL60. *J Biol Chem*, 264(9), 5159-63.

[104] Takahashi, N., & Breitman, T. R. Retinoylation of HL-60 proteins. Comparison to labeling by palmitic and myristic acids. *J Biol Chem*, 265(31), 19158-62.

[105] Takahashi, N., & Breitman, T. R. Retinoylation of proteins in leukemia, embryonal carcinoma, and normal kidney cell lines: differences associated with differential responses to retinoic acid. *Arch Biochem Biophys*, 285(1), 105-10.

[106] Takahashi, N., Liapi, C., Anderson, W. B., & Breitman, T. R. Retinoylation of the cAMP-binding regulatory subunits of type I and type II cAMP-dependent protein kinases in HL60 cells. *Arch Biochem Biophys*, 290(2), 293-302.

[107] Takahashi, N., Jetten, A. M., & Breitman, T. R. Retinoylation of cytokeratins in normal human epidermal keratinocytes. *Biochem Biophys Res Commun*, 180(1), 393-400.

[108] Djakoure, C., Guibourdenche, J., Porquet, D., Pagesy, P., Peillon, F., Li, J. Y., et al. Vitamin A and retinoic acid stimulate within minutes cAMP release and growth hormone secretion in human pituitary cells. *J Clin Endocrinol Metab*, 81(8), 3123-6.

[109] Varani, J., Burmeister, B., Perone, P., Bleavins, M., & Johnson, K. J. All-trans retinoic acid inhibits fluctuations in intracellular Ca2+ resulting from changes in extracellular Ca2+. *Am J Pathol*, 147(3), 718-27.

[110] Hensel, J., Hintz, M., Karas, M., Linder, D., Stahl, B., & Geyer, R. Localization of the palmitoylation site in the transmembrane protein p12E of Friend murine leukaemia virus. *Eur J Biochem*, 232(2), 373-80.

[111] De Mar, J. C., Jr , , & Anderson, R. E. Identification and quantitation of the fatty acids composing the CoA ester pool of bovine retina, heart, and liver. *J Biol Chem*, 272(50), 31362-8.

[112] Hang, H. C., Geutjes, E. J., Grotenbreg, G., Pollington, A. M., Bijlmakers, MJ, & Ploegh, HL. Chemical probes for the rapid detection of Fatty-acylated proteins in Mammalian cells. *J Am Chem Soc*, 129(10), 2744-5.

[113] Adams, S. R., Campbell, R. E., Gross, L. A., Martin, B. R., Walkup, G. K., Yao, Y., et al. New biarsenical ligands and tetracysteine motifs for protein labeling in vitro and in vivo: synthesis and biological applications. *J Am Chem Soc*, 124(21), 6063-76.

[114] Adams, S. R., Lev-Ram, V., & Tsien, R. Y. (1997). A new caged Ca2+, azid-1, is far more photosensitive than nitrobenzyl- based chelators. *Chem Biol*, 4(11), 867-78.

[115] Griffin, B. A., Adams, S. R., Jones, J., & Tsien, R. Y. (2000). Fluorescent labeling of recombinant proteins in living cells with FlAsH. *Methods Enzymol*, 327, 565-78.

[116] Nagai, T., Sawano, A., Park, E. S., & Miyawaki, A. (2001). Circularly permuted green fluorescent proteins engineered to sense Ca2+. *Proc Natl Acad Sci U S A*, 98(6), 3197-202.

[117] Gaietta, G. M., Giepmans, B. N., Deerinck, T. J., Smith, W. B., Ngan, L., Llopis, J., et al. Golgi twins in late mitosis revealed by genetically encoded tags for live cell imaging and correlated electron microscopy. *Proc Natl Acad Sci U S A*, 103(47), 17777-82.

[118] Martin, B. R., Giepmans, B. N., Adams, S. R., & Tsien, R. Y. Mammalian cell-based optimization of the biarsenical-binding tetracysteine motif for improved fluorescence and affinity. *Nat Biotechnol*, 23(10), 1308-14.

[119] Ju, W., Morishita, W., Tsui, J., Gaietta, G., Deerinck, T. J., Adams, S. R., et al. Activity-dependent regulation of dendritic synthesis and trafficking of AMPA receptors. *Nat Neurosci*, 7(3), 244-53.

[120] Stults, J. T., & Arnott, D. (2005). Proteomics. Methods Enzymol.; , 402, 245-89.

[121] Kenyon GL, Bruice TW. (1977). Novel sulfhydryl reagents. *Methods Enzymol*, 47, 407-30.

[122] Qanbar, R., & Bouvier, M. Determination of protein-bound palmitate turnover rates using a three-compartment model that formally incorporates [3H]palmitate recycling. *Biochemistry*, 43(38), 12275-88.

[123] Ducker, C. E., Draper, J. M., Xia, Z., & Smith, C. D. In vitro and cellular assays for palmitoyl acyltransferases using fluorescent lipidated peptides. *Methods*, 40(2), 166-70.

[124] Kenworthy, A. K. Fluorescence-based methods to image palmitoylated proteins. *Methods*, 40(2), 198-205.

[125] Resh, M. D. Use of analogs and inhibitors to study the functional significance of protein palmitoylation. *Methods*, 40(2), 191-7.

[126] Ducker, C. E., Griffel, L. K., Smith, R. A., Keller, S. N., Zhuang, Y., Xia, Z., et al. Discovery and characterization of inhibitors of human palmitoyl acyltransferases. *Mol Cancer Ther*, 5(7), 1647-59.

[127] Varner, A. S., Ducker, C. E., Xia, Z., Zhuang, Y., De Vos, M. L., & Smith, C. D. Characterization of human palmitoyl-acyl transferase activity using peptides that mimic distinct palmitoylation motifs. *Biochem J*, 373(Pt1), 91-9.

[128] Schmidt, M., Schmidt, M. F., & Rott, R. Chemical identification of cysteine as palmi-
       toylation site in a transmembrane protein (Semliki Forest virus E1). *J Biol Chem*,
       263(35), 18635-9.

[129] Drisdel, R. C., & Green, W. N. Labeling and quantifying sites of protein palmitoyla-
       tion. *Biotechniques*, 36(2), 276-85.

[130] Drisdel, R. C., Manzana, E., & Green, W. N. The role of palmitoylation in functional
       expression of nicotinic alpha7 receptors. *J Neurosci*, 24(46), 10502-10.

[131] Wan, J., Roth, A. F., Bailey, A. O., & Davis, N. G. Palmitoylated proteins: purification
       and identification. 2(7), 1573-84.

[132] Liu, H., Lin, D., & Yates, J. R. 3rd. Multidimensional separations for protein/peptide
       analysis in the post-genomic era. *Biotechniques*, 32(4), 898 -900, 2 passim.

[133] Roth, A. F., Wan, J., Green, W. N., Yates, J. R., & Davis, N. G. Proteomic identification
       of palmitoylated proteins. *Methods*, 40(2), 135-42.

[134] Schweizer, A., Rohrer, J., Jeno, P., De Maio, A., Buchman, T. G., & Hauri, H. P. A re-
       versibly palmitoylated resident protein (63 of an ER-Golgi intermediate compart-
       ment is related to a circulatory shock resuscitation protein. *J Cell Sci*, 104(Pt 3),
       685-94.

[135] Zhang, J., & Zacharias, D. A. Global Analysis of the Dynamic Palmitoylosome. *Lipid
       Rafts and Cell Funciton*, 23-28, Steamboat Springs, Colorado: Keystone Symposia.

[136] Kostiuk, M. A., Corvi, M. M., Keller, B. O., Plummer, G., Prescher, J. A., Hangauer,
       M. J., et al. Identification of palmitoylated mitochondrial proteins using a bio-orthog-
       onal azido-palmitate analogue. *FASEB J*, 22(3), 721-32.

[137] Saxon, E., & Bertozzi, C. R. (2000). Cell surface engineering by a modified Staudinger
       reaction. Science. Mar 17 , 287(5460), 2007-10.

[138] Jennings, B. C., Nadolski, M. J., Ling, Y., Baker, M. B., Harrison, M. L., Deschenes, R.
       J., et al. 2bromopalmitate and 2-(2-Hydroxy-5-nitro-benzylidene)-benzo[b]thio-
       phen-3-one inhibit DHHC-mediated palmitoylation in vitro. *J Lipid Res.*

[139] Mikic, I., Planey, S., Zhang, J., Ceballos, C., Seron, T., Massenbach, Bv., et al. (2006). A
       live-cell, image based approach to understanding the enzymology and pharmacolo-
       gy of 2bromopalmitate and palmitoylation. *Methods in enzymology*, 414.

[140] Chase, J. F., & Tubbs, P. K. Specific inhibition of mitochondrial fatty acid oxidation
       by2-bromopalmitate and its coenzyme A and carnitine esters. *The Biochemical journal*,
       129(1), 55-65.

[141] Coleman, R. A., Rao, P., Fogelsong, R. J., & Bardes, E. S. Bromopalmitoyl-CoA and 2-
       bromopalmitate: promiscuous inhibitors of membrane-bound enzymes. *Biochimica et
       biophysica acta*, 1125(2), 203-9.

[142] Draper, J. M., & Smith, C. D. (2009). Palmitoyl acyltransferase assays and inhibitors (Review). Mol Membr Biol. Jan , 26(1), 5-13.

[143] Fabian, M. A., Biggs, W. H. 3.r.d, Treiber, . D. K., Atteridge, C. E., Azimioara, M. D., Benedetti, M. G., et al. A small molecule-kinase interaction map for clinical kinase inhibitors. *Nature biotechnology*, 23(3), 329-36.

[144] Karaman, M. W., Herrgard, S., Treiber, D. K., Gallant, P., Atteridge, C. E., Campbell, B. T., et al. A quantitative analysis of kinase inhibitor selectivity. *Nature biotechnology*, 26(1), 127-32.

[145] Feng, Y., Yin, Y., Weiser, A., Griffin, E., Cameron, Lin. L., et al. Discovery of substituted 4-(pyrazol-4-yl)-phenylbenzodioxane-2-carboxamides as potent and highly selective Rho kinase (ROCK-II) inhibitors. *Journal of medicinal chemistry*, 51(21), 6642-5.

[146] Huang, K., Sanders, S., Singaraja, R., Orban, P., Cijsouw, T., Arstikaitis, P., et al. Neuronal palmitoyl acyl transferases exhibit distinct substrate specificity. *Faseb J*, 23(8), 2605-15.

[147] Prigozhina, N. L., Zhong, L., Hunter, E. A., Mikic, I., Callaway, S., Roop, D. R., et al. Plasma membrane assays and three-compartment image cytometry for high content screening. *Assay and drug development technologies*, 5(1), 29-48.

[148] Morelock, M. M., Hunter, E. A., Moran, T. J., Heynen, S., Laris, C., Thieleking, M., et al. Statistics of assay validation in high throughput cell imaging of nuclear factor kappaB nuclear translocation. *Assay and drug development technologies*, 3(5), 483-99.

[149] Wolff, M., Kredel, S., Wiedenmann, J., Nienhaus, G. U., & Heilker, R. Cell-based assays in practice: cell markers from autofluorescent proteins of the GFP-family. *Combinatorial chemistry & high throughput screening*, 11(8), 602-9.

[150] Collins, M. A. Generating'omic knowledge: The Role of Informatics in High Content Screening. *Combinatorial chemistry & high throughput screening*.

[151] Shaner, N. C., Campbell, R. E., Steinbach, P. A., Giepmans, B. N., Palmer, A. E., & Tsien, R. Y. Improved monomeric red, orange and yellow fluorescent proteins derived from Discosoma sp. red fluorescent protein. *Nature biotechnology*, 22(12), 1567-72.

[152] Inglese, J., Auld, Jadhav. A., Johnson, R. L., Simeonov, A., Yasgar, A., et al. Quantitative high-throughput screening: a titration-based approach that efficiently identifies biological activities in large chemical libraries. *Proceedings of the National Academy of Sciences of the United States of America*, 103(31), 11473-8.

[153] Chung, C. C., Ohwaki, K., Schneeweis, J. E., Stec, E., Varnerin, J. P., Goudreau, P. N., et al. A fluorescence-based thiol quantification assay for ultra-high-throughput screening for inhibitors of coenzyme A production. *Assay and drug development technologies*, 6(3), 361-74.

[154] Lazo, P.A. Functional implications of tetraspanin proteins in cancer biology. *Cancer Sci*; 98: 1666-77.

[155] Patra, S.K. Dissecting lipid raft facilitated cell signaling pathways in cancer. *Biochimica et biophysica acta*; 1785: 182-206.

Chapter 3

Air, Water and Soil: Resources for Drug Discovery

Luis Jesús Villarreal-Gómez,
Irma Esthela Soria-Mercado, Ana Leticia Iglesias and
Graciela Lizeth Perez-Gonzalez

Additional information is available at the end of the chapter

1. Introduction

Drug discovery is the process by which new candidate drugs are discovered. The chemical compounds that are present in plants and animals have been an important source of new bioactive compounds. Also, we can found organisms that live in air, water and soil that we don`t see, but posses a great variety of chemical that we can use to create new medicines. Bioactive compounds offer an enormous diversity of chemical structures with strong biologic effect; this is one of the reasons why natural products research cannot be replaced by synthesis chemistry as a source for new bioactive compounds. Actually, more than the half of currently used medicines came from natural sources or are related to them, specifically in the situation of anticancer drugs that more than 60% belongs from nature [1].

Based on the experience in this field, it is considered that a chemical compound isolated from natural origin should be fully assessed in order to be used to combat diseases; in this manner is important to consider the type of new chemical entities potentially applicable for partial or total synthesis, as well as its use in different kind of diseases that are treatable with these compounds (2); Therefore is very important continue the search for new secondarymetabolites potentially usable as drugs by human.

2. Importance of drug discovery

The importance of look for new bioactive compounds to synthesize new drugs it's based by a main objective of saving human life that it's lose by illness. Also, it is important to recognized that the drug discovery projects, help those countries that target their efforts in this area to economically and sociality develop themselves, because when chemical compounds are discovered from microorganism that lives in natural environments, this chemical can be exploited industrially and generate more jobs.

Now, the new drugs and innovative procedures are usually able to keep people alive for a long time with better conditions that would have previously been rapidly fatal, such as cancer and end-stage heart, liver, lung, kidney, and neurologic diseases. As a result, most people in modern countries die from long-term chronic conditions that are characterized by a prolonged period of distressing symptoms and progressive loss of function.

According with World Health Organization (WHO) of "*57 million global deaths in the last report in 2008, 36 million (63%), were due to no communicable diseases (NCDs). The four main NCDs reported are cardiovascular diseases, cancers, diabetes and chronic lung diseases. The burden of these diseases is rising disproportionately among lower income countries and populations. In 2008, nearly 80% of no communicable disease deaths -- 29 million -- occurred in low- and middle-income countries with about 29% of deaths occurring before the age of 60 in these countries. The leading causes of NCD deaths in 2008 were cardiovascular diseases (17 million deaths, or 48% of all NCD deaths), cancers (7.6 million, or 21% of all NCD deaths), and respiratory diseases, including asthma and chronic obstructive pulmonary disease (4.2 million). Diabetes caused another 1.3 million deaths*" [3]. As we can see, in the WHO's statistic data, there are less number of people that die with microbial infection, it can be said to thanks to the constant development of pharmaceutical drugs.

The discovery of new bioactive compounds from microorganism present in the ambient, needs the previously determination of diversity, because by knowing the kind of microbes that live in a certain site, we can be able to design strategies and culture methods adapted for the different types of microorganism present in nature [4]. We can be able to screen chemical bioactivity only if we can culture the microorganism, because we need the microbial biomass to obtain the compounds. To culture microorganism from natural sources is not an easy topics, because, when we try to cultivate bacteria or fungi from substrates and conditions that are in constant change, and incubate them in a static temperature and nutrients; many microbes don't resist this transformation of circumstances and die.

3. Drug resistance bacteria

Some Bacteria can innately be resistant to one or more types of antimicrobial compounds and other can be capable of acquired. In actuality, it is well know the factors that provoke mutations in bacteria that create stronger species that are able to survive to the effects of currents drugs. Examples of these factors are the unnecessary use of antibiotics by humans, the use in animal feeds in low doses, availability over-the-counter in many countries, misuse by health professionals, patient failure to follow prescribed treatment, antibiotic use in agriculture, aquaria and family pets, eating raw or undercooked foods.

It can be describe several strategies of antibiotics resistance in different bacterial genera. Pathogens bacteria that have become resistant to the current antibiotic drug are an increasing public health problem. Some examples of diseases that have become very hard to treat with the current drugs are wound infections, septicemia, tuberculosis, pneumonia, and gonorrhea, to name a few. One part of the problem is that bacteria and other microbes that cause infections are remarkably adaptable and have developed several mechanisms to be immune to antibiotics and other antimicrobial drugs.

Also, it`s been reported that over-prescription and the improper use of antibiotics has led to the generation of antibiotic resistance bacteria that use to be susceptible at those antibiotics [5].

4. Mechanisms of bacteria to become antibiotics resistant

a. **Avoiding entrance of antibiotic into the bacteria cell:** Bacteria and other microbes can actually change the properties of its membrane by changing its grade of permeability by reducing the number of ion channels which are the entrance of some drugs to diffuse into the cells. Another way to get rid of antibiotics in some bacteria is use adenosine triphosphate (ATP) to obtain energy to activate this ion channels and pump it out of the cells.

b. **Editing transmembrane protein expression:** The mechanism of several antibiotics it`s to interact specifically with molecules in the membrane of the microbes and preventing it from interacting with other molecules (usually proteins) inside the cell. Some bacteria respond by changing the chemical structure or the expression of the molecule (replacing it with another molecule) so that the antibiotic can no longer recognize it or bind to it.

c. **Bacterial enzymes that destroy antibiotics:** Some bacteria can be resistant to antibiotics by neutralizing them directly. For example, some organisms may obtain new genes that encode proteins like enzymes that neutralize antibiotics agents before they get to their targets. An example of this enzymes can be found in the β–lactamases like penicillinases, cephalosporinases, carbenicillinase, cloxacilanase, carbapenamase, metalloenzyme that destroy the β-lactamics (penicillins, monobactams, carbapenems, and cephalosporins). The β–lactamases can be isolated from Gram Negative Bacteria: *Escherichia coli, Enterobacter cloacae, Citrobacter freundii, Serrati amarcescens*, and *Pseudomona aeruginosa*. The mechanism of action of β–lactamases is the breaking of β-lactam ring of the antibiotic, thus destroying the drug [6]. Other example of this is *Pseudomona sp.* erithromycinesterases that degrade erythromycin by hydrolysis of the lactone ring of erythromycin [7].

5. Cancer

Cancer is an illness that comprises more than hundred types. This disease appears when old cells are not replaced by new cells and are accumulated in a mass of tissue known as tumor" [4]. To cite some statistics data; cancer is responsible for one of every four deaths in the United States.

It's second only after heart disease as a cause of death in this country. About 1.2 million Americans were diagnosed with cancer in 1998. Of that number, more than 500,000 are expected to die of this disease. Cancer can attack anyone, but the chances of getting the disease increase with age. The most common forms of cancer are skin, lung, colon, breast and prostate cancer. Cancer is a disorder that affects the genes. There were an estimated 12.7 million cancer cases around the world in 2008, of these 6.6 million cases were in men and 6.0 million in women. This number is expected to increase to 21 million by 2030. Lung cancer is the most common cancer worldwide contributing nearly 13% of the total number of new cases diagnosed in 2008. Breast cancer (women only) is the second most common cancer with nearly 1.4 million new cases in 2008 and colorectal cancer (Figure 1) is the third most common cancer with over 1.2 million new cases in 2008 [8].

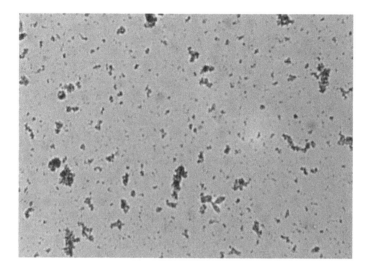

Figure 1. Cancer Colorectal HCT-116 cell culture in McCoy medium at 40 X amplification

6. Natural source for drug discovery

6.1. Drug discovery from air microorganisms

The atmosphere its well characterized for possess a good light intensity, extreme temperature variations, low concentration of organic matter and water, hence become a very hostile place for microorganism. However, there are a numerous quantity of microbes founded in the atmosphere, most of them introduced by human activity.

Bioaerosols are airborne particles that are biological in foundation. Bioaerosols can be formed from nearly any process that involves biological materials and generates enough energy to separate small particles from the larger substance, such as wind, water, air, or mechanical movement. Plants, soil, water, and animals (including humans) all serve as sources of bioaerosols and are present in most places where any of these sources live.

Microorganisms are frequently considered passive habitants of the air, dispersing via airborne dust particles (Figure 2). However, latest studies suggest that many airborne microorganisms are metabolically active, even up to altitudes of 20,000 m. Also, it has been suggested, that some airborne microbes may modify atmospheric conditions [9].

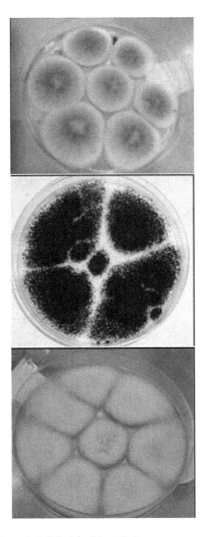

Figure 2. Fungal strains from air samples in Valle de las Palmas, Mexico.

Several studies reported a great variety of microorganism present in air samples, for example, a study realized in Mexico, in 2007, showed 21 species of bacteria founded in air samples from landfill, some of them are pathogenic and opportunistic bacteria, the most abundant are *Pasteurella haemolytica, Serratia plymuthica, Escherichia coli* y *Klebsiella pneumonia* and 19 fungal species, 7 of them allergenic, *Cladosporium herbarum, Aspergillus* sp y *Penicillium* sp. [10]. Despite this, *Serratia plymuthica*it's well known to possess 2-amino-3-(oxirane-2,3-dicarboxamido)-propanoyl-valine has been shown to inhibit the growth of the human pathogen *Candida albicans* efficiently [11].

Another studies found airborne microbes collected at indoor air with filters installed in two shopping centers in Singapore. The most common microorganism appears to be several species of *Brevundimonas* (50%) [12] other study has identified *Brevundimonas diminuta*as producer of a nematicidal metabolite known as (R)-(-)-2-ethykhexan-1-ol which have a strong activity against *C. elegans* and *B. xylophilus* [13].

6.2. Drug discovery from soil microorganisms

Soil microorganisms (Figure 3), such as bacteria and fungi, play central roles in soil fertility and promotion of plant health. It is assessed that in 1 g of soil there are 4000 different bacterial "genomic units" based on culture independent identification methods. In the other hand, an estimated 1,500,000 species of fungi, but they are more difficult to cultivated by standard methods [14].

In soil there is a constant exchange of organic substances and flow of energy. Feeding, predation, degradation of macromolecular substrates and absorption of nutrients have been important in chemical processes in soil. One of the most important microorganism in drug discovery found in natural habitat mainly in soil are the actinomycetes which are very diverse family of bacteria, they are an important source of bioactive compounds with high value in pharmaceutical industry. It's have been reported that almost 80% of the world`s antibiotics come from the genera *Micromonospora* and *Streptomyces*. Beside this, the majority of the actinomycetes in soil that are potential drug sources remain uncultivable, and therefore in cannot be screened for novel antibiotic discovery [5].

Has been reported that microorganisms found in soil are a plentiful source of chemically diverse bioactive compounds, and have been an important source for the discovery of antibacterial agents including penicillins, cephalosporins, aminoglycosides, tetracyclines, and polyketides [2].

Also, from 117 actinomycetes strains isolated from the wasteland alkaline and garden soil samples in India, were found 15 actinomycetes strain that showed antimicrobial activity against at least two pathogen bacteria between them *Staphylococcus aureus*[5].

According to reference [15], environmental factors, such as carbon and energy sources, mineral nutrients, growth factors, ionic composition, available water, temperature, pressure, air composition, electromagnetic radiation, pH, oxidation–reduction potential, surfaces, spatial relationships, genetics of the microorganisms and interaction between microorganisms, can alter the microbial diversity, activity and population dynamics of microorganisms in soil. It is important to mention that almost 80–90% of the microorganisms habiting soil are on solid surfaces [15].

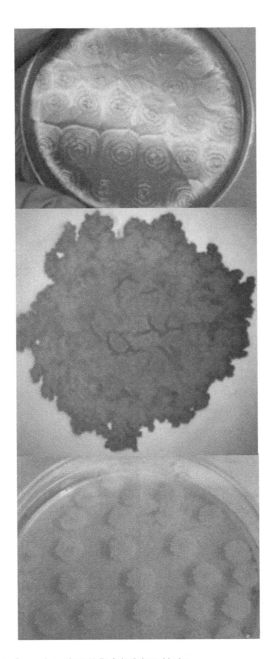

Figure 3. Bacteria strains from soil samples in Valle de las Palmas, Mexico.

6.3. Drug discovery from water microorganisms

The world's oceans comprise about 70 % of the earth's surface, where the extensive drug discovery efforts involving soil bacteria have not been extended to this ecosystem [16]. This environment have special attention since is known that typical microbial abundance of 10^6 per ml in the water column and 10^9 per ml in ocean bottom sediments. Actinobacteria is among the most dominant population and successful phyla of all environments [17]. This class takes into account 5 subclasses, 9 orders, 55 families, 240 genera and 3000 species [18].

From all actinobacteria, Marine Actinobacteria have become the most important source of secondary metabolites with medical application, such as anticancer, antibiotics, antitumor, anti-inflammatory, and antifungal compounds [16-17, 19].

Actinobacteria, called commonly actinomycetes are Gram positive bacteria having a higher guanine plus cytosine (G+C) percentage in its DNA than any other bacteria. Most of these organisms are aerobic (oxidative), some are facultative or forced anaerobes (fermentation) [20]. These microorganisms grow as networks called mycelium. They structures are filamentous. Sometimes are on the surface, for that is called aerial mycelium, or substrate mycelium if it attaches to the substrate surface [21]. The individual filaments of the mycelium or hyphae are divided into units as a result of growth of the cell wall into the hyphae at regular intervals along this structure. This process is called septation and each of the resulting septa contains one DNA molecule. The mycelium bacterium is analogous to the mycelium forming filamentous fungi [22]. Actinobacteria produce spores in specialized hyphae many of which are developed on the aerial filament, sometimes these spores are flagellated. The Actinobacteria inhabit the soil where play an important role in soil chemistry, the characteristic odor of soil is due to special metabolites that are known as Geominas [23]. Actinobacteria also inhabit aquatic environments including those marine. Actinomycetes are the most economically and biotechnologically valuable prokaryotes [24].

Almost 60 years in actinomycetes researches, more than 15000 bioactive compounds have been discovery for academic and pharmaceutical researchers many of which are used as drugs today. Fact more than half of the antibiotics discovered to date are obtained from the soil-derived actinomycete bacteria *Streptomyces* and *Micromonospora* genus spores [25].

The majority of the actinomycetes isolated from marine sources was largely of terrestrial origin and had been washed to shore and existed in the ocean as metabolically inactive spores [25]. Recently, phylogenetic analyses of the 16S rRNA genes indicate that existing new taxa widely distributed in ocean sediments [26], including some that appear to be unique and obligate marine actinomycete bacteria [27]. These strains represent the most significant source of naturally occurring microbial antibiotics [17, 28- 30] and antitumor compounds [28- 30] with specific metabolic and physiological capabilities that had not been observed in terrestrial microorganisms before [31-32]. Members of this group are producers of clinically useful antitumor drugs such as anthracyclines, glycopeptides, aureolic acids, enediynes, antimetabolites, carzinophilin, mitomycins and others [19].

The studies related with new biodiversity and drugs discovery had been examined from waters all around the world such as San Diego Bay, Bahamas, Fiji and Guam Islands among others. Recently, one study in the Gulf of California [32] found Operational Taxonomic Units (OTUs) belonging *Streptomyces* and *Actinomadura* genus and a potentially represent a new genus-level taxon in the family *Streptomycetaceae*. In addition, several previously descri-bed marine species were isolated including *Micromonospora krabiensis*, *Saccharomonospora marina*, *Streptomyces fenhuangensis*, *Verrucosispora maris* and *Verrucosispora sediminis* suggest-ing that these species may have broad geographic distributions.

The genes involved in secondary metabolism are responsible for the biosynthesis of small molecules that mediate important functional traits such as allelopathy, chemical communi-cation and iron acquisition [33]. These compounds have been used to assess biogeographical patterns among bacteria [34].

Polyketide synthase (PKSI) genes are called Type I and are responsible for the production of many important secondary metabolites including the antibiotic erythromycin [35] and the anticancer agent epothilone [35-36].

Bacteria can maintain complex assemblies of PKS genes [37], many of which are not ex-pressed under normal laboratory conditions [38]. Recently, a study found that HGT plays an important role in the evolution of PKSI genes and that ketosynthase (KS) domains within polyketide synthase genes are phylogenetically important making predictions about pro-duction of secondary metabolites by complex biosynthetic pathways [39-40]. Other method used for providing further evidence for endemism associated with secondary metabolites [33], is the terminal restriction fragment length polymorphism (T-RFLP) used to demon-strate that subpopulations of bacteria cluster together based on collection site [41].

According to [32] targeting KS domains provides a rapid method to assess PKS diversity and novelty within individual strains. The results revealed evidence of common pathways shared with other *Salinispora* strains but also sequences that share low levels of identity with any characterized pathways and thus may be associated with the production of new secon-dary metabolites. It is noteworthy that the new sequence type "L" also possesses a KS se-quence that has not previously been observed in "*S. pacifica*".

Secondary metabolites are linked to an organism's fitness and therefore represent an emerg-ing marker to study population structure and function, taxonomically meaningful patterns of secondary metabolite production have been detected in bacteria [42] and fungi [43].

Progress has also been made in drug discovery from actinomycetes by using high through-put screening and fermentation, metabolic profiling technologies, genome scanning, mining genomes for cryptic pathways, and combinatorial biosynthesis to generate new secondary metabolites related to existing pharmacophores [17, 44]. Metagenomic screening of DNA from environmental samples [45-46] provides an alternative way of discovering new antibi-otic biosynthetic genes.

According to [47] recently published new web tools that provide automated methods to assess the secondary metabolite gene diversity; those are the Natural Product Domain Seeker (NaP-DoS) analysis based on the phylogenetic relationships of sequence tags derived from polyketide synthase and non-ribosomal peptide synthethase (NRPS) genes. These results are compared with an internal experimentally database. NaPDoS provides a rapid mechanism used to infer the generalized structures of secondary metabolites biosynthetic gene richness and diversity within a genome or environmental sample by extract and classification of ketosynthase and condensation domains from PCR products, genomes, and metagenomic datasets increasing exponentially the investigations in this field of science with benefits in the field of drug discovery.

Table 1 shows a list of microorganisms isolated from different sources which produce antioxidant, antibacterial, anticoagulant, antiviral, anti-inflammatory, immune system, antidiabetic and nematicidal activities, as well as their action mechanisms.

Microorganism	Bioactive Compounds	Bioactivity	Mechanism	Reference	Natural Source
Brevundimonas diminuta	(R)-(-)-2-ethylhexan-1-ol	Nematicidal	Inhibitor against *C. elegans* and *B. xylophilus*	[48]	Air
Pasteurella haemolytica	A1-Derived Leukotoxin and Endotoxin	Inmune system	Induce Intracellular Calcium Elevation in Macrophages	[49]	Air
Streptomyces strain PM0324667	NFAT-133	Antidiabetic	induced glucose uptake in L6 skeletal muscle cells	[50]	Soil
Clostridium cellulolyticum	Closthioamide	Antibiotic	*Staphylococci* Multiresistente inhibition	[51]	Soil
Gordonia sputi DSM 43896	G48 JF905613 Compound	Antimicrobial	*C. albicans, S. aureus* inhibition	[52]	Soil
Actinomycetes	3Ba3 Compound	Antibacterial	E. amylovora, P. viridiflova, A. tumefaciens, B. subtilis ATCC 663, E. coli ATCC 29998 3 inhibition	[53]	Soil
Micromonospora sp.	Diazepinomicin/ ECO-4601	Antimicrobial	Unespecific	[54]	Soil
Eurotium Herbariorum	E. Herbariorum NE-4	Antioxidant	Antioxidant *in vitro*	[55]	Water
Sponge	Batzelladine L y M	Antibacterial	*S. aureus* and methicillinresistant, *S. aureus* inhibition	[56]	Water
Bivalve mollucs	Anticoagulant polypeptide (TGAP)	Anticoagulant	Inhibition of factor II tolla conversion	[56]	Water
Fungus	8'-O-Demethylnigerone	Antituberculosis	M. tuberculosis inhibition	[56]	Water
Algae	Dolabelladienetriol	Antiviral	Inhibition of HIV-1 replication	[56]	Water
Soft coral	Durumolides A-C	Anti-inflammatory	Modulation of LPS-activated murine macrophage cell line	[56]	Water
Sea cucumber	Frondoside A	Immune system	Lysosomal activity, phagocytosis and ROS activation	[56]	Water

Table 1. Microorganism isolated from natural sources that produce bioactive compounds

7. Conclusion

Bioactive compounds isolated from aerial, terrestrial and marine organisms have extensive past and present use in the treatment of many diseases and serve as compounds of interest both in their natural form and as templates for synthetic modification. To found new compounds useful to develop new pharmaceutical drugs, a good potential source and diverse bioactive chemicals is microorganism present in natural sources as air, soil and water.

Chemical compounds from natural sources are the major protagonists in chemical diversity for pharmaceutical discovery over the past century. The interesting chemicals identified as natural products are derived from the biodiversity in which the interactions between microbial entities and their environment formulate the diverse complex chemical entities within the organisms that enhance their survival and competitiveness. Hence, it is important to study inter and intraspecific interactions between microorganism in natural environments, this will make the screening for bioactive compounds in microbes easier.

Microbial interactions can influence the secretion of bioactive compound. Has been reported, various types of contacts among bacterial species and other organism. For example, these relations can be negative (parasitism, competition and predation) or positive (metabiosis and symbiosis) for these microorganisms. Between interactions in microorganism we can emphasize competition. Some bacteria are reduced by different species when the environmental resources are limited; therefore they produce compounds that impress negatively in their competitors [4].

Finally, air, soil and water are the home of microorganism that compete all the time to survive, resist changes in temperature, pressure, nutrient, carbon and nitrogen content, microorganisms that are obligated to produce weapons against predators, change and mutate to scape of detection of other microbes. All this, are the reason why we can find an unimaginable number and variety of chemical that are effective to be part of a pharmaceutical drug formulation.

Author details

Luis Jesús Villarreal-Gómez[1*], Irma Esthela Soria-Mercado[2], Ana Leticia Iglesias[3] and Graciela Lizeth Perez-Gonzalez[3]

*Address all correspondence to: luis.villarreal@uabc.edu.mx

1 Center of Engineering and Technology, University Autonomous of Baja California, Tijuana, BC., México

2 Marine Science Faculty, University Autonomous of Baja California, Ensenada, BC., México

3 Center of Engineering and Technology, University Autonomous of Baja California, Tijuana, BC., México

References

[1] Gordaliza M. Los compuestos naturales en el descubrimiento de fármacos. Institut ode Estudios de la Ciencia y la Tecnología. Universidad de Salamanca. 2009. http:// gredos. usal. es/jspui/bitstream/10366/22600/1/DQFA_Compuestosnaturales.pdf.

[2] Chin Y-W, Balunas MJ, Chai HB, Kinghorn AD. Drug Discovery from Natural Sources. AAPS Journal. 2006; 8(2): E239-E253. DOI: 10. 1208/aapsj080228.

[3] World Health Organization. Global Health Observatory (GHO). 2008. http://www. who. int/gho/ncd/mortality_morbidity/en/index. html.

[4] Soria-Mercado IE, Villarreal-Gómez, LJ, Guerra-Rivas, G, Ayala-Sánchez, NE. Bioactive Compounds from Bacteria Associated to Marine Algae. Biotechnology. Molecular Studies and Novel Application for Improved Quality of Human Life INTECH. 2012; 3: 25-44.

[5] Kumar N, Singh RK, Mishra SK, Singh AK, Pachouri UC. Isolation and screening of soil Actinomycetes as source of antibiotics active against bacteria. International Journal of Microbiology Research. 2010; 2(2): 12-16.

[6] Tenover FC. Mechanisms of Antimicrobial Resistance in Bacteria. The American Journal of Medicine. 2006; 119(6A): 53-510.

[7] Kim YH, Cha CJ, Cerniglia CE. Purification and Characterization of an erythromycin esterase from an erythromycin-resistant Pseudomonas sp. FEMS Microbiology Letters. 2012; 210: 239-244.

[8] http://www. wcrf. org/cancer_statistics/world_cancer_statistics. php.

[9] Bowers RM, Lauber CL, Wiedinmyer C, Hamady M, Hallar AG, Fall R, Knight R, Fierer N. Characterization of Airborne Microbial Communities at a High-Elevation Siteand Their Potential To Act as Atmospheric Ice Nuclei. Applied and Environmental Microbiology. 2009; 75 (15): 5121–5130.

[10] Flores-Tena FJ, Pardave LM, Valenzuela-Cárdenas IC. Estudio Aerobiológico de la Zona Aledaña al Relleno Sanitario "San Nicolás", Municipio de Aguascalientes. Investigacióny Ciencia. 2007; 37: 13-18.

[11] Sammer UF, Völksch B, Möllmann U, Schmidtke M, Spiteller P, Spiteller M, SpitellerD. 2-Amino-3-(Oxirane-2,3-Dicarboxamido)-Propanoyl-Valine, an Effective PeptideAntibiotic from the Epiphyte Pantoea agglomerans 48b/90. 2009; Applied Enviromental Microbiology. 1-30. doi:10. 1128/AEM. 01244-09.

[12] Tringe SG, Zhang T, Liu X, Yu Y, Lee WH, Yap J, Yao F, Suan ST, Ing SK, Haynes M, Rohwer F, Lin Wei C, Tan P, Bristow J, Rubin EM, Ruan Y. The Airborne Metagenomein an Indoor Urban Environment. PLoS ONE. 2008; 3(4): e1862. doi:10. 1371/journal. pone. 0001862.

[13] Zheng L, Li G, Wang X, Pan W, Li L, Lv H, Liu F, Dang L, Mo M, Zhang K. Nematici-da lendophytic bacteria obtained from plants. Annals of Microbiology. 2008; 58 (4): 569-572.

[14] Kirk JL, Beaudettea LA, Hartb M, Moutoglisc P, Klironomosb JN, Lee H, Trevors JT. Methods of studying soil microbial diversity. Journal of Microbiological Methods. 2004; 58:169– 188.

[15] Nannipieri P, Ascher J, Ceccherini MT, Landi L, Pietramellara G, Renella G. Microbi-al diversity and soil functions. European Journal of Soil Science. 2003; 54: 655–670. doi: 10. 1046/j. 1365-2389. 2003. 00556. x

[16] Fenical W, Jensen PR. Developing a new resource for drug discovery: marine actino-mycete bacteria. Natural Chemical Biology. 2006; 2(12): 666-673.

[17] Bull AT, Stach JEM. Marine actinobacteria: new opportunities for natural product search and discovery. Trends Microbiology. 2007; 15:491–499.

[18] Goodfellow M. Selective isolation of actinobacteria. In: Manual of industrial microbi-ology and biotechnology, 3rd edn. Baltz RH, Davies J, Demain AL (volume eds) Sec-tion1: Isolation and screening of secondary metabolites and enzymes, Bull AT, Davies JE (section eds). ASM Press, Washington, DC, 2010. pp 13–27.

[19] Olano C, Méndez C, Salas JA. Antitumor compounds from actinomycetes from gen-eclusters to new derivatives by combinatorial synthesis. Natural Products Report. 2009b;. 26:628–660.

[20] Logan N. Bacterial systematic. Blackwell scientific publications, oxford. 1994; pp. 272.

[21] Torres-Beltrán M, Cardoso-Martínez F, Millán-Aguiñaga N, Becerril-Espinosa A, So-ria-Mercado IE. Evaluation of the Gulf of California as a potential source of bioactive marine actinobacteria. Ciencias Marinas (2012), 38(4):1CM DOI:10. 7773/cm. v38i4. 2131.

[22] Nathan A, Magarvey KJM, Bernan V, Dworkin M. Isolation and characterization of-novel marine-derived Actinomycete taxa rich in bioactive metabolites. Applied Envi-ronmental Microbiology. 2004; 70:7520–7529.

[23] Bull AT, Ward AC, Goodfellow M. Microbiology and Molecular Biology Reviews. 2000; 64:573-604.

[24] Jemimah N, Mohana-Srinivasan SV, Subathra-Devi C. Novel anticancer compounds from marine actinomycetes: A Review Journal of Pharmacy Research. 2011; 4(4): 1285-1287. ISSN: 0974-6943.

[25] Goodfellow M, Haynes JA. In Bilogical, Biochemical, and Biomedical Aspects of Acti-nomycetes; Ortíz-Ortíz, L., Bojalil, L. F., Yakoleff, V., Editorals. Academic Press: Or-lando. 1984. Pp 453-472.

[26] Mincer TJ, Jensen PR, Kauffman CA, Fenical, W. Widespread and persistent populations of a major new marine actinomycetes taxon in ocean sediments. Applied Environmental Microbiology. 2002. 68:5,005–5, 2011.

[27] Feling RH, Buchanan GO, Mincer TJ, Kauffman CA, Jensen PR, Fenical W. Salino-
sporamideA: A Highly Cytotoxic proteasome inhibitor from a novel microbia
lsource, a marine bacterium of the new genus Salinospora. Angewandte Chemie International Edition 2003; 42(3) 355-357.

[28] Bhatnagar I. Immense essence of excellence: Marine microbial compounds, Mar.
Drugs. 2008; 8, 2673-2701.

[29] Soria-Mercado IE, Prieto-Davó, A, Jensen PR, Fenical W. Antibiotic Terpenoid-
Chloro Dihydroquinones from a new Marine Actinomycete. Journal of Natural Products. 2005; 68: 904-910.

[30] Strohl WR. In Microbial Diversity and Bioprospecting. Antimicrobials. Edited by Bul-
lAT. ASM Press; 2004; 336-355.

[31] Blunt JW, Copp BR, Munro MH, Northcote PT, Prinsep MR. Marine natural products. Natural Products Reports. 2006; 23: 26-78.

[32] Magarvey NA, Keller JM, Bernan V, Dworkin M, Sherman DH. Isolation and characterization of novel marine-derived actinomycete taxa rich in bioactive metabolites.
Applied Environmental Microbiology. 2004; 70:7520-7529.

[33] Becerril-Espinosa A. Actinobacterias aisladas del sedimento marino del Golfo de California y de Bahía Todos Santos: diversidad, bioactividad y dominios cetosintetasa.
PhD Dissertation, Universidad Autónoma de Baja California, México. 2011. 114 pp.

[34] Wawrik B, Kutliev D, Abdivasievna UA, Kukor JJ, Zylstra GJ, Kerkhof L. Biogeogra-
phy of Actinomycete Communities and Type II Polyketide Synthase Genes in Soils
Collected in New Jersey and Central Asia. Applied Environmental Microbiology.
2007; 73(9):2982. DOI:10. 1128/AEM. 02611-06.

[35] Freel KC, Edlund A, Jensen PR. Microdiversity and evidence for high dispersal rates
in the marine actinomycete"Salinispora pacifica". Enviromental Microbes. 2012; 14(2):
480-493.

[36] Cortes J, Haydock SF, Roberts GA, Bevitt DJ, Leadlay PF. An unusually large multi-
functional polypeptide in the erythromycin-producing polyketide synthase of Saccha-
ropolyspora erythraea. Nature. 1990; 348: 176–178.

[37] Bollag DM, McQueney PA, Zhu J, Hensens O, Koupal L, Liesch J. Epothilones, a new
class of microtubule-stabilizing agents with a taxol-like mechanism of action. Cancer
Research. 1995; 55: 2325-2333.

[38] Fischbach MA, Walsh CT. Assembly-line enzymology for polyketide and nonriboso-
mal peptide antibiotics: logic, machinery, and mechanisms. Chemistry Reviews.
2006;106:3468–3496.

[39] Bentley SD, Chater KF, Cerdeno-Tarraga AM, Challis GL, Thomson NR, James KD. Complete genome sequence of the model actinomycete Streptomyces coelicolor A3(2). Nature. 2002; 417: 141–147.

[40] Ginolhac A, Jarrin C, Robe P, Perriëre G, Vogel T, Simonet P, Nalin R. Type I polyketidesynthases may have evolved through horizontal gene transfer. Journal of Molecular Evolution. 2005; 60: 716–725.

[41] Gontang EA, Gaudíncio S, Fenical W, Jensen PR. Sequence-based analysis of secondary-metabolite biosynthesis in marine actinobacteria. Applied Environmental Microbiology. 2012; 76:2487–2499.

[42] Edlund A, Loesgen S, Fenical W, Jensen PR. Geographic distribution of secondary metabolite genes in the marine actinomycete *Salinispora arenicola*. Applied Environmental Microbiology. 2011; 77:5916–5925.

[43] Jensen PR, Williams PG, Oh DC, Zeigler L, Fenical W. Species-specific secondary metabolite production in marine actinomycetes of the genus Salinispora. Applied Environmental Microbiology. 2007; 73:1146–1152.

[44] Larsen TO, Smedsgaard J, Nielson KF, Hansen ME, Frisvad JC. Phenotypic taxonomyand metabolite profiling in microbial drug discovery. Natural Products Reports. 2005; 22:672–695.

[45] Baltz RH. Renaissance in antibacterial discovery from actinomycetes. Current Opinion in Pharmacology 2008; 8:557–563.

[46] Handelsman J. Soils—the metagenomics approach. In: Bull AT (ed) Microbial diversity and bioprospecting. ASM Press, Washington, 2004; pp 109–119.

[47] Schloss PD, Handelsman J. Metagenomics for studying unculturable microorganisms: cutting the Gordian knot. Genome Biology. 2005; 6:229–232.

[48] McAlpine JB, Banskota AH, Charan RD, Schlingmann G, Zazopoulos E, Piraee M, Janso J, Bernan VS, Aouidate M, Farnet CM, Feng X, Zhao Z, Carter GT. Biosynthesis of Diazepinomicin/ECO-4601, a *Micromonospora* Secondary Metabolite with a Novel Ring System. Journal of Natural Products. 2008; 71, 1585–1590.

[49] Zheng L, Li G, Wang X, Pan W, Li L, Lv H, Liu F, Dang L, Mo M, Zhang K. Nematicidal endophytic bacteria obtained from plants. Annals of Microbiology. 2008; 58 (4) 569-572.

[50] Mayer AMS, Rodríguez AD, Berlinck RGS, Fusetani N. Marine compounds with antibacterial, anticoagulant, antifungal, anti-inflammatory, antimalarial, antiprotozoal, antituberculosis, and antiviral activities; is affecting the immune and nervous system, and other miscellaneous mechanisms of action. Comparative Biochemistry and Physiology, Part C. Marine pharmacology in 2007–8: 2011; 153 191–222.

[51] Kulkarni-Almeida AA, Brahma MK, Padmanabhan P, Mishra PD, Parab RR, Gaikwad NV. Fermentation, Isolation, Structure, and antidiabetic activity of NFAT-133 produced by Streptomyces strain PM0324667. AMB Express. 2011; 21;1(1):42.

[52] Lincke T, Behnken S, Ishida K, Roth M, Hertweck C. Closthioamide: an unprecedented polythioamide antibiotic from the strictly anaerobic bacterium *Clostridium cellulolyticum*. Angewandte Chemie International Edition. 2010; 8; 49(11):2011-3. Air, Water and Soil: Resources for Drug Discovery http://dx. doi. org/10. 5772/52659.

[53] Lee LH, Cheah YK, Sidik SM, Ab Mutalib NS, Tang YT, Lin HP, Hong K. Molecular characterization of Antarctic actinobacteria and screening for antimicrobial metabolite production. World Journal Microbiology Biotechnology. 2012; 28:2125–2137.

[54] Oskay M, Üsame Tamer A, Azeri C. Antibacterial activity of some actinomycetes isolated from farming soils of Turkey. African Journal of Biotechnology. 2004; 3 (9): 441-446.

[55] Ziemert N, Podell S, Penn K, Badger JH, Allen E, Jensen PR. The Natural Product Domain Seeker NaPDoS: A Phylogeny Based Bioinformatic Tool to Classify Secondary Metabolite Gene Diversity. Plos one/www.plosone. org: 2012; 7(3): e34064. 9 pp.

[56] Miyake Y, Ito C, Itoigawa M, Osawa T. Antioxidants produced by *Eurotium herbariorum* of filamentous fungi used for the manufacture of karebushi, dried bonito (Katsuobushi). Bioscience Biotechnology and Biochemistry. 07/2009; 73(6):1323-7.

[57] Hsuan SL, Kannan MS, Jeyaseelan S, Y. S. Prakash, G. C. Sieck, and S. K. Maheswaran. *Pasteurella haemolytica*A1-Derived Leukotoxin and Endotoxin Induce Intracellular Calcium Elevation in Bovine Alveolar Macrophages by Different Signaling Pathways. Infection and Immunity. 1998; 66(6): 2836–2844.

Suppression of Pro-Inflammatory Cytokines via Targeting of STAT-Responsive Genes

Charles J. Malemud

Additional information is available at the end of the chapter

1. Introduction

The Janus Kinase/Signal Transducers and Activators of Transcription (JAK/STAT) signaling pathway play a fundamental role in regulating chronic systemic inflammatory responses in rheumatoid arthritis (RA) [1-5], based on compelling evidence that JAK/STAT is activated by many of the pro-inflammatory cytokines such as interleukin-1β (IL-1β), IL-2, IL-3, IL-6, IL-12, IL-17, IL-18, IL-19/IL-20, interferon-α/γ (IFN-α/γ) and oncostatin M (OSM) which are well-known to regulate, in part, immune-mediated inflammation in several autoimmune diseases, including RA [6-10]. However, complicating matters is the fact that some of the anti-inflammatory cytokines, which are known to dampen inflammatory responses induced by pro-inflammatory cytokines, including, IL-4, IL-10 and IL-13 also activate JAK/STAT [11-14]. In this regard, Müller-Ladner *et al.* [15] showed that synovial tissue obtained from RA patients contained significant amounts of constitutively activated IL-4/STAT. Therefore it will be necessary to understand more precisely the extent to which pro- and/or anti-inflammatory cytokine gene expression is deregulated in RA and which of the STAT-responsive genes known to alter immune-mediated inflammation in response to these cytokines may be amenable to therapeutic intervention.

2. JAKs

JAKs are non-receptor tyrosine kinases that are pre-associated with the membrane-proximal site of cytokine receptors [16]. Four mammalian JAK isoforms, JAK1, JAK2 and JAK3 and TYK2 have been described to date mainly from the results of gene structural analysis [17]. All of the JAK isoforms share a common structure known as the JAK homology (JH) domain. Leonard and O'Shea [18] identified a proline-rich conserved region in the cytokine receptors, called Box1, that associated with JH7 whereas the catalytic phosphotyrosine kinase site, called YY was determined to correspond to the other JH domains (Figure 1).

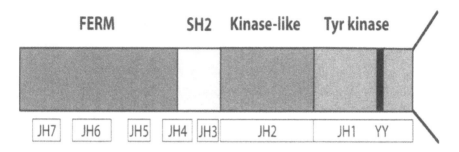

Figure 1. JH domains and phosphorylation sites of JAK3: Structural analysis combined with functional studies of JAK3 showed that the JH4-JH7 region contained band 4.1 also known as the Four-point-one, Ezrin, Radixin, Moesin (FERM) domain. Reprinted by permission from [16].

Additional structural analysis predicted that the JH2 domain was more than likely to be a pseudosubstrate domain [19]. In view of this latter finding the structural requirements for JAK activation was further clarified. Thus, the JH3-JH4 domain which shows a Src-homology-2-like structure had a shared homology with JH2. This finding indicated that the JH4-JH7 domains were, indeed, the critical regions required for regulating the interactions between the various JAK isoforms and other protein kinases. JH4-JH7 were also found to be essential for receptor binding, catalytic function, JAK autophosphorylation and even in some cases, inhibition of JAK activity.

3. Stat proteins

Gene analysis has revealed the existence of at least 6 STAT protein isoforms, namely, JAK1, JAK2, JAK3, JAK5A, JAK5B and JAK6 [20]. In normal homeostasis, phosphorylation of these STAT proteins is achieved via phosphorylation (i.e. activation) of specific JAK isoforms following the interaction of various cytokines and growth factors with their specific receptors [16, 21]. In this manner, cytokine receptor-mediated JAK activation results in the conversion of latent cytoplasmic un-phosphorylated STAT (U-STAT) proteins into phosphorylated STAT (p-STAT) proteins which can form homo- or heterodimers and are then translocated to the nucleus where these activated STAT protein dimers act as potent transcription factors [17-20]. Although phosphorylation of specific STAT-tyrosine residues remains the primary requisite mechanism for p-STAT protein dimer formation, a second phosphorylation site was also recognized at a serine in the C-termini domain of the STAT protein [20, 22].

An amplification loop with potential major clinical significance in RA involves the transcriptional activity of p-STAT proteins which further regulate the expression of pro-inflammatory and anti-inflammatory cytokine genes as well as other genes of significance in cancer and autoimmune diseases [23-28]. In addition, p-STAT proteins can regulate other signaling pathways necessary for lymphocyte development, as well as the aberrant survival of activated dendritic cells, monocytes, lymphocytes and synoviocytes in disorders of the immune system [29-33].

It is noteworthy that during normal homeostasis, activation of STAT proteins induced the expression of Suppressor of Cytokine Signaling (SOCS) and Cytokine-Inducible SH-2 (CIS) proteins and it has been concluded that this is the negative feedback loop that underlies one of the mechanisms responsible for inhibiting JAK-mediated signaling by cytokines [34-38]. Thus, results of recently published experiments with human endothelial cells are germane to this point since the data in this paper provided a direct connection between the silencing of STAT3 with STAT3-specific silencing RNA and the suppression of SOCS3 [39].

The extent to which negative regulation of JAK-mediated signaling by SOCS/CIS may be inactivated in autoimmune diseases is a focus of current studies. In that regard, recent advances in unraveling the details of mechanism(s) governing negative regulation of cytokine signaling by SOCS/CIS proteins have shed additional light on the extent to which SOCS/CIS-mediated down-regulation of pro- and/or anti-inflammatory cytokine JAK/STAT signaling may be compromised in inflammatory arthritis [40]. However, the results of some recent studies with osteoarthritic human cartilage have not clarified this issue. For example, one study showed that the level of SOCS2 and CIS-1, but not SOCS1 and SOCS3, were reduced in femoral head cartilages from subjects with osteoarthritis [41], whilst the results of another study [42] indicated that SOCS3, but not SOCS1 expression, was elevated in chondrocytes obtained from osteoarthritic cartilage compared to chondrocytes from cartilage obtained from patients who had femoral neck fracture.

The status of the activity of certain other negative regulators such as protein tyrosine phosphatases, including SHP-1,-2 [43] and CD45 [44] and the 'Protein Inhibitor of Activated STAT' (PIAS) proteins [16, 45, 46] are also not precisely known in autoimmune diseases. These proteins could very likely suppress the activity of phosphorylated JAKs and p-STAT proteins by dephosphorylation or by interacting with p-STAT proteins in normal cells. However, these pathways may be compromised or markedly suppressed in arthritis.

It is also critical for gaining a further understanding of what alterations may occur in cytokine signaling in RA to recognize the fact that activation of JAK/STAT by any of the relevant cytokines can also activate other intracellular signaling pathways via the "cross-talk" mechanism. Thus, "cross-talk" between JAK/STAT and other signaling pathways [16] can cause activation of the Stress-Activated Protein Kinase/Mitogen-Activated Protein Kinase (SAPK/MAPK) pathway, the Phosphatidylinositol-3-Kinase/Akt/mammalian Target of Rapamycin (PI3K/Akt/mTOR) pathway [47], activation of signaling via Toll-like receptors [47, 48] and immunoreceptor tyrosine-based activation motifs (ITAMs) [49] as well as the NF-κB pathway [50]. These alternative signaling pathways which are all connected to inflammation have also been shown to significantly modulate many of the survival and/or apoptosis-signals required to perpetuate abnormal proliferation and/or to cause the death of activated dendritic cells, lymphocytes, macrophages, synoviocytes and chondrocytes.

Evidence from a genome-wide analysis study (GWAS) of STAT-target genes showed that many of these genes regulated cellular proliferation, angiogenesis and metastasis in cancer cells [51]. These results when coupled with the data from another recent study [52] which highlighted the nature of the several forms of STAT-interacting proteins that bind to DNA suggested that GWAS could be employed to identify pro-inflammatory and/or anti-inflammatory cytokine STAT-target gene structures and potentially additional STAT-interacting proteins present in RA joint tissues. Thus GWAS may be considered the next step in the development of future therapies for RA based on targeting STAT-responsive genes. This could be especially useful depending on the status of the activity of the SOCS/CIS protein family acting on cytokine-receptor-mediated signaling. For example, if SOCS/CIS activity is dampened or deregulated in RA then it would be unlikely that this negative regulator pathway for controlling cytokine signaling would be able to inhibit the amplification of pro-inflammatory cytokine-induced JAK/STAT signaling. To illustrate this point, Isomäki et al. [40] showed that although SOCS-1 and SOCS-2 were up-regulated in T-cells recovered from peripheral blood, that SOCS-3 was found in peripheral blood monocytes and a significant number of synovial tissue macrophages expressed SOCS-1 and SOCS-3 proteins, the majority of T-cells in RA synovium were 'SOCS negative.'

For further discussion, this chapter will focus on the recent progress that has been made in furthering our understanding of how cytokine gene expression is regulated by both U-STAT and p-STAT proteins. The long-term prospect arising from the results of these studies would be to exploit this new knowledge to reduce the level of pro-inflammatory cytokines or to raise the level of anti-inflammatory cytokines in RA. By doing so this could potentially restore the balance between these cytokine families and retard ongoing synovial joint damage whilst also ameliorating RA clinical signs and symptoms.

4. Stat-DNA promoter-binding motifs

Defining transcription factor binding sites was critical for revealing the structure of cis-regulatory motifs that regulated transcriptional activity [53]. However, microarray analysis using different cell types determined that although several hundred genes were potential STAT3-target gene sites, only a small fraction of those STAT3-target gene sites turned out to be true direct STAT3-target genes [54].

As previously indicated, p-STAT proteins do not act independently of one another and U- and p-STAT-protein interactions take various forms which enable them to bind efficiently to DNA [55]. These activated STAT-protein interaction types include, 1) the direct binding of activated STAT homodimers to DNA; 2) the interaction of activated STATs with non-STAT proteins to form activated STAT/non-STAT protein complexes which bind to DNA; and 3) activated STAT proteins interacting with other non-STAT transcription factors or co-activator proteins which bind to DNA [16, 53]. In addition, several novel mechanisms were described for the binding of U-STAT3 and U-STAT1 to DNA [54, 55]. In that regard, Cheon et al. [56] showed that U-STAT3 can drive expression of proteins not induced by p-STAT3, whereas U-STAT1 was shown to extend and up-regulate the expression of a subset of genes initially responsive to p-STAT1 (e.g., interferon, IL-6), that result in more prolonged antiviral and/or immune responses. Thus, the results of these studies provided novel information regarding the functional significance for U-STAT1 and U-STAT3 acting as transcriptional activators and organizers of chromatin. These events have been shown to be important cellular mechanisms for regulating gene transcription in the nuclei of cells of the immune system and cancer cells.

The results of DNA sequencing studies originally demonstrated specific DNA-binding sites for STAT1 and STAT3 [57]. Boucheron et al. [58] then demonstrated that specific DNA binding sites existed for STAT5A and STAT5B homodimers despite the fact that STAT5A and STAT5B are evolutionarily conserved and encoded by 2 genes with a 91% homology in amino acid structure [59]. Moreover, targeted gene deletion of STAT5A and STAT5B in mice resulted in distinctive phenotypes [60]. This finding suggested a structural dissimilarity in the DNA-binding motifs for these two STAT proteins. The results of studies reported in [60] were later confirmed using the IL-3-dependent early pre-B cell line, Ba/F3 [61]. Here it was shown that both STAT isoforms bound to all of the promoters tested, but STAT5A and STAT5B bound with differing kinetics [62]. This result suggested that DNA binding activity was likely at the root of any differences in the biological activity of these two STAT protein isoforms.

Ehret et al. [63] compared the specificity of STAT-DNA binding sites in specific STAT gene knockout mice showing distinct phenotypes with the STAT-DNA binding sites in a variety of cultured cells. From the *in vitro* analysis, Ehret et al. [63] also demonstrated that DNA binding site motifs for STAT1, STAT5A, STAT5B and STAT6 were essentially the same with only minor differences in DNA binding site specificity. However, STAT5A DNA-binding specificity was much more similar to STAT6 than was the preferential DNA-binding site for STAT1. Thus, the preferential DNA binding site for STAT6 contained a 4 base pair spacer (i.e. TTCNNNNGAA) (N_4) which was defined as the weak DNA binding site. However, additional analyses showed that STAT6 bound to TTCNNNG-AA (N_3) sites (i.e. the strong binding site) as well [63]. The binding of STAT1 and STAT5 to the N_3 site was distinct from STAT5A which preferred N_4. Of note, most of the STAT6 binding sites were found in IL-4 responsive promoters in the N_4 sites [64-67]. These results reported by Ehret et al. [63] were extended by the findings of Moucadel and Constantinescu [64] who showed that STAT5B bound to chromatin at both the N_3 and the N_4 site.

5. Stat-responsive cytokines genes

This overview covering the specificity of STAT-DNA binding becomes especially important for improving our understanding of which cytokine gene expressional events are altered by p-STAT and U-STAT proteins. This section analyzes our current interpretation of several cytokines relevant to RA and other autoimmune diseases, namely, IL-2, IL-3, IL-4, IL-6, IL-15, IL-17, IL-19 and INF-γ, all of which have been shown to activate the JAK/STAT pathway [16]. Moreover, activation of JAK/STAT signaling by these cytokines was shown to result in altered patterns of transcriptional activity which lead to changes in the expression of the following cytokine or cytokine-related genes, IL-2R, IL-3, IL-4, IL-6, IL-6ST (gp130), IL-10, IL-18R1, INF-γ, oncostatin M (OSM) and TNF-α (Table 1).

Charles J. Malemud: Suppression of Pro-Inflammatory Cytokines via Targeting of STAT-Responsive Genes

STAT Responsive Cytokine/Protein	STAT Activator[1]	Activated STAT(s)[2]	Major Function(s) of STAT-Responsive Genes[3]	Involvement of STAT activator in RA	Representative Reference
IL-2Rα	IL-4	STAT6	Complexes with IL-2Rβ/IL-2Rγ→high affinity IL-2R	Anti-inflammatory Cytokine	[81]
IL-10	IL-2, IL-3	STAT5, STAT5A, STAT5B	Activator of JAK3, I-SRE-4/IL-10 gene	↑ T-Cell Growth ↑ T-Cell Development	[73] [207] [127]
IL-18R1	IL-4	STAT6	↑ T_reg Cell Development IL18/IL-18R1	Inducer of TNF-α, GM-CSF, IFN-γ	
IL-6	IL-6/IL-17 IL-3 IL-12	STAT3/STAT1 STAT5 STAT4	Activator of JAK3	Promotes T_h17 Cell Production;	[9] [174] [140]
	IL-19 IL-10/IL-13	STAT3 STAT4		↑MMP Synthesis ↑MMP Synthesis	[207] [140]
IL-6ST(gp130)[4]	IL-6/IL-17/OSM	STAT3/STAT4/STAT5A	Heterodimer between gp130/LIFR[5] forms the OSMR[6]	Promotes T_h17 Cell Production	[100]
IL-4	IL-2	STAT3/STAT4/STAT5A	↑T_h2 Differentiation		[118]
INF-γ	IFN-γ	STAT1/STAT4/STAT5/STAT6	Activator of multiple protein kinases	Inhibitor of Anti-Inflammatory Cytokine IL-4 and IL-10 Production	[86]
	IL-3 IL-2 IL-12	STAT5 STAT5 STAT4			[207] [207] [113]
OSM	IL-2/IL-3	STAT5 STAT3	Activator of JAK2	↑ Monocyte Trafficking ↑ MMP-2 ↑ VEGF	[122] [125]
TNF-α	IL-3 IL-6/IL-19	STAT5 STAT3/STAT5	Activator of JAK3;	Activator of NF-κB	[200] [86]
	IL-15 IL-22	STAT1/STAT3/STAT5	Activator of p38[7], JNK[8]		[186]

[1]Cytokines that activate this STAT protein

[2]Activated STAT that becomes a transcription factor for the STAT-responsive cytokine/protein

[3]Function(s) of STAT-responsive cytokine/protein

[4]IL-6 Signal Transducer

[5]Leukemia Inhibitory Factor Receptor

[6]Oncostatin M Receptor

[7]p38 kinase

[8]C-Jun-N-terminal kinase

Table 1. STAT-Responsive Pro-Inflammatory Cytokine Gene Expression

6. T_h1/T_h2 Cells, T_{reg} Cells, IL-2R, and IL-15

Up-regulation of the T_h1 and T_h17 T-cell subsets and reduced levels of human T-regulatory (T_{reg}) cells are known to occur in autoimmune diseases [16, 68]. In addition, T_{reg} cells are a critical contributor to T-cell development in the thymus as well as being the T-cell subset that regulates the genesis and maintenance of immune tolerance [16].

The IL-2Rα/IL-2Rβ subunits in complex with the common IL-2γ subunit make up the high-affinity IL-2 receptor, whereas homodimeric IL-2Rα results in a low-affinity receptor [69]. The functional significance of blocking the high-affinity IL-2R with the small molecule inhibitor (SMI), SP4206 (K_d ~70nM) in response to IL-2 (K_d~10nM) was that JAK/STAT activation was inhibited [70]. This result could provide the impetus for development of the next generation SMI designed to efficiently inhibit the IL-2/IL-2R pathway and this task should be facilitated by employing recently developed technologies based on the principles of protein-protein interactions [71].

As indicated previously, the interaction of IL-2 with the high-affinity IL-2R causes activation of JAK/STAT with STAT5A and STAT5B, the principally activated STAT proteins. However, the eventual change in STAT5-gene responsiveness following IL-2 activation of STAT5 was shown to be dependent on the complexity of the promoter regions of those STAT5-target genes [72]. Interestingly, Tsuji-Takayama et al. [73] showed that IL-2-mediated JAK/STAT activation up-regulated the production of IL-10 by T_{reg} cells. The production of IL-10 arose from the interaction of STAT5 with a STAT5-responsive element within intron 4, designated I-SRE-4 of the IL-10 locus which was considered to be an interspecies conserved enhancer sequence (Table 1). Of note, the clustered CpG regions around I-SRE-4 were under-methylated in IL-10-producing T_{reg} cells, but not in other T-cell subsets. This result confirmed previous results which showed that expression of Foxp3, a member of the forkhead/winged-helix family of transcription factors and a biomarker for the development and function of T_{reg} cells [47, 74] was also IL-2/STAT5-dependent [75]. Thus, development of T_{reg} cells was regulated by the methylation status of CpG residues because methylation of CpG residues suppressed Foxp3 expression [76].

Chen et al. [77] identified a novel set of IL-4/STAT6-target genes in mice that regulated the proliferation of activated T-cells. In addition, these genes were shown to regulate the production of the T_h2 lineage as evinced by the finding that the cells isolated from wild-type mice produced T_h2 whereas cells from STAT6$^{-/-}$ mice did not. Later, Lund et al. [78] showed that the IL-4/STAT6 pathway was also critical for the commitment of naïve T-cells to become either the T_h1 or T_h2 subset. In that regard, the ratio of T_h1 to T_h2 produced from naïve T-cells was found to be dependent on a set of STAT6-responsive genes which included the transcription factors STATB1, Bcl-6, and TCF7 [78, 79]. Moreover, the IL-4/STAT6-mediated pathway was also shown to be a strong modulator of human T_{reg} cell production from either T_h1 or T_h17 cells [80].

Wurster et al. [81] were among the first to demonstrate that IL-4-mediated activation of STAT6 could also up-regulate IL-2Rα gene expression (Table 1). Because IL-2 is the major growth-promoting cytokine for T-cells [81], elevated production of IL-2Rα in response to activated STAT6 is considered instrumental in facilitating the proliferation of activated T-cells in cancer as well as in several types of autoimmune diseases. In that regard, the high level of expression of IL-2Rα in tumors correlated with a poor prognosis in cancer patients [82]. Thus, it will be interesting to determine if the same relationship holds true for RA patients as well, including what role IL-2Rα polymorphisms [83, 84] might play in determining the level of the expression of IL-2Rα. For example, IL-15, a pro-inflammatory cytokine which interacts with two receptor subunits similar to IL-2Rα/β drives the production of the memory CD8+ T-cell phenotype [85]. Experimental therapies focusing on inhibiting the binding of IL-15 to the IL-2Rα/β receptor complex were a decade ago considered to be a potential target for autoimmune diseases [85]. However, since then considerable evidence has accumulated showing a robust relationship between IL-15/IL-2Rα/β-mediated signaling, osteoclastogenesis and boney erosions in RA joints [3]. In addition, González-Alvaro et al. [86] showed that IL-15 stimulated production of TNF-α by monocytes derived from RA patients including, the induction of the CD69 monocyte biomarker, and synthesis of IFN-γ protein by natural killer (NK) cells. Of note, the results of a clinical study showed that IL-15 expression in RA synovial tissue persisted even after TNF-α blockade, the latter treatment resulting in a positive clinical response and reduced disease activity [87]. However, treating mononuclear cells *in vitro* with HuMax-IL-15 f (ab')$_2$ neutralized the effect of IL-15 on these cells. Furthermore, treatment with HuMax-IL-15 f(ab')$_2$ caused a significant improvement in RA disease activity as measured by the American College of Rheumatology (ACR) clinical response criteria [88]. This finding may be particularly important for future drug development because the results of a recently completed clinical trial showed that high levels of serum IL-15 in patients with early arthritis predicted a more progressive and severe clinical course which may call for early and aggressive drug therapy [89].

6.1. IL-6/gp130/IL-17

The IL-6/IL-6R/gp130 pathway is one of the strongest inducers of STAT3 activation [9] (Table 1) so much so that many studies have been devoted to the activation of the JAK/STAT pathway by IL-6 because IL-6 is critical to the progression of joint damage in RA [16]. In fact, the development of the anti-IL-6R monoclonal antibody, tocilizumab, appears to have been predicated on this emerging evidence such that this drug is now considered useful in the armamentarium of drug therapies for RA [90, 91]. Most compelling was recent evidence that tocilizumab in conjunction with methotrexate retarded the progression of joint damage in RA patients [92], an effect of this drug regimen that was apparently independent of the capacity of tocilizumab to modify several clinical biomarkers of inflammation and concomitant RA disease activity.

Recent results have also emerged which have focused attention on the extent to which other pro-inflammatory cytokines, such as IL-17, activate JAK/STAT and the mechanism by which IL-17 modifies the production of IL-6 and other pro-inflammatory cytokines [9]. In that regard, the results of a study by Jovanovic et al. [93] was extremely informative because it provided evidence that IL-17 was capable of activating additional signaling pathways other than JAK/STAT which resulted in elevated production of IL-1β and TNF-α. Therefore, it has become obvious that suppressing the activity of IL-17 could bring about a reduction of these pro-inflammatory cytokines as well, although this point must be rigorously reexamined in view of the results from Dragon et al. [94] who showed that IL-17A significantly decreased GM-CSF-induced neutrophil/granulocyte apoptosis by suppressing activation of p38 kinase, extracellular-regulated kinase 1/2 and STAT5B.

Inhibiting aberrant T-cell survival in RA may ultimately hinge on the development of a therapeutic strategy directed specifically at STAT3 since STAT3 was shown to inhibit T-cell proliferation by up-regulating the Class O Forkhead transcriptions factors (Fox) via the binding of STAT3 to FoxO1and FoxO3a promoters [95]. Potentially, STAT3 may also protect T-cells from apoptosis [30, 96] in RA by suppressing IL-2 activity, although the results [95] indicated that STAT3 increased T-cell proliferation and their survival through the up-regulation of OX-40 (CD134), a member of the TNFR-superfamily of receptors and bcl-2 and by suppressing FasL and Bad expression.

Perhaps the most intriguing aspect of the clinical studies with tocilizumab performed in RA patients is the extent to which neutralization of the IL-6/IL-6R/gp130 pathway using this drug together with the putative suppression of IL-6 and gp130 gene expression in response to inhibition of the STAT3 activation rebalances the skewed ratio of T_h17/T_{reg} in favor of T_{reg} [97, 98], the elevated serum levels of T_h17-associated cytokines, IL-17, IL-23, IL-6 and TNF-α, and the depressed level of T_{reg} cells with its associated growth factor, transforming growth factor-β (TGF-β) [99]. What is pertinent to these events are the results of a recent study which showed that treatment of RA patients with tocilizumab in combination with methotrexate resulted in a significant decrease in the percentage of T_h17 cells (from 0.9% at baseline to 0.45%) and a significant increase in T_{reg} cells (from 3.05% to 3.94%) whilst maintaining their functional activity [98].

The extent to which gp130 gene expression is altered in response to inhibition of the JAK/STAT pathway activation is also an area of immense importance because deregulated over-expression of gp130 in RA patients should not be neutralized by anti-IL-6R therapy. Importantly, O'Brien and Manolagas [100] showed that IL-6 or oncostatin M (OSM), a member of the IL-6 protein superfamily, stimulated the activity of the gp130 (Table 1) promoter in which the cytokine response element contained a cis-acting motif for activated STAT complexes, including activated STAT1 and STAT3 homo- and heterodimers. Furthermore, it can be conjectured that other pro-inflammatory cytokine members of the IL-6 protein superfamily, such as ciliary neutrotrophic factor (CNTF), leukemia inhibitory factor (LIF) and cardiotropin-1 which use gp130 as their primary signal transducer protein [9, 101] may provide an alternate mechanism resulting in constitutive JAK/STAT activation. Under those conditions STAT protein activation may not be inhibited any of the anti-IL-6R agents which retain up-regulated gp130 gene expression. Of note, constitutive activation of STAT proteins is one of the signature events in the development and progression of various cancers [102, 103] with a similar phenomenon having been described in RA synovial tissue [15]. Constitutively activated STAT proteins could also be predictive of a more aggressive form of RA [96].

6.2. INF-α/IFN-γ

The interferon protein family in conjunction with the interferon-regulated gene (IRG) pathway plays an important role in RA, SLE and other autoimmune diseases because the IRG pathway is a critical mediator of autoimmune-dependent inflammation [104-106]. INF-γ is known to be one of the strongest activators of JAK/STAT and Tyk2 resulting in IRG-mediated responses [16, 107, 108]. INF-γ has also been shown to play a role in the epigenetic regulation of specific gene activation as evinced by the finding of an association of pJAK2 and IFN-γ receptor in the nucleus with histone H3 in IFN-γ-treated human amnionic (WISH; American Tissue Culture Collection; CCL 25) cells *in vitro* [109]. AG-490 a JAK2 inhibitor, also down-regulated STAT1 gene expression and AG-490 inhibited prolactin-induced IFN-γ, TNF-α, IL-1β and IL-12p40 synthesis in mouse peritoneal macrophages *in vitro* [110]. Of note, inhibition of JNK activity with the SMI, SP600125, also resulted in down-regulating IFN-γ and TNF-α indicating that both the JAK/STAT and MAPK pathways contributed to alterations in the expression of these cytokines. Although the importance of these results in providing a rationale for manipulating signal transduction pathways in human RA remains to be fully elucidated, the fact that the expression of several pro-inflammatory cytokines relevant to RA pathology are potentially controlled by cross-talk between JAK/STAT and MAPK appears to be significant [47, 111, 112].

Three DNA-binding sites related to STAT protein-DNA binding have been recognized within the IFN-γ promoter. These DNA binding sites include an IL-12-mediated STAT4/DNA binding site, an IL-2-induced STAT5/DNA binding site and a CD2-mediated STAT/IFN-γ binding site [113]. Thus, CD2-mediated activation of human peripheral blood mononuclear cells was shown to result in STAT/DNA binding to a 3.6kb DNA motif within the IFN-γ promoter which occurred principally via STAT5A binding and less so by STAT5B, with both being independent of IL-2.

Induction of some of the IFN-regulatory factors (Irfs), including those gene responses brought about by activation of irf9 via IFN-α were found to be STAT protein-independent [114]. In addition, results from other studies showed that Akt activity was also involved in key IFN-α, -γ gene responses [115]. Moreover, regulation of IFN-α, -γ-mediated responses required the direct control of mTOR [116] beginning with the initiation of protein translation [117].

In RA, the depressed level of IL-4 and IL-10 in mononuclear phagocytes is, in part, responsible for the imbalance in T_h1/T_h2 cytokines [3, 16]. The primary model employed to describe the relationship between IFN-γ and IL-4/IL-10 is dependent on several factors. This view was originally proposed by Hamilton et al. [118] as follows; IL-4 was shown to markedly suppress the transcriptional activity of IFN-γ because the promoter sequence between IL-4 and IFN-γ were essentially identical. Proof of this came from the results of experiments that showed that IFN-γ/STAT1 and IL-4/STAT6 both formed complexes at the same regulatory sequence, but whereas activated STAT1 promoted IFN-γ transcription, activated STAT6 did not. However, activated STAT6 was required to suppress the transcriptional up-regulation of IL-4. Thus, in the model, IL-4 appeared to be necessary to reduce IFN-γ gene expression (Table 1) and was related to a competition between activated STAT1 and activated STAT6 for binding to the IFN-γ promoter. In keeping with this model, the expression of IL-10 is also known to be suppressed by INF-γ

[119]. Thus, it was shown that when transfected RPMI 8226.1 B-cells were incubated with IFN-γ followed by lipopolysaccharide (LPS), IFN-γ reduced LPS-induced IL-10 promoter activity which was independent of the irf, but dependent on an activated STAT-motif. Further analyses indicated that IFN-γ down-regulated IL-10 gene expression via displacement of the trans-activated STAT3 by STAT1 induced by IFN-γ.

Experimental strategies could be designed to increase the mononuclear cell expression of IL-4/IL-10 by manipulating the ultra-sensitive INF-γ promoter region with various activated STAT protein types. Another strategy for potentially improving the level of IL-10 in RA would involve manipulating natural T_{reg} cells in a cell-based therapy mode because T_{reg} cells are a rich source of IL-10 [120, 121]. However, as pointed out by Nandakumar et al. [121] one must be mindful that the antigen specificity of natural T_{reg} cells must be carefully regulated to protect against the development of self-reactive effector T-cells or for that matter, T_{reg} cells with inappropriate antigen specificity.

6.3. OSM

Recent advances have assigned OSM, a member of the IL-6 protein superfamily an important role in the pathogenesis and progression of RA and OA [101]. In that regard, one of the more important experimental results involving OSM were reported by Hams et al. [122] who compared the inflammatory responses in wild-type mice to IL-6-deficient and mice deficient in the OSM receptor β (OSMRβ). They showed that the OSMRβ knockout mice showed enhanced trafficking of monocytes to sites of inflammation when these mice were compared to the wild-type or IL-6-knockout mice. However, the OSMRβ knockout mice did not demonstrate any differences in neutrophil or lymphocyte migration to inflamed tissue when compared to their wild-type or IL-6-deficient counterparts. These results suggested that the OSM/OSMRβ-pathway probably regulated chemokine production and chemokine function. Indeed this proved to be the case when the up-regulated chemokine in response to the activation of the OSMRβ-pathway was eventually identified as CCL5. CCL5 has been shown to be a critical chemokine for regulating the recruitment and retention of monocytes in inflamed RA synovial joints [3]. Although the evidence was indirect, these results suggested that a drug with the capacity to neutralize the interaction between IL-6 and IL6R in arthritic joints would not alter OSM/OSMRβ-mediated STAT activation [9]. This view was supported by the results from several previous studies which showed that 1) although the OSMR consisted of a heterodimer of the LIF receptor and gp130, the alternative form of OSMR, namely, OSMRβ, was activated only by OSM and not by LIF [123]; 2) OSM, but neither IL-6 nor LIF induced tyrosine phosphorylation in the Shc adaptor protein p52 and p66 isoforms which in association with growth factor receptor-bound protein 2 (Grb2) were both recruited to OSMR, but not to gp130 [124]; and 3) at least in human or canine osteosarcoma cell lines, treatment with OSM phosphorylated JAK2/STAT3 and Src, each of which was shown to be involved in an OSM dose-dependent-mediated increase in expression of the MMP-2 gene (i.e. 72kDa gelatinase) and vascular endothelial growth factor (VEGF) gene [125]. Of note, the STAT3 SMI, LLL3, inhibited MMP-2 and VEGF gene expression indicating that MMP-2 and VEGF were genes targeted by activated STAT3. Importantly, Clarkson et al. [126] showed that another one of the activated STAT-responsive genes in mammary epithelial cells was OSMR. This finding was critical for completing the circle which showed that activation of OSMRβ was central to the upstream activation of the OSM-mediated pathway as well as to the downstream increase in the expression of the OSMRβ gene, both events involving STAT proteins.

7. Other cytokines/cytokine receptors

The role played by activated STAT proteins in various aspects of autoimmune diseases and in oncogenesis is best exemplified by the many genes and transcription factors that have been shown to be STAT protein-responsive [51, 127]. Many of these STAT-regulated genes include additional pro-inflammatory cytokine and cytokine receptor genes besides those previously discussed. In this section we will analyze the contributions of these cytokine and cytokine receptor genes to the pathology of RA.

7.1. IL-18

IL-18 is structurally similar to IL-1 and the IL-18 receptor is a member of the IL-1R/TLR protein superfamily [128]. However, the function of IL-18 differs considerably from that of IL-1 and, in fact unlike IL-1, IL-18 is produced by a variety of immune as well as non-immune cells. Although IL-18 in its role as a stimulator of T_h1 responses is well known by its activity as an immune defense cytokine against microbial infection, the over-production of IL-18 can result in autoimmune disease via its capacity to modify and accentuate adaptive immunological responses such as those seen in RA [129-132]. However, paradoxically IL-18 can also stimulate T_h2-related cytokine responses as well [128]. Thus, its putative role in altering the T_h1/T_h2 cytokine repertoire cannot be dismissed.

Particularly important with regard to the role played by IL-18 in RA were results of a study by Gracie et al. [133] who first identified abundant IL-18 in RA synovial tissue. These findings are relevant when coupled with those from other studies by Tanaka et al. [134] who also found elevated IL-18 and the IL-18 receptor α/β in RA synovial tissue. They also demonstrated that IL-18 was a co-factor and regulatory cytokine in stimulating the synthesis of IFN-γ by T-cells in RA synovial tissue, the latter also requiring IL-12, thus implicating the up-regulation of IL-18 gene expression as an important component of RA disease progression.

Activated STAT3 was identified as the JAK/STAT-related transcription factor responsible for the increased synthesis of IL-18 [127]. In that regard, TNF-α was shown to increase IL-18 gene expression in RA synoviocyte cultures suggesting the possibility that TNF-α, a known activator of p38 kinase and JNK may also activate STAT3 in synoviocyte and chondrocyte cultures. Indeed, recent results from our laboratory showed that recombinant human TNF-α activated STAT3 in normal human chondrocyte cultures and TNF-α activated STAT3, p38 kinase and JNK in cultured chondrocytes derived from human osteoarthritic knee cartilage [Malemud et al. submitted]. Thus, it was instructive to learn that treating RA patients with the combination therapy of infliximab and methotrexate reduced the level of IL-18 in serum whilst the level of the chemokine, CXCL12 was unaltered [135]. Moreover, synovial fluid from these RA patients had higher levels of IL-18 (as well as TNF-α and IL-15) prior to beginning combination therapy with infliximab and methotrexate compared to the level of these cytokines in a patient's sera. In addition, the level of IL-18/TNF-α in synovial fluid was strongly correlated with a patient's high Disease Activity Score-28 [136]. Thus, it may be informative going forward to assess the level of activated STAT3 and IL-18 in the synovial fluid and sera of RA patients before and after treatment with TNF antagonists or other biological drugs that neutralize the activation of JAK/STAT and MAPK pathways to determine the extent to which the level of activated STAT3, p38 kinase or JNK is correlated with IL-18 gene expression by synovium and cartilage *ex vivo*.

7.2. IL-12

IL-12 is made up of 2 disulfide-linked protein subunits, termed IL-12p35 and IL-12p40 linked in a heterodimer configuration [137, 138]. Whilst the IL-12p40 subunit has structural similarities with cytokine receptors, the IL-12p35 component is structurally similar to IL-6 and granulocyte-colony stimulating factor (G-CSF) [139]. Of note, if IL-12p35 and IL-12p40 are produced by the same cell, the bioactive heterodimer is termed, IL-12p70 [140].

IL-12 is synthesized by many cell types of the innate and adaptive immune systems, including, monocytes, macrophages, dendritic cells and neutrophils. IL-12 is a minor product of B-cells [140]. Although IL-12p35 is constitutively expressed at low levels by many of these cells, the expression of IL-12p40 is limited to those phagocytic cells that synthesize IL-12p70.

The connection between IL-12 and activation of the JAK/STAT pathway stems from the finding that IL-12 production was positively regulated by IFN-γ, the latter cytokine which is also induced by IL-12. Thus, IFN-γ regulates IL-12 gene expression and vice versa. By contrast, two of the anti-inflammatory cytokines, namely, IL-10 and IL-13 which also activate JAK/STAT, suppressed IL-12 production [140] (Table 1). In addition, the type I interferon proteins, exemplified by IFN-β, which activates STAT1 [141] was shown to inhibit IL-12 gene expression in mice [142].

The main immune functions of IL-12 involve the regulation of T_h1 differentiation via the activation of STAT4 which induces the synthesis of the T-bet transcription factor [143]. T-bet was shown to regulate IFN-γ expression and CD8$^+$ suppressor T-cell development which had been characterized as principally IFN-γ/STAT1-dependent, and IL-12/STAT4 independent. In fact, expression of T-bet was shown to require activated STAT4 to achieve total IL-12-dependent T_h1 cell-fate determination [143]. However, Yang et al. [144] showed that the effect of IL-12/STAT4 was more complex. Thus, IL-12 -induced activated STAT4 bound to a distant but highly conserved STAT-responsive T-bet enhancer region where it induced IFN-γ-activated STAT1 independent T-bet gene expression in CD8$^+$ cells. Importantly, IL-4-induced STAT6 activation regulates the development and effector functions, not of T_h1 cells, but rather of T_h2 cells in peripheral tissues such as skin, lung and gut [145]. However, T_h2 cell produced in lymph nodes did not require IL-4-mediated activation of STAT6 [145].

In summary, cell-fate determination induced by the IL-12-mediated activation of STAT4, IL-4-mediated activation of STAT6, transforming growth factor-β (TGF-β), IL-6 plus TGF-β and IL-27 activation of STAT3 profoundly influence the balance of T_h1 and T_h2 cells, T_h17 cells and T_{reg} cell production, respectively [80, 146-149]. This conclusion must, however, be tempered by results of recent studies which also showed that formal interplays occurred between IL-4-induced STAT6 phosphorylation, the GATA-binding protein-3 (GATA₃) zinc-finger transcription factor [150] and the T_{reg} cell transcription factor, FoxP3 as well. Importantly, GATA₃ was revealed as the key transcription factor in this complex interplay because GATA₃ could 1) directly inhibit T_h1 differentiation through its capacity to block up-regulation of the IL-12β2 receptor; 2) inhibit the activity of STAT4; and 3) neutralize the activity of runt-related transcription factor 3 (runx3), via its capacity to induce protein-protein interactions [150]. Thus, by modulating the activities of IL-4/STAT6, GATA₃/STAT4 and runx3 one could potentially alter the activity of pro-inflammatory and anti-inflammatory cytokines as well as overcome immune tolerance.

7.3. IL-21

IL-21 is a member of the Type I cytokine superfamily of cytokine receptors. In this group, the common γ cytokine receptor complex is the functional component for receptor-mediated signal transduction of IL-2, IL-4, IL-7, IL-9 and IL-15 [151-153]. Although IL-21 has strong structural homology to IL-15, IL-21 interacts with a unique receptor, termed, IL-21Rα, which pairs with the γ-common cytokine receptor chain (i.e. CD132) to form the active IL-21 receptor complex [154].

IL-21-mediated events affect the functions of NK cells, T-cells and B-cells. Although development of T_{reg} cells from the T_h17 lineage is generally considered to require IL-6 because IL-6 reciprocally controls T_h17 and T_{reg} cell development through its ability to inhibit TGF-β-induced FoxP3 and by inducing RORγ, in fact, IL-21 can also induce RORγ and T_h17 development in the absence of IL-6. However, evidence also showed that the number of T_h17 cells, the recruitment of T_h17 cells to inflamed tissues and the development of autoimmune encephalitis and myocarditis did not differ between IL-21R and IL-21 deficient mice compared to their wild-type counterparts [155, 156]. More importantly, IL-6 was the more potent inducer of T_h17 differentiation compared to IL-21 thus calling into question, whether IL-21 was even required for T_h17 development.

Despite the emerging controversies regarding how important IL-21 is in T-cell development and immune responses, a therapeutic intervention designed to limit the responses of immune cells to IL-21 has long been considered for treating cancer and autoimmune diseases [157]. In addition, because the binding of IL-21R induces activation of several of the JAK isoforms [153], it became apparent that it would be necessary to elucidate which cellular events were controlled by STAT proteins activated by phosphorylated JAKs in response to IL-21/IL-21R. Attempting to address this point, Habib et al. [151] found that IL-21 induced proliferation of pro-B-lymphoid cells *in vitro* which was dependent on both γc and the γc-associated JAK3 complex. However, a monoclonal antibody reactive only with γc was effective in limiting the proliferation of BaF3/IL21R α cells [151] indicating that neutralization of γc alone could cause inhibition of JAK activation by IL-21/IL-21R.

Implying a role for IL-21 in the development and progression of RA would also depend on finding an elevated level of IL-21 in human RA tissues and by demonstrating an involvement of IL-21 in the pathogenesis of CIA or inflammatory arthritis in other animal models. Thus the results of a study by Young et al. [158] were noteworthy in this regard for several reasons. First and foremost, treating DBA mice with CIA with an antibody to IL-21R (i.e. IL-21R.Fc) reduced the severity of arthritis. The reduction in hind paw swelling was accompanied by lower levels of IL-6 in the hind paw but also in the sera of mice treated with IL-21R.Fc suggesting that one of the downstream events regulated by IL-21 was IL-6 gene expression. Of note, the level of INF-γ was increased in the hind paws of mice with CIA. Furthermore, the cultured cells from the lymph nodes of mice with CIA treated with IL-21R.Fc showed an increased level of IFN-γ *ex vivo*. These findings (i.e. reduced IFN-γ; increased IL-6) were mirrored *ex vivo* using Type II collagen-specific spleen cells from CIA mice treated with IL-21R.Fc. Most importantly from the perspective of potentially using an anti-IL-21R antibody as a therapeutic agent for RA was the finding that treating Lewis rats with adjuvant –induced arthritis therapeutically with IL-21R.Fc "reversed" the swelling in inflamed joints and tissues from these joints whilst the tissues showed improvement using a well-validated histological scoring system. More recently, Yuan et al. [159] showed that IL-21R mRNA was found in human RA synovial tissue samples. In addition, this group also confirmed the results of the Young et al. study [158] since they showed that an anti-IL-21R antibody ameliorated the severity of arthritis in CIA which was accompanied by reduced cytokine levels in cells derived from the anti-IL-21R antibody-treated mice. Interestingly, IL-21R-deficient K/BxN mice [160] failed to develop arthritis; a result which suggested that IL-21R played a critical role in the pathogenesis of K/BxN serum-induced arthritis.

There now are several lines of evidence that showed that the IL-21/IL-21R pathway plays a functional role in regulating inflammatory responses in autoimmune arthritis. In that regard, anti-IL-21 blockade should also be considered for future drug development for RA. However, what would also be crucial to improving our understanding of the role of IL-21 in RA would be to discover which pro-inflammatory cytokine levels are altered in response to the JAK/STAT activation by IL-21/IL21R. This could provide a novel paradigm for reducing pro-inflammatory cytokine levels in RA.

8. The extended IL-10 cytokine superfamily

IL-19, IL-20, IL-22, IL-24 (melanoma differentiation-associated gene 7; mda-7), and IL-26 (AK155) are all structurally similar to IL-10 and these interleukins constitute members of the extended IL-10 cytokine superfamily [161-163]. Three additional members of the IL-10 cytokine superfamily have recently been added to this list, namely, IL-28A, IL-28B and IL-29 which now comprise the IFN-λ cytokine subfamily [164-166].

IL-19 and IL-20 are α-helical proteins. They have similar cysteine sites; their amino acid sequences are approximately 30% identical. In the human genome, the genes encoding these IL-10 superfamily members are located in two clusters; one cluster comprises the genes for

IL-10, IL-19, IL-20, and IL-24/mda-7 which are located on chromosome 1q31-32 [167]. IL-19 and IL-20 were predominately expressed in monocytes, as well as non-immune cells under inflammatory conditions [168], whereas IL-22 and IL-26 was only produced by T-cells, especially T_h1 cells and NK cells, whilst IL-24 synthesis was restricted to monocytes and T-cells [169].

Both IL-20 and IL-24 bind to the IL-20R complex which is made up of the cytokine receptor family 2-8/IL-20Rα (IL-20R1) [170], although it was previously shown that IL-19/IL-19 receptor binding was similar to IL-20/IL-24 receptor binding [170]. IL-19 was also shown to interact with a DIRS1-like element which is composed of tyrosine recombinase-encoding transposons/IL-20Rβ (IL-20R2) [170-172].

In all cases, the binding of IL-19, IL-20 or IL-24 to these receptors caused activation of STAT3 and activation of a minimal promoter region containing those sequences identified as STAT-binding sites. Importantly, absent either of the R1 proteins in the two types of receptor complexes, IL-20R1/IL-20R2 and IL-22R1/IL-22R2 reduced the affinity of IL-19 or IL-24 for these receptors. Furthermore, IL-20R2, and not IL-20R1, was identified as the high affinity receptor chain for these cytokines [173].

The functional significance of the IL-10-related cytokines, IL-19, IL-20, IL-21, IL-22 and IL-24 in terms of the pathophysiology of RA and other autoimmune diseases is systematically being elucidated. In most cases, the role played by these cytokines has been inferred from measurements in sera of RA patients before and/or after medical therapy.

8.1. IL-19

Sakurai et al. [174] showed that IL-19 was produced by cells of human RA synovial tissue. The majority of IL-19 positive cells were vimentin- and CD68-positive, indicating that fibroblasts and macrophages were the main sources of IL-19 in RA synovium. From a functional perspective, synovial tissue lining and sublining layers were both identified with anti-IL-20R1 and anti-IL-20R2 antibodies.

IL-19 activated synoviocyte STAT3 and, downstream, STAT3 activation caused up-regulation of IL-6 and IL-19 gene expression whilst decreasing synoviocyte apoptosis induced by serum-starvation [174], a change which may predict the role of IL-19 in the development of synovial hyperplasia [30, 96]. However, the role of IL-19 in RA relative to its activation of signal transduction was further complicated by the findings of Alanärä et al. [175] who showed that IL-1β, an activator of the MAPK pathway [176], also increased the level of IL-19 in peripheral blood mononuclear cells *in vitro*. Combined with other data this result showed that in RA joints IL-19 expression was the highest of all of the IL-10 family cytokines. Furthermore, these results suggested that IL-19 played a significant role in synovial tissue inflammation, with the caveat that further consideration of IL-19 as a target for intervention in in RA must focus on the relative level of JAK/STAT activation of JAK/STAT versus activation of the other signaling pathways.

IL-19 was highly expressed in synovial tissue and, in particular, expressed in fibroblasts isolated from rats with collagen-induced arthritis (CIA) [177]. Of note, treating these rats with a anti-IL-19 antibody, 1BB1, reduced arthritis severity which was accompanied by the lower level of boney erosions and an improvement in the quality of subchondral bone. Moreover, treatment of rats with CIA with 1BB1 reduced the expression of TNF-α, IL-1β, IL-6 and Receptor Activator of Nuclear Factor Kappa-B Ligand (RANKL) genes in synovial tissue and also lowered IL-6 levels in serum. Synovial fibroblasts isolated from rats with CIA responded to treatment with IL-19 in a similar fashion seen with synovial tissue *in situ* where increased synthesis of TNF-α, IL-1β, IL-6 and RANKL was detected.

There is now compelling evidence that IL-19-mediated activation of STAT3 was associated with the development and progression of inflammatory arthritis which was characterized by the elevated expression of many of the pro-inflammatory cytokines pertinent to human RA joint destruction. These data also showed that the rat CIA model could be further exploited to determine the extent to which specific dampening or up-regulation of STAT-responsive cytokine genes would ameliorate inflammatory responses associated with CIA.

8.2. IL-20

IL-20 interacts with IL-20R1/IL-20R2 to activate the JAK/STAT pathway [166] and IL-20 has been implicated in the pathogenesis of autoimmune diseases [178]. However, IL-20R2 signaling was shown to blunt mouse CD4 and CD8 T-cell responses to antigen *in vitro* and *in vivo* [179]. Thus, it remains to be determined the extent to which IL-20 promotes or suppresses immune-mediated inflammation.

In the CIA model in the rat, treatment with an anti-IL-20 antibody 7E, either alone, or in combination with the TNF blocker, etanercept was compared to etanercept alone for their capacity to 1) ameliorate cartilage damage; 2) stabilize bone mineral density; and 3) alter cytokine production [180]. In addition, the effect of antibody 7E on expression of various genes implicated in the progression of CIA was evaluated on rat synovial fibroblasts *in vitro*. Treatment with 7E or etanercept or the combination of 7E and etanercept significantly reduced the severity of arthritis as measured by rat hind paw thickness and swelling. These treatments also prevented cartilage degradation and bone loss whilst reducing the level of synovial tissue IL-20, IL-1β, IL-6, RANKL and MMPs. Of note, IL-20 induced the expression of TNF-α in synovial fibroblasts isolated from rats with CIA. Moreover, IL-20 induced RANKL production in synovial fibroblasts, osteoblasts and T$_h$17 cells. In another study, antibody 7E was shown to inhibit mouse osteoclast differentiation induced by macrophage-CSF and RANKL [181]. These results [181] coupled with results from the CIA model [180] indicated that IL-20 was likely to have promoted the increased bone loss in CIA by promoting osteoclast differentiation and the activity of osteoclast-mediated bone resorption.

Correlative human studies of IL-20-mediated responses in RA are just emerging. However, the results have differed somewhat from those seen in the CIA model. Thus, Kragstrup et al. [182] showed that plasma IL-20 levels were increased in RA compared to OA patients with the elevated level of IL-20 primarily localized to mononuclear cells and neutrophils. Stimulating mononuclear cells isolated from RA synovium with recombinant IL-20 resulted in the increased secretion of the chemoattractant CCL2/MCP-1. However, at variance with findings in the CIA model, recombinant IL-20 did not alter the expression of TNF-α or IL-6 by mononuclear cells *in vitro*.

8.3. IL-22

IL-22 binds to the class II cytokine receptor family, IL-22R and IL-10Rβ [183]. IL-22 was shown to activate STAT-1, -3 and -5 in H4IIE rat hepatoma cells by inducing the phosphorylation of JAK1 and Tyk2, but not JAK1 [184]. However, H4IIE failed to respond to IL-10 via activation of JAK1 and Tyk2 indicating a distinct signaling pathway for IL-22 versus IL-10. IL-22 also failed to inhibit pro-inflammatory cytokine gene expression by monocytes in response to LPS although IL-22 did blunt the inhibitory effects of IL-4 produced from T_h2 cells, a finding distinct from the activity of IL-10.

A role for IL-22 in inflammation was inferred from its involvement as an inducer of pancreatitis-associated protein by pancreatic acinar cells [185] and by the elevated serum levels of IL-22 in patients with active Crohn's disease [186]. With regard to activating various signaling mechanisms, Lejeune et al. [187] showed that IL-22 activated JAK/STAT. However, IL-22 also activated ERK, JNK and p38 kinase indicating that IL-22 could activate all of the 3 major MAPK pathways. Brand et al. [186] then showed that treating intestinal epithelial cells with TNF-α, IL-1β or LPS significantly increased IL-22R1 gene expression without altering IL-10R2 mRNA. IL-22 also activated STAT1/STAT3, Akt, ERK 1/2 and JNK and, most importantly IL-22 increased the expression of SOCS3, TNF-α, IL-8 and human-defensin-2 mRNAs. Because IL-22 was shown to activate several disparate signaling pathways it is conjecture that up-regulation of pro-inflammatory gene mRNAs by IL-22 involves 'cross-talk' between all three pathways. Thus, experiments employing specific SMIs added either individually or together to cells in culture will have to be performed to determine the extent to which any or all of these signaling pathways are involved in regulating TNF-α, IL-8 or IL-1β gene expression in response to IL-22.

IL-22 is elevated in RA synovial tissue with the lining and sublining layers of RA synovium expressing the highest levels of IL-22R1 [188]. Recently, Leipe et al. [189] showed that about 50% of the RA patients studied had elevated serum IL-22 compared to a group of healthy subjects. The level of serum IL-22 closely correlated with the extent of bone erosions as determined from radiographic analysis. However serum IL-22 did not correlate with the presence or absence of either rheumatoid factor (RF) or anti-cyclic citrullinated peptide antibodies nor was IL-22 associated with disease activity. CD4 T-cells were identified as the main source of IL-22 in these RA patients. However, in another study, de Rocha Jr et al. [190] showed that elevated serum IL-22 did correlate with the Disease Activity Score-28 (DAS-28) and the Clinical Disease Activity Index, a positive titer for RF and the extent to which bone was eroded. The findings from this study [190] agreed with the results from another recently published study [191] the latter showing that plasma IL-22 was increased in 30 patients with established RA (i.e. mean disease duration of 10.7 years), even in those patients receiving immunomodulatory therapy. Thus, any discrepancies between the results of these various clinical studies relative to establishing a relationship between IL-22, RA disease activity and RF levels may involve differences in terms of the types and duration of the immunotherapies employed or in the proportion of RA patients who were in the early or late stage of disease. The relationship between IL-22 and the presence of RF could also correlate with the immunological status of B-cells since, unlike IL-10, IL-22 does apparently not regulate the induction of Ig by activated B-cells [192].

8.4. IL-24/mda-7

The apoptosis-inducing activity of IL-24/mda-7 has made this unique member of the extended IL-10 cytokine family a target for cancer therapeutics [193-195] in view of the finding that IL-24/mda-7 could kill cancer cells specifically without affecting the vitality off normal cells or tissues [196]. Receptor binding of IL24/mda-7 to IL-20R activates STAT1 and STAT3 although additional signaling pathways have been shown to be modulated by cells over-expressing IL-24/mda-7 which did not involve JAK/STAT activation [193]. Besides the interest in IL-24/mda-7 as a tumor suppressor cytokine, mda-7/IL-24 has also been implicated in regulating some of components of RA and psoriasis immunopathology [197]. However, some of the details of the mechanism(s) by which IL-24/mda-7 could alter pro-inflammatory cytokine gene expression in RA via JAK/STAT have not been fully elucidated, although epigenetic and other transcriptional factor activity beyond activated STAT proteins have been postulated to play critical roles. Thus, it is of interest that Sahoo et al. [198] recently showed that STAT6 and c-Jun binding to the IL-24 promoter locus in T_h2 cells caused trans-activation of the IL-24 gene. Finding a relationship between the activators of STAT6 and c-Jun that are relevant to RA which leads to IL-24 gene transcription may hold the key to increasing local IL-24/mda-7 levels by T_h2 cells. This, in turn, could help overcome the 'apoptosis-resistance' of RA synovium [96].

8.5. IL-3

IL-3 is one of several major cytokines that drive the differentiation of cells of the hematopoietic lineage. The interaction between IL-3 and its cognate receptor activates several signaling pathways, including, JAK/STAT, PI3K/Akt/mTOR and the Ras/Raf/MAPK pathways [199]. Downstream events that are regulated by IL-3 which are germane to RA and autoimmunity, in general, include the findings that depending on the conditions in the microenvironment, IL-3 can alter cell proliferation, survival or induce cell death by apoptosis [30].

IL-3 was identified as an activator of JAK2 and STAT5 [200] and the expression of the pro-apoptotic protein, c-myc. This finding provided the initial evidence that cell proliferation and apoptosis was regulated, in part, by activated STAT5. However, a subsequent study by Chaturvedi et al. [201] provided evidence to the contrary in that the interaction of IL-3 with its receptor activated STAT3 via the phosphorylation of tyr[701]. Moreover, the results of this study [201] also showed that myeloid cell proliferation was regulated by IL-3-activated Src kinase and not by IL-3-actiivated JAK3. This conclusion was based on the following results. Inhibition of c-Src kinase activation using a dominant-negative (dn) Src mutant also blocked STAT3 activation and, this in turn, inhibited proliferation of the 32Dcl3 myeloid cell line in response to IL-3. Moreover, expression of a dn-JAK2 mutation increased apoptosis in 32Dcl3 cells in the absence of IL-3 which also involved the concomitant down-regulation of ERK-2. Taken together these results indicated that Src kinase activation of STAT proteins regulated myeloid cell proliferation whereas JAKs controlled the activation of ERK-2 and associated anti-apoptotic signals [202].

The results of another study [203] showed that IL-3 played an important role in regulating SOCS3 and PIAS proteins [16, 20, 21] both of which are important in regulating cytokine signaling as well as the fine-tuning of the survival and/or cell death pathways for immune and non-immune cells in general. IL-3 plays a particularly critical role in regulating these events in mast cells [203], plasmacytoid dendritic cells [204], osteoclast-like cells, [205] and osteoclasts [206, in particular. All of these cell types are involved in some aspect of RA pathology.

To further illustrate this point, Gupta et al. [206] showed that osteoclasts treated with IL-3 were diverted to the dendritic cell lineage which may also be related to the finding that that IL-3 dampened human osteoclast-mediated bone resorption. Most recently, Srivastava et al. [207] showed that IL-3 increased the number of functionally active T_{reg} cells by stimulating the production of IL-2 by non-T_{reg} cells the latter being dependent on the dose of IL-3. Of note, treating mice with CIA with IL-3 significantly reduced the severity of arthritis and also increased the frequency of T_{reg} cells found in the thymus, lymph nodes and spleen. Although this study [207] did not directly measure the status of activated STAT proteins in the CIA mice treated with IL-3, these additional results showed that treatment of CIA with IL-3 decreased production of IL-6, IL-17A, TNF-α and IL-1 whilst increasing IFN-γ and IL-10 (Table 1).

8.6. IL-7

IL-7 was shown to be a fundamental contributor to thymocyte development as well as a regulator of T-cell homeostasis in peripheral blood. IL-7 activates both the PI3K/Akt/mTOR and JAK/STAT pathways suggesting that IL-7 regulates the survival and/or death of T-cells [208].

The IL-7 receptor provides an indicator of the biological activity of IL-7. IL-7R is composed of a γC and Rα polypeptide. JAK3 associates with γC. The binding of JAK3 to γC allows IL-7 dimer formation to occur between γC and Rα so that JAK3 can phosphorylate Rα and/or JAK1 [209]. In most cases, activation of JAK3 causes STAT5 to be phosphorylated.

With respect to relationship between IL-7 and RA, Kim et al. [210] showed that the levels of IL-1β and TNF-α found in the synovial fluid of RA patients could typically increase IL-7 production by stromal cells in culture. In addition, IL-7 was also a strong inducer of RANKL production by T-cells, independent of TNF-α [210]. Interestingly, van Roon et al. [211] showed that TNF-α blockade in RA patients reduced IL-7 production. However, high levels of IL-7 persisted in RA patients who failed to respond to antagonists of TNF-α.

Hartgring et al. [212] found significantly higher amounts of IL-7Rα in the synovial fluid of RA patients as well as in synovial fluid from patients with undifferentiated arthritis. IL-7 level strongly correlated with the number of activated CD3$^+$ T-cells. IL-7Rα was also identified on B-cells and macrophages from RA patients, but importantly IL-7Rα-expressing T-cells did not co-express, FoxP3. *Ex vivo* studies performed on monocytes collected from RA patients revealed that recombinant human IL-7Rα inhibited IL-7 induced T-cell proliferation and IFN-γ production suggesting that blockade of IL-7Rα in RA patients reduced the expression of the STAT-responsive gene, IFN-γ.

With respect to the putative role of IL-7 in regulating certain aspects of cartilage responses in arthritis, Yammani et al. [213] reported that IL-7, IL-6 or IL-8 stimulated the production of the Ca^{2+}-binding protein, S100A4, by cultured human articular chondrocytes. Importantly, IL-7 increased the synthesis of S100A4 to a greater extent than either IL-6 or IL-8 with IL-7-stimulated S100A4 resulting from JAK3/STAT3 activation. In that regard, pre-treating chondrocytes with the experimental JAK3, inhibitor, WHI-P154, or with cyclohexamide blocked S100A4 synthesis which also inhibited the production of MMP-13. Because S100A4 has been implicated as significantly contributing to pannus-mediated destruction of cartilage in RA inflammation [214], blockade of IL-7R may be useful for down-regulating the expression of S100A4 and MMP-13 with associated blunting of pannus invasion into cartilage.

The interaction between S100A4 and the tumor suppressor p53 protein was purported to be related to the role of S100A4 as a promoter of cancer metastasis [215]. IL-7 via S100A4 was also shown to induce the expression of MMP-13 as well as MMP-1, MMP-9 and S100A4 was also shown to be involved in the neoangiogenesis and aberrant cell proliferation of rheumatoid synovium [216]. Importantly a selective inhibitor of MMP-13 reduced the level of cartilage destruction in 2 of 3 animal models of RA, including the SCID-mouse co-implantation model and CIA, but not adjuvant arthritis. [217]. Thus, evidence has gradually accumulated to show that up-regulation of S100A4 via activation of STAT3 significantly alters the progression of inflammatory arthritis.

9. Experimental therapies that inhibit activated stat proteins: Is cytokine gene expression altered?

The results of a Phase 2B RA clinical trial have recently been published which showed that the JAK3-specific SMI, tofacitinib (CP690, 550) had clinical efficacy as measured by the ACR response criteria [218]. However, there has been less progress on developing novel strategies to directly inhibit activated STAT proteins or dampen STAT gene responses. Noteworthy have been proof-of-principle studies that activated STAT proteins can be experimentally 'deactivated' which result in the inhibition of STAT/DNA binding. Thus, JNK-mediated phosphorylation of the STAT6 ser[707] decreased the DNA binding capacity of IL-4-stimulated STAT6 resulting in the inhibition of STAT6-responsive genes [219]. Using immunosuppressive STAT oligodeoxynucleotides (ODN) to inhibit activated STAT proteins have also been relatively successful. These ODN have been shown to interfere with the phosphorylation of STAT1 and STAT4 [220] and STAT1 and STAT3 [221]. Lastly, administration of a single dose of a STAT1 decoy ODN suppressed joint swelling and the histological appearance of acute and chronic adjuvant-induced experimental arthritis in the mouse [222]. Electrophoretic mobility shift analysis of the nuclear extracts from synoviocytes from the STAT1 decoy ODN-treated animals incubated with the STAT-1 decoy ODN inhibited STAT-1 binding to DNA. Of note, STAT-1 decoy ODN also inhibited the expression of macrophage CD40 suggesting that interference with CD40-mediated signaling by macrophages may be the mechanism responsible for the attenuation of arthritis by the STAT-1 decoy ODN.

10. Conclusion

The medical therapy of RA was revolutionized with the introduction of biological drugs, including TNF antagonists, the IL-6R antagonist, tocilizumab, the T-cell co-stimulatory factor inhibitor, abatacept, the B-cell inhibitor, rituximab and the IL-1 receptor antagonist, anakinra as well as the use of first-line therapy with disease-modifying anti-rheumatic drugs (DMARDs) such as methotrexate and anti-malarial drugs [223]. Nevertheless, the long-term and chronic use of these drugs for treating RA patients is not without potential deleterious consequences for those RA patients who use them. Thus, RA patients prescribed DMARDs and/or biological drugs need to be continuously monitored for changes in liver enzyme levels, ocular and/or kidney toxicities, infections and to a lesser extent malignancies such as lymphoma [224]. Just as important is the fact that some RA patients fail to respond to one or several of these biological drugs or become refractory to their action [225].

Development of JAK-specific SMIs was originally predicated on their use as a treatment for suppressing organ transplant rejection. However, JAK-SMIs were also considered as a potential adjunctive therapy for overcoming issues of long-term use of biological drugs for the therapy of RA [7, 11, 16, 17]. Now only time will tell whether or not the JAK-specific SMI, tofacitinib [218, 225], will be aggressively employed in the treatment of RA, or whether tofacitinib will be used in RA patients who only have exhibited a moderate or inadequate response to biological drugs or DMARDs.

Presently, there has been little attention paid, comparatively speaking, on acquiring data from RA patients in the general population who have been treated over several years with biological drugs to determine the extent to which the pro-inflammatory and/or anti-inflammatory cytokine repertoires have been altered from baseline. In addition, there are hardly any systematic studies, with the exception of some analyses conducted (often as a minor component of an RA clinical trial) with respect to which of several biological drugs restore the imbalance between T_h1 and T_h2 cytokines, suppress the activity of T_h17-producing cytokines, or improve the biological activity of dysfunctional T_{reg} cells [225]. Truly, the possibility exists that treating RA patients with biological drugs only partially inhibit over-expression of the pro-inflammatory cytokines that have been shown to mainly contribute to the progression of RA, namely, IL-6, IFN-γ and TNF-α (Table 1). This 'take-home' point appears to adequately justify a continual search for alternative cellular mechanisms that are active in determining whether clinical remission in RA patients is sustained or not. In conclusion, determining how STAT-responsive cytokine genes are regulated at the molecular and cellular level offers the potential going forward for developing yet another treatment modality designed to suppress the clinical activity and progression of RA pathology.

Acknowledgments

The Arthritis Research Laboratory at Case Western Reserve University School of Medicine was supported by an investigator-initiated project grant from Takeda Pharmaceuticals of North America (Deerfield, IL) and is presently supported by an investigator-initiated project grant from Genentech/Roche Group, (South San Francisco, CA).

Author details

Charles J. Malemud*

Address all correspondence to: cjm4@cwru.edu

Arthritis Research Laboratory, Division of Rheumatic Diseases, Case Western Reserve University School of Medicine, Cleveland, Ohio, USA

The author declares no conflict of interest.

References

[1] Ivashkiv LB, Hu X. Signaling by STATs. Arthritis Research & Therapy 2004; 6(4) 159-168.

[2] Walker JG, Ahern MJ, Coleman M et al. Expression of Jak3, STAT1, STAT4 and STAT6 in inflammatory arthritis: unique Jak3 and STAT4 expression in dendritic cells in seropositive rheumatoid arthritis. Annals of the Rheumatic Diseases 2006; 65(2) 149-156.

[3] Malemud CJ, Reddy SK. Targeting cytokines, chemokines and adhesion molecules in rheumatoid arthritis. Current Rheumatology Reviews 2008; 4(4) 219-234.

[4] Imboden JB. The immunopathogenesis of rheumatoid arthritis. Annual Review of Pathology 2009; 4 417-434.

[5] Stritesky GL, Kaplan MH. Changing the STATus quo in T helper cells. Transcription 2011; 2(4) 179-182.

[6] Hanada T, Yoshimura A. Regulation of cytokine signaling and inflammation. Cytokine & Growth Factor Reviews 2002; 13(4-5) 413-421.

[7] Hebenstreit D, Horejs-Hoeck J, Duschl A. JAK/STAT-dependent gene regulation by cytokines. Drug News Perspective 2005; 18(4) 243-249.

[8] Schindler C, Plumlee C. Interferons pen the JAK-STAT pathway. Seminars in Cell and Developmental Biology 2008; 19(4) 311-318.

[9] Malemud CJ. Recent advances in neutralizing the IL-6 pathway in arthritis. Open Access Rheumatology Research & Reviews 2009; 1: 133-150.

[10] Goenka S, Kaplan MH. Transcriptional regulation by STAT6. Immunologic Research 2011; 50(1) 87-96.

[11] Heim MH. The Jak-STAT pathway: cytokine signalling from the receptor to the nucleus. Journal of Receptor Signal Transduction Research 1999; 19(1-4) 75-120.

[12] Jiang H, Harris MB, Rothman P. IL-4/IL-13 signaling beyond JAK/STAT. Journal of Allergy & Clinical Immunology 2000; 105(6 Pt 1) 1063-1070.

[13] Hebenstreit D, Wirnsberger G, Horejs-Hoeck J, Duschl A. Signaling mechanisms, interaction partners, and target genes of STAT6. Cytokine & Growth Factor Reviews 2006; 17(3) 173-188.

[14] Tuomela S, Rautajoki KJ, Moulder R, Nyman TA, Lahesmaa R. Identification of novel Stat6 regulated proteins in IL-4-treated mouse lymphocytes. Proteomics 2009; 9(4): 1087-1098.

[15] Müller-Ladner U, Judex M, Ballhorn W et al. Activation of the IL-4 STAT pathway in rheumatoid synovium. Journal of Immunology 2000; 164(7) 3894-3901.

[16] Malemud CJ, Pearlman E. Targeting JAK/STAT signaling pathway in inflammatory diseases. Current Signal Transduction Research 2009; 4 201-221.

[17] Darnell JE Jr. STATS and gene regulation. Science 1997; 277(5332) 1630-1635.

[18] Leonard WJ, O'Shea JJ. Jaks and STATs: biological implications. Annual Review of Immunology 1998; 16 293-322.

[19] Giordanetto F, Kroemer RT. Prediction of the structure of human Janus kinase2 (JAK2) comprising JAK homology domains 1 through 7. Protein Engineering 2002; 15(9) 727-737.

[20] Decker T, Korvarik P. Serine phosphorylation of STATs. Oncogene 2000; 19(21) 2628-2637.

[21] Malemud CJ. Differential activation of JAK enzymes in rheumatoid arthritis and autoimmune disorders by pro-inflammatory cytokines: potential drug targets. International Journal of Interferon, Cytokine & Mediator Research 2010; 2(1) 97-111.

[22] Zhu J, Cote-Sierra J, Guo L, Paul WE. Stat5 activation plays a critical role in Th2 differentiation. Immunity 2003; 19(5) 739-748.

[23] Hennighausen L, Robinson GW. Interpretation of cytokine signaling through the transcription factors STAT5A and STAT5B. Genes & Development 2008; 22(6) 711-721.

[24] Radtke S, Wüller S, Xang XP et al. Cross-regulation of cytokine signalling: pro-inflammatory cytokines restrict IL-6 signalling through receptor internalisation and degradation. Journal of Cell Science 2010; 123 (Pt 6) 947-959.

[25] Santos CI, Costa-Pereira AP. Signal transducers and activators of transcription-from cytokine signaling to cancer biology. Biochimica et Biophysica Acta 2011; 1816(1) 38-49.

[26] Stark GR, Darnell JE Jr. The JAK-STAT pathway at twenty. Immunity 2012; 36(4) 503-514.

[27] Wang X, Liu Q, Ihsan A et al. JAK/STAT pathway plays a critical role in the proin-flammatory gene expression and apoptosis of RAW264.7 cells induced by trichothe-cenes as DON and T-2 toxin. Toxicological Sciences 2012; 127(2) 412-424.

[28] Buitenhuis M, Coffer PJ, Koenderman L. Signal transducer and activator of transcrip-tion 5 (STAT5). International Journal of Biochemistry & Cell Biology 2004; 36(11) 2120-2124.

[29] Kasperkovitz PV, Verbeet NL, Smeets TJ et al. Activation of the STAT1 pathway in rheumatoid arthritis. Annals of the Rheumatic Diseases 2004; 63(3) 233-239.

[30] Malemud CJ, Gillespie HJ. The role of apoptosis in arthritis. Current Rheumatology Reviews 2005; 1(1) 131-142.

[31] Walker JG, Ahern MG, Coleman M et al. Changes in synovial tissue Jak-STAT ex-pression in rheumatoid arthritis in response to successful DMARD treatment. Annals of the Rheumatic Diseases 2006; 65(12) 1558-1564.

[32] Walker JG, Ahern MG, Coleman M et al. Characterisation of a dendritic cell subset in synovial tissue which strongly expresses Jak/STAT transcription factors from pa-tients with rheumatoid arthritis. Annals of the Rheumatic Diseases. 2007; 66 (8) 992-999.

[33] Stritesky GL, Muthukrishnan R, Sehra S et al. The transcription factor STAT3 is re-quired for T helper 2 cell development. Immunity 2011; 34(1) 39-49.

[34] Krebs DL, Hilton DJ. SOCS proteins: negative regulators of cytokine signaling. Stem Cells 2001; 19(5) 378-387.

[35] Giordanetto F, Kroemer RT. A three-dimensional model of Suppressor of Cytokine Signaling 1 (SOCS-1). Protein Engineering 2003; 16(2) 115-124.

[36] Yoshimura A, Naka T, Kubo M. SOCS proteins, cytokine signalling and immune reg-ulation. Nature Reviews Immunology 2007; 7(6) 454-465.

[37] van de Geijn GJ, Gits J, Touw IP. Distinct activities of suppressor of cytokine signal-ing (SOCS) proteins and involvement of the SOCS box in controlling G-CSF signal-ing. Journal of Leukocyte Biology 2004; 76(1) 237-244.

[38] Bruun C, Heding PE, Rønn SG et al. Suppressor of cytokine signalling-3 inhibits tu-mor necrosis factor-alpha induced apoptosis and signalling in beta cells. Molecular & Cellular Endocrinology 2009; 311(1-2) 32-38.

[39] Pirvulescu M, Manduteanu I, Gan AM et al. A novel pro-inflammatory mechanism of action of resistin in human endothelial cells: upregulation of SOCS3 expression

through STAT3 activation. Biochemical & Biophysical Research Communications 2012; 422(2) 321-326.

[40] Isomäki P, Alanärä T, Isohanni P et al. The expression of SOCS is altered in rheumatoid arthritis. Rheumatology (Oxford) 2007; 46(10) 1538-1546.

[41] de Andrés MC, Imagawa K, Hashimoto K et al. Suppressors of cytokine signaling (SOCS) are reduced in osteoarthritis. Biochemical & Biophysical Research Communications 2011; 407(1) 54-59.

[42] van de Loo FA, Veenbergen S, van den Brand B et al. Enhanced suppressor of cytokine signaling-3 in arthritic cartilage dysregulates human chondrocyte function. Arthritis & Rheumatism 2012; 64(10) 3313-3323.

[43] Zhang J, Somani AK, Siminovitch KA. Roles of SHP-1 tyrosine phosphatases in the negative regulation of cell signaling. Seminars in Immunology 2000; 12 (4) 361-378.

[44] Alexander DR. The CD45 tyrosine phosphatase: a positive and negative regulator of immune cell function. Seminars in Immunology 2000; 12(4) 349-359.

[45] Shuai K. Regulation of cytokine signaling pathways by PIAS proteins. Cell Research 2006; 16(2) 196-202.

[46] Tahk S, Liu B, Chernishof V, Wong KA, Wu H, Shuai K. Control of specificity and magnitude of NF-κB and STAT1-mediated gene activation through PIASy and PIAS1 cooperation. Proceedings of the National Academy of Sciences United States of America 2007; 104(28) 11643-11648.

[47] Malemud CJ. Dsyfunctional immune-mediated inflammation in rheumatoid arthritis dictates that development of anti-rheumatic drugs target multiple intracellular signaling pathways. Anti-Inflammatory & Anti-Allergy Agents in Medicinal Chemistry 2011; 10(1) 78-84.

[48] Hu X, Chen J, Wang L, Ivashkiv LB. Crosstalk among JAK-STAT, Toll-like receptor, and ITAM-dependent pathways in macrophage activation. Journal of Leukocyte Biology 2007; 82(2) 237-243.

[49] Ivashkiv LB. Cross-regulation of signaling by ITAM-associated receptors. Nature Immunology 2009; 10(4) 340-347.

[50] Lawrence T. The nuclear factor NF-κB pathway in inflammation. Cold Spring Harbor Perspectives in Biology 2009; 1(6) e001651.

[51] Alvarez JV, Frank DA. Genome-wide analysis of STAT target genes. Elucidating the mechanism of STAT-mediated oncogenesis. Cancer Biology & Therapy 2004; 3(11) 1045-1050.

[52] Oh YM, Kim JK, Choi S, Yoo JY. Identification of co-occurring transcription factor binding sites from DNA sequence using clustered position weight matrices. Nucleic Acids Research 2012; 40(5) e38.

[53] Snyder M, Huang XY, Zhang JJ. Identification of novel direct Stat3 target genes for control of growth and differentiation. Journal of Biological Chemistry 2008; 283(7) 3791-3798.

[54] Shuai K. Modulation of STAT signaling by STAT-interacting proteins. Oncogene 2000; 19(21) 2638-2644.

[55] Timofeeva OA, Chasovskikh S, Lonskaya I et al. Mechanisms of unphosphorylated STAT3 transcription factor binding to DNA. Journal of Biological Chemistry 2012; 287(17) 14192-14200.

[56] Cheon H, Yang J, Stark GR. The functions of signal transducers and activators of transcriptions 1 and 3 as cytokine-inducible proteins. Journal of Interferon & Cytokine Research 2011; 31(1) 33-40.

[57] Horvath CM, Wen Z, Darnell JE Jr. A STAT protein domain that determines DNA sequence recognition suggests a novel DNA-binding domain. Genes & Development 1995; 9(8) 984-994.

[58] Boucheron C, Dumon S, Santos SC et al. A single amino acid in the DNA binding regions of STAT5A and STAT5B confers distinct DNA binding specificities. Journal of Biological Chemistry 1998; 273(51) 33936-33941.

[59] Basham B, Sathe M, Grein J et al. In vivo identification of novel STAT5 target genes. Nucleic Acids Research 2008; 36(11) 3802-3818.

[60] Grimley PM, Dong F, Rui H. Stat5a and Stat5b: fraternal twins of signal transduction and transcription activation. Cytokine & Growth Factor Reviews 1999; 10(2) 131-157.

[61] Chang Y, Spicer DB, Sonenshein GE. Effects of IL-3 on promoter usage, attenuation and antisense transcription of the c-myc oncogene in the IL-3-dependent Ba/F3 early pre-B cell line. Oncogene 1991; 6(11) 1979-1982.

[62] Nelson EA, Walker SR, Alvarez JV, Frank DA. Isolation of unique STAT5 targets by chromatin immunoprecipitation-based gene identification. Journal of Biological Chemistry 2004; 279(52) 54724-54730.

[63] Ehret GB, Reichenbach P, Schindler U et al. DNA binding specificity of different STAT proteins. Comparison of *in vitro* specificity with natural target sites. Journal of Biological Chemistry 2001; 276(9) 6675-6688.

[64] Moucadel V, Constantinescu SN. Differential STAT5 signaling by ligand-dependent and constitutively active cytokine receptors. Journal of Biological Chemistry 2005; 280(14) 13364-13373.

[65] Rickert M, Wang X, Boulanger MJ, Goriatcheva N, Garcia KC. The structure of interleukin-2 complexed with its alpha receptor. Science 2005; 308(5727) 1477-1480.

[66] Kanai A, Suzuki K, Tanimoto K, Mizushima-Sugano J, Suzuki Y, Sugano S. Characterization of STAT6 target genes in human B cells and lung epithelial cells. DNA Research 2011; 18(5) 379-392.

[67] Thanos CD, DeLano WL, Wells JA. Hot-spot mimicry of a cytokine receptor by a small molecule. Proceedings of the National Academy of Sciences of the United States of America. 2006; 103(42) 15422-15427.

[68] Quaglino P, Bergallo M, Ponti R et al. Th1, Th2, Th17 and regulatory T cell patterns in psoriatic patients: modulation of cytokines and gene targets induced by etanercept treatment and correlation with clinical responses. Dermatology 2011; 223(1) 57-67.

[69] Delphin S, Stavnezer J. Characterization of an interleukin 4 (IL-4) responsive region in the immunoglobulin heavy chain germline epsilon promoter: regulation by NF-IL-4, a C/EBP family member and NF-kappa B/p50. Journal of Experimental Medicine 1995; 181(1) 181-192.

[70] Kotanides H, Reich NC. Interleukin-4-induced STAT6 recognizes and activates a target site in the promoter of the interleukin-4 receptor gene. Journal of Biological Chemistry 1996; 271(41) 25555-25561.

[71] Morelli X, Bourgeas R, Roche P. Chemical and structural lessons from recent successes in protein-protein interaction inhibition (2P2I). Current Opinion in Chemical Biology 2011; 15(4) 475-481.

[72] Lin JX, Leonard WJ. The role of Stat5a and Stat5b in signaling by IL-2 family cytokines. Oncogene 2000; 19(21) 2566-2576.

[73] Tsuji-Takayama K, Suzuki M, Yamamoto M et al. The production of IL-10 by human regulatory T cells is enhanced by IL-2 through a STAT5-responsive intronic enhancer in the IL-10 locus. Journal of Immunology 2008; 181(6) 3897-3905.

[74] Ochs HD, Gambineri E, Torgerson TR. IPEX, FOXP3 and regulatory T-cells: a model for autoimmunity. Immunologic Research 2007; 38(1-3) 112-121.

[75] Murawski MR, Litherland SA, Clare-Salzler MJ, Davoodi-Semiromi A. Upregulation of Foxp3 expression in mouse and human Treg is IL-2/STAT dependent: implications for the NOD STAT5B mutation in diabetes pathogenesis. Annals of the New York Academy of Sciences 2006; 1079 198-204.

[76] Lai G, Bromberg JS. Epigenetic mechanisms of regulation of Foxp3 expression. Blood 2009; 114(18) 3727-3735.

[77] Chen Z, Lund R, Aittokallio T, Kosonen M, Nevalainen O, Lahesmaa R. Identification of novel IL-4/STAT6-regulated gene in T lymphocytes. Journal of Immunology 2003; 171(7) 3627-3635.

[78] Lund R, Ahlfors H, Kainonen E, Lahesmaa AM, Dixon C, Lahesmaa R. Identification of genes involved in the initiation of human Th1 or Th2 cell commitment. European Journal of Immunology 2005; 35(11) 3307-3319.

[79] Maier E, Hebenstreit D, Posselt G, Hammerl P, Duschl A, Horejs-Hoeck J. Inhibition of suppressive T cell factor (TCF-1) isoforms in naïve CD_4^+ T cells is mediated by IL-$_4$/STAT6 signaling. Journal of Biological Chemistry 2011; 286(2) 919-928.

[80] Chapoval S, Dasgupta P, Dorsey NJ, Keegan AD. Regulation of the T helper cell type 2 (Th2/T regulatory cell (Treg) balance by IL-4 and STAT6. Journal of Leukocyte Biology 2010; 87(6) 1011-1018.

[81] Wurster AL, Tanaka T, Grusby MJ. The biology of Stat4 and Stat6. Oncogene 2000; 19(21) 2577-2584.

[82] Kuhn DJ, Dou QP. The role of interleukin-2 receptor alpha in cancer. Frontiers in Bioscience 2005; 10 1462-1474.

[83] Kurreeman FA, Daha NA, Chang M et al. Association of IL2RA and IL2RB with rheumatoid arthritis: a replication study in a Dutch population. Annals of the Rheumatic Diseases 2009; 68(11) 1789-1790.

[84] Raychaudhuri S. Recent advances in the genetics of rheumatoid arthritis. Current Opinion in Rheumatology 2010; 22(2) 109-118.

[85] Waldmann TA. The IL-2/IL-15 receptor systems: targets for immunotherapy. Journal of Clinical Immunology 2002; 22(2) 51-56.

[86] González-Álvaro I, Domínguez-Jiménez C, Ortiz AM et al. Interleukin-15 and interferon-γ participate in the cross-talk between natural killer and monocytic cells required for tumor necrosis factor production. Arthritis Research & Therapy 2006; 8(4) R88.

[87] Ernestam S, af Klint E, Catrina AI et al. Synovial expression of IL-15 in rheumatoid arthritis is not influenced by blockade of tumor necrosis factor. Arthritis Research & Therapy 2006; 8(1) R18.

[88] Baslund B, Tvede N, Danneskiold-Samsoe B et al. Targeting interleukin-15 in patients with rheumatoid arthritis: a proof-of-concept study. Arthritis & Rheumatism 2005; 52(9) 2686-2692.

[89] González-Álvaro I, Ortiz AM, Álvaro-Gracia JM et al. Interleukin-15 levels in serum may predict a severe disease course in patients with early arthritis. Public Library of Science One 2011; 6(12) e29492.

[90] Navarro-Millán I, Singh JA, Curtis JR. Systematic review of tocilizumab for rheumatoid arthritis: a new biologic agent targeting the interleukin-6 receptor. Clinical Therapy 2012; 34(4) 788-802.e3.

[91] Ogata A, Hirano T, Hishitani Y, Tanaka T. Safety and efficacy of tocilizumab for the treatment of rheumatoid arthritis. Clinical Medicine Insights in Arthritis & Musculoskeletal Disorders 2012; 5 27-42.

[92] Smolen JS, Avila JC, Aletaha D. Tocilizumab inhibits the progression of joint damage in rheumatoid arthritis irrespective of its anti-inflammatory effects: dissociation of the link between inflammation and destruction. Annals of the Rheumatic Diseases 2012; 71(5) 687-693.

[93] Jovanovic DV, Di Battista JA, Martel-Pelletier J et al. IL-17 stimulates the production and expression of proinflammatory cytokines, IL-1β and TNF-α, by human macrophages. Journal of Immunology 1998; 160(7) 3513-3521.

[94] Dragon S, Saffar AS, Shan L, Gounni AS. IL-17 attenuates the anti-apoptotic effects of GM-CSF in human neutrophils. Molecular Immunology 2008; 45(1) 160-168.

[95] Oh HM, Yu CR, Golestaneh N et al. STAT3 protein promotes T-cell survival and inhibits interleukin-2 production through up-regulation of Class O Forkhead transcription factors. Journal of Biological Chemistry 2011; 286(35) 30888-30897.

[96] Malemud CJ. Apoptosis-resistance in rheumatoid arthritis synovial tissue. Journal of Clinical & Cellular Immunology 2012; S3-006; doi: 10.4172/21559899.

[97] Kimura A, Kishimoto T. IL-6: regulator of Treg/Th17 balance. European Journal of Immunology 2010; 40(7) 1830-1835.

[98] Samson M, Audia S, Janikashvili N et al. Inhibition of IL-6 function corrects Th17/Treg imbalance in patients with rheumatoid arthritis. Arthritis & Rheumatism 2012; 64(8) 2499-2503

[99] Niu Q, Cai B, Huang ZC, Shi YY, Wang LL. Disturbed Th17/Treg balance in patients with rheumatoid arthritis. Rheumatology International 2012; 32(9) 2731-2736.

[100] O'Brien CA, Manolagas SC. Isolation and characterization of the human gp130 promoter. Regulation by STATs. Journal of Biological Chemistry 1997; 272(23) 15003-15010.

[101] Malemud CJ. Anticytokine therapy for osteoarthritis. Evidence to date. Drugs & Aging 2010; 27(2) 95-115.

[102] Wang T, Niu G, Kortylewski M et al. Regulation of the innate and adaptive immune responses by Stat-3 signaling in tumor cells. Nature Medicine 2004; 10(1) 48-54.

[103] Costa-Pereira AP, Bonito NA, Secki MJ. Dysregulation of janus kinases and signal transducers and activators of transcription in cancer. American Journal of Cancer Research 2011; 1(6) 806-816.

[104] Sozzani D, Bosisio D, Scarsi M, Tincani A. Type I interferons in systemic autoimmunity. Autoimmunity 2010; 43(3) 196-203.

[105] Biswas PS, Bhagat G, Pernis AB. IRF4 and its regulators: insights into the pathogenesis of inflammatory arthritis? Immunologic Reviews 2010; 233(1) 79-96.

[106] Pramanik R, Jørgensen TN, Xin H, Kotzin BL, Choubey D. Interleukin-6 induces expression of Ifi202, an interferon-inducible candidate gene for lupus susceptibility. Journal of Biological Chemistry 2004; 279(16) 16121-16127.

[107] Christova R, Jones T, Wu PJ et al. P-STAT1 mediates higher-order chromatin remodeling of the human MHC response to IFNγ. Journal of Cell Science 2007; 120(Pt 18) 3262-3270.

[108] Vogl C, Flatt T, Fuhrmann B et al. Transcriptosome analysis reveals a major impact of JAK protein tyrosine kinase (Tyk2) on the expression of interferon-responsive and metabolic genes. Biomedical Central Genomics 2010; 11 199.

[109] Noon-Song EN, Ahmed CM, Dabelic R, Canton J, Johnson HM. Controlling nuclear JAKs and STATs for specific gene activation by IFNγ. Biochemical & Biophysical Research Communications 2011; 410(3) 648-653.

[110] Tripathi A, Sodhi A. Prolactin-induced production of cytokines in macrophages in vitro involves JAK/STAT and JNK MAPK pathways. International Immunology 2008; 20(3) 327-336.

[111] David M, Petricoin E III, Benjamin C, Pine R, Weber MJ, Larner AC. Requirement of MAP kinase (ERK2) activity in interferon α and interferon β-stimulated gene expression through STAT proteins. Science 1995; 269(5231) 1721-1723.

[112] Aznar S, Valéron PF, del Rincon SV, Peréz LF, Perona R, Lacal JC. Simultaneous tyrosine and serine phosphorylation of STAT3 transcription factor is involved in Rho A GTPase oncogenic transformation. Molecular & Cellular Biology 2001; 12(10) 3282-3294.

[113] Gonsky R, Deem RL, Bream J, Young HA, Targan SR. Enhancer role of STAT5 in CD2 activation of IFN-γ gene expression. Journal of Immunology 2004; 173(10) 6241-6247.

[114] Tsuno T, Mejido J, Zhao T, Schmeisser H, Morrow A, Zoon KC. IRF9 is a key factor for eliciting the antiproliferative activity of IFN-α. Journal of Immunotherapy 2009; 32(8) 803-816.

[115] Kaur S, Uddin S, Platanias LC. The PI3' kinase pathway in interferon signaling. Journal of Interferon & Cytokine Research 2005; 25(12) 780-787.

[116] Kaur S, Sassano A, Dolniak B et al. Role of the Akt pathway in mRNA translation of interferon-stimulated genes. Proceedings of the National Academy of Sciences of the United States of America 2008; 105(12) 4808-4813.

[117] Kaur S, Katsoulidis E, Platanias LC. Akt and mRNA translation by interferons. Cell Cycle 2008; 7(14) 2112-2116.

[118] Hamilton TA, Ohmori Y, Tebo JM, Kishore R. Regulation of macrophage gene expression by pro- and anti-inflammatory cytokines. Pathobiology 1991; 67(5-6) 241-244.

[119] Schaefer A, Unterberger C, Frankenberger M et al. Mechanism of interferon-gamma mediated down-regulation of interleukin-10 gene expression. Molecular Immunology 2009; 46(7) 1351-1359.

[120] Torgerson GR. Regulatory T cells in human autoimmune diseases. Springer Seminars in Immunopathology 2006; 28(1) 63-76.

[121] Nandakumar S, Miller CW, Kumaraguru U. T regulatory cells: an overview and intervention techniques to modulate allergy outcome. Clinical & Molecular Allergy 2009; 12(7) 5.

[122] Hams E, Colmont CS, Dioszeghy V et al. Oncostatin M receptor-β signaling limits monocyte cell recruitment in acute inflammation. Journal of Immunology 2008; 181(3) 2174-2180.

[123] Mosley B, De Imus C, Friend D et al. Dual oncostatin M (OSM) receptors. Cloning and characterization of an alternative signaling subunit conferring OSM-specific receptor activation. Journal of Biological Chemistry 1996; 271(51) 32635-32643.

[124] Hermanns HM, Radkte S, Schaper F, Heinrich PC, Behrmann I. Non-redundant signal transduction of interleukin-6-type cytokines. The adaptor protein Shc is specifically recruited to the oncostatin M receptor. Journal of Biological Chemistry 2000; 275(52) 40742-40748.

[125] Fossey SL, Bear MD, Kisseberth WC, Pennell M, London CA. Oncostatin M promotes STAT3 activation, VEGF production and invasion of osteosarcoma cell lines. Biomedical Central Cancer 2011; 11 125.

[126] Clarkson RWE, Boland MP, Kritikou EA et al. The genes induced by signal transducers and activators of transcription (STAT)3 and STAT5 in mammary epithelial cells define the roles of these STATs in mammary development. Molecular Endocrinology 2006; 20(3) 675-685.

[127] STAT Gene Regulatory Network. rulai/cshl.edu/TRED/GRN/STAT.htm

[128] Nakanishi K, Yoshimoto T, Tsutsui H, Okamura H. Interleukin-18 regulates both Th1 and Th2 responses. Annual Review of Immunology 2001; 19 423-474.

[129] Liew FY, McInnes IB. Role of interleukin 15 and interleukin 18 in inflammatory response. Annals of the Rheumatic Diseases 2002; 61(Suppl 2) ii100-ii102.

[130] McInnes IB, Liew FY, Gracie JA. Interleukin-18: a therapeutic target in rheumatoid arthritis? Arthritis Research & Therapy 2005; 7(1) 38-41.

[131] Matsui K, Tsutsui H, Nakanishi K. Pathophysiological roles for IL-18 in inflammatory arthritis. Expert Opinion on Therapeutic Targets 2003; 7(6) 701-724.

[132] Lotito AP, Silva CA, Mello SB. Interleukin-18 in chronic joint diseases. Autoimmunity Reviews 2007; 6(4) 253-256.

[133] Gracie JA, Forsey RJ, Chan WL et al. A proinflammatory role for IL-18 in rheumatoid arthritis. Journal of Clinical Investigation 1999; 104(10) 1393-1401.

[134] Tanaka M, Harigai M, Kawaguchi Y et al. Mature form of interleukin-18 is expressed in rheumatoid arthritis synovial tissue and contributes to interferon-gamma production by synovial T-cells. Journal of Rheumatology 2001; 28(8) 1779-1787.

[135] Van Oosterhout M, Levarht EWN, Sont JK, Huizinga TWJ, Toes REM, van Laar JM. Clinical efficacy of infliximab plus methotrexate in DMARD naïve and DMARD re-

fractory rheumatoid arthritis is associated with decreased synovial expression of TNFα and IL-18 but not CXCL12. Annals of the Rheumatic Diseases 2005; 64(4) 537-543.

[136] Petrovic-Rackov I, Pejnovic N. Clinical significance of IL-18, IL-15, IL-12 and TNF-α measurement in rheumatoid arthritis. Clinical Rheumatology 2006; 25(4) 448-452.

[137] Trinchieri G, Scott P. Interleukin-12: a proinflammatory cytokine with immunoregulatory functions. Research in Immunology 1995; 146(7–8) 423–431.

[138] Trinchieri G, Scott P. Interleukin-12: basic principles and clinical applications. Current Topics in Microbiology & Immunology 1999; 238 57–78.

[139] Merberg DM, Wolf SF, Clark SC. Sequence similarity between NKSF and the IL-6/G-CSF family. Immunology Today 1992; 13(2) 77–78.

[140] Watford WT, Moriguchi M, Morinobu A, O'Shea JJ. Mini review. The biology of IL-12: coordinating innate and adaptive immune responses. Cytokine & Growth Factor Reviews 2003; 14 361–368.

[141] Yen JH, Kong W, Ganea D. IFN-β inhibits dendritic cell migration through STAT-1-mediated transcriptional suppression of CCR7 and matrix metalloproteinase 9. Journal of Immunology 2010; 187(7) 3478-3486.

[142] Tuohy VK, Yu M, Yin L, Mathisen PM, Johnson JM, Kawczak JA. Modulation of the IL-10/IL-12 cytokine circuit by interferon-β inhibits the development of epitope spreading and disease progression in murine autoimmune encephalomyelitis. Journal of Neuroimmunology 2000; 111(1-2) 55-63.

[143] Thieu VT, Yu Q, Chang HC et al. Signal transducer and activator of transcription 4 is required for the transcription factor T-bet to promote T helper 1 cell-fate determination. Immunity 2008; 29(5) 679-690.

[144] Yang Y, Ochando JC, Bromberg JS, Ding Y. Identification of a distant T-bet enhancer responsive to IL-12/Stat4 and IFNγ/Stat1 signals. Blood 2007; 110(7) 2494-2500.

[145] Forbes E, van Panhuys N, Min B, Le Gros G. Differential requirements for IL-4/STAT6 signalling in CD4 T-cell fate determination and the Th2-immune effector responses. Immunology and Cell Biology 2010; 88(3) 240-243.

[146] Huber M, Steinwald V, Guralnik A et al. IL-27 inhibits the development of regulatory T cells via STAT3. International Immunology 2008; 20(2) 223-234.

[147] Afzali B, Lombardi G, Lechler RI, Lord GM. The role of T helper 17 (Th17) and regulatory T cells (Treg) in human organ transplantation and autoimmune disease. Clinical & Experimental Immunology 2007; 148(1) 32-46.

[148] Peck A, Mellins ED. Plasticity of the T-cell phenotype and function: the T helper type 17 example. Immunology 2010; 129(2) 147-153.

[149]   Chen Z, O'Shea JJ. Th17 cells: a new fate for differentiating helper T cells. Immunologic Research 2008; 41(2) 87-102.

[150]   Yagi R, Zhu J, Paul WE. An updated view on transcription factor $GATA_3$-mediated regulation of T_h1 and T_h2 cell differentiation. International Immunology 2011; 23(7) 415-420.

[151]   Habib T, Senadheera S, Weinberg K, Kaushansky K. The common γ chain (γc) is a required signaling component of the IL-21 receptor and supports IL-21-induced cell proliferation via JAK3. Biochemistry 2002; 41(27) 8725-8731.

[152]   Mehta DS, Wurster AL, Grusby MJ. Biology of IL-21 and the IL-21 receptor. Immunologic Reviews 2004; 202 84-95.

[153]   Ma J, Ma D, Ji C. The role of IL-21 in hematological malignancies. Cytokine 2011; 56(2) 133-139.

[154]   Collins M, Whitters MJ, Young DA. IL-21 and IL-21 receptor: a new cytokine pathway modulates innate and adaptive immunity. Immunologic Reviews 2003; 28(2) 131-140.

[155]   Sonderegger I, Kisielow J, Meier R, King C, Kopf M. IL-21 and IL-21R are not required for development of Th17 cells and autoimmunity in vivo. European Journal of Immunology 2008; 3897 1833-1838.

[156]   Coquet JM, Chakravarti S, Smyth MJ, Godfrey DI. Cutting edge: IL-21 is not essential for Th17 differentiation or experimental autoimmune encephalomyelitis. Journal of Immunology 2008; 180(11) 7097-7101.

[157]   Davis ID, Skak K, Smyth MJ, Kristjansen PE, Miller DM, Sivakumar PV. Interleukin-21 signaling: functions in cancer and autoimmunity. Clinical Cancer Research 2007; 13(23) 6926-6932.

[158]   Young DA, Hegen M, Ma HL et al. Blockade of the interleukin-21/interleukin-21 receptor pathway ameliorates disease in animal models of rheumatoid arthritis. Arthritis & Rheumatism 2007; 56(4) 1152-1163.

[159]   Yuan FL, Hu W, Lu WG et al. Targeting interleukin-21 in rheumatoid arthritis. Molecular Biology Reports 2011; 38(3) 1717-1721.

[160]   Wooley PA. What animal models are best to test novel rheumatoid arthritis therapies? Current Rheumatology Reviews 2008; 4(4) 277-287.

[161]   Dumoutier L, Louahed J, and Renauld JC. Cloning and characterization of IL-10-related T cell-derived inducible factor (IL-TIF), a novel cytokine structurally related to IL-10 and inducible by IL-9. Journal of Immunology 2000; 164(4) 1814-1819.

[162]   Blumberg H, Conklin D, Xu WF et al. Interleukin 20: discovery, receptor identification and role in epidermal function. Cell 2001; 104(1) 9-19.

[163] Zenewicz LA, Flavell RA. Recent advances in IL-22 biology. International Immunology 2011 23(3) 159-163.

[164] Donnelly RP, Sheikh F, Kotenko SV, Dickensheets H. The expanded family of class II cytokines that share the IL-10 receptor-2 (IL-10R2) chain. Journal of Leukocyte Biology 2004; 76(2) 314-321.

[165] Commins S, Steinke JW, Borish L. The extended IL-10 superfamily: IL-10, IL-19, IL-20, IL-22, IL-24, IL-26, IL-28 and IL-29. Journal of Allergy & Clinical immunology 2008; 121(5) 1108-1111.

[166] Trivella DB, Ferreira-Júnior JR, Dumoutier L, Renauld JC, Polikarpov I. Structure and function of interleukin-22 and other members of the interleukin-10 family. Cellular & Molecular Life Sciences 2010; 67(17) 2909-2935.

[167] Asadullah K, Sterry W, Volk HD. Interleukin-10 therapy – review of a new approach. Pharmacological Reviews 2003; 55(2) 241-269.

[168] Sabat R, Wallace E, Endesfelder S, Wolk K. IL-19 and IL-20: two novel cytokines with importance in inflammatory diseases. Expert Opinion on Therapeutic Targets 2007; 11(5) 601-612.

[169] Wolk K, Kunz S, Asadullah K, Sabat R. Cutting edge: Immune cells as sources and targets of the IL-10 family members. Journal of Immunology 2002; 168(11) 5397-5402.

[170] Parrish-Novak J, Xu W, Brender T et al. Interleukins 19, 20, and 24 signal through two distinct receptor complexes. Differences in receptor-ligand interactions mediate unique biological functions. Journal of Biological Chemistry 2002; 277(49) 47517-47523.

[171] Dumoutier L, Leemans C, Lejeune D, Kotenko SV, Renauld JC. Cutting edge: STAT activation by IL-19, IL-20 and mda-7 through IL-20 receptor complexes of two types. Journal of Immunology 2001; 167(7) 3545-3549.

[172] Kunz S, Wolk K, Witte E et al. Interleukin (IL)-19, IL-20 and IL-24 are produced and act on keratinocytes and are distinct from classical ILs. Experimental Dermatology 2006; 15(12) 991-1004.

[173] Zdanov A. Structural features of the interleukin-10 family of cytokines. Current Pharmaceutical Design 2004; 10(31) 3873-3884.

[174] Sakurai N, Kuroiwa T, Ikeuchi H et al. Expression of IL-19 and its receptors in RA: potential role for synovial hyperplasia formation. Rheumatology (Oxford) 2008; 47(6) 815-820.

[175] Alanärä T, Karstila A, Moilanen T, Silvennoinen O, Isomäki P. Expression of IL-10 family cytokines in rheumatoid arthritis: elevated levels of IL-19 in joints. Scandinavian Journal of Rheumatology 2010; 39(2) 118-126.

[176] Malemud CJ. MAP kinases. In: OA, Inflammation and Degradation: A Continuum: Biomedical and Health Research - Vol 70. Buckwalter J, Lotz M, Stoltz J-F. (eds). Amsterdam: IOS Press; 2007. p 99-117.

[177] Hsu YH, Hsieh PP, Chang MS. Interleukin-19 blockade attenuates collagen-induced arthritis in rats. Rheumatology (Oxford) 2012; 51(3) 434-442.

[178] Leng RX, Pan HF, Tao JH, Ye DQ. IL-19, IL-20 and IL-24: potential therapeutic targets for autoimmune diseases. Expert Opinion on Therapeutic Targets 2011; 15(2) 119-126.

[179] Wahl C, Müller W, Leithäuser F et al. IL-20 receptor signaling down-regulates antigen-specific T cell responses. Journal of Immunology 2009; 182(2) 802-810.

[180] Hsu YH, Chang MS. Interleukin-20 antibody is a potential therapeutic agent for experimental arthritis. Arthritis & Rheumatism 2010; 62(11) 3311-3321.

[181] Hsu YH, Chen WY, Chan CH, Wu CH, Sun ZJ, Chang MS. Anti-IL-20 monoclonal antibody inhibits the differentiation of osteoclasts and protects against osteoporotic bone loss. Journal of Experimental Medicine 2011; 208(9) 1849-1861.

[182] Kragstrup TW, Otkjaer K, Holm C et al. The expression of IL-20 and IL-24 and their shared receptors are increased in rheumatoid arthritis and spondyloarthropathy. Cytokine 2008; 41(1) 16-23.

[183] Kotenko SV, Izotova LS, Mirochnitchenko OV et al. Identification of the functional Interleukin-22 (IL-22) receptor complex. The IL-10R2 chain (IL-10Rβ) is a common chain of both the IL-10 and IL-22 (IL-10-related T cell-derived inducible factor, IL-TIF) receptor complexes. Journal of Biological Chemistry 2001; 276(4) 2725-2732.

[184] Xie MH, Aggarwal S, Ho WH et al. Interleukin (IL)-22, a novel human cytokine that signals through the interferon receptor-related proteins CRF2-4 and IL-22R. Journal of Biological Chemistry 2000; 275(40) 31335-31339.

[185] Aggarwal S, Xie MH, Maruoka M, Foster J, Gurney AL. Acinar cells of the pancreas are a target of interleukin-22. Journal of Interferon & Cytokine Research 2001; 21(12) 1047-1053.

[186] Brand S, Beigel F, Olszak T et al. IL-22 is increased in active Crohn's disease and promotes proinflammatory gene expression and intestinal cell migration. American Journal of Physiology-Gastrointestinal and Liver Physiology 2006; 290(4) G827-G-838.

[187] Lejeune D, Dumoutier L, Constantinescu S, Kruijer W, Schuringa JJ, Renauld J-C. Interleukin-22 (IL-22) activates the JAK/STAT, ERK, JNK, and p38 MAP kinase pathways in a rat hepatoma cell line. Pathways that shared with and distinct from IL-10. Journal of Biological Chemistry 2002; 277(37) 33676-33682.

[188] Ikeuchi H, Kuroiwa T, Hiramatsu N et al. Expression of interleukin-22 in rheumatoid arthritis. Potential role as a proinflammatory cytokine. Arthritis & Rheumatism 2005; 52(4) 1037-1046.

[189] Leipe J, Schramm MA, Grunke M et al. Interleukin 22 serum levels are associated with radiographic progression in rheumatoid arthritis. Annals of the Rheumatic Diseases 2011; 70(8) 1453-1457.

[190] da Rocha LF Jr, Duarte AL, Dantas AT et al. Increased serum interleukin-22 in patients with rheumatoid arthritis and correlation with disease activity. Journal of Rheumatology 2012; 39(7) 1320-1325.

[191] Zhang L, Li JM, Liu XG et al. Elevated Th22 cells correlated with Th17 cells in patients with rheumatoid arthritis. Journal of Clinical Immunology 2011; 31(4) 606-614.

[192] Lécart S, Morel F, Noraz N et al. IL-22, in contrast to IL-10, does not induce Ig production, due to absence of a functional IL-22 receptor on activated human B cells. International Immunology 2002; 14(11) 1351-1356.

[193] Gopalkrishnan RV, Sauane M, Fisher PB. Cytokine and tumor cell apoptosis inducing activity of mda-7/IL-24. International Immunopharmacology 2004; 4(5) 635-647.

[194] Dent P, Yacoub A, Hamed HA et al. The development of MDA-7/IL-24 as a cancer therapeutic. Pharmacology & Therapeutics 2010; 128(2) 375-384.

[195] Dent P, Yacoub A, Hamed A et al. MDA-7/IL-24 as a cancer therapeutic: from bench to bedside. Anticancer Drugs 2010; 21(8) 725-731.

[196] Dash R, Bhutia SK, Azab B et al. mda-7/IL-24: a unique member of the IL-10 gene family promoting cancer-targeted toxicity. Cytokine & Growth Factor Reviews 2010; 21(5) 381-391.

[197] Sahoo A, Sim SH. Molecular mechanism governing IL-24 gene expression. Immune Network 2012; 12(1) 1-7.

[198] Sahoo A, Lee CG, Jash A et al. Stat6 and c-Jun mediate Th2 cell-specific IL-24 gene expression. Journal of Immunology 2011; 186(7) 4098-4109.

[199] Yen JJ, Yang-Yen HF. Transcription factors mediating interleukin-3 survival signals. Vitamins & Hormones 2006; 74 147-163.

[200] Mui AL, Wakao H, Kinoshita T, Kitamura T, Miyajima A. Suppression of interleukin-3-induced gene expression by a c-terminal Stat5. European Molecular Biology Organization Journal 1996; 15(10) 2425-2433.

[201] Chaturvedi P, Reddy MV, Reddy EP. Src kinases and not JAKs activates STATs during IL-3-induced myeloid cell proliferation. Oncogene 1998; 16(13) 1749-1758.

[202] Reddy EP, Korapati A, Chaturvedi P, Rane S. IL-3 signaling and the role of Src kinases, JAKs and STATs: a covert liaison unveiled. Oncogene 2000; 19(21) 2532-2547.

[203] Morales JK, Falanga YT, Depcrynski A, Fernando J, Ryan JJ. Mast cell homeostasis and the JAK-STAT pathway. Genes & Immunity 2010; 11(8) 599-608.

[204] Cavanagh LL, Boyce A, Smith L et al. Rheumatoid arthritis synovium contains plasmacytoid dendritic cells. Arthritis Research & Therapy 2005; 7(2) R230-R240.

[205] Barton BE, Mayer R. IL-3 induces differentiation of bone marrow precursor cells to osteoclast-like cells. Journal of Immunology 1989; 143(10) 3211-3216.

[206] Gupta N, Barhanpurkar AP, Tomar GB et al. IL-3 inhibits human osteoclastogenesis and bone resorption through downregulation of c-Fms and diverts the cells to dendritic cell lineage. Journal of Immunology 2010; 185(4) 2261-2272.

[207] Srivastava RK, Tomar GB, Barhanpurkar AP et al. IL-3 attenuates collagen-induced arthritis by modulating the development of Foxp3+ regulatory T cells. Journal of Immunology 2011; 186(4) 2262-2267.

[208] Khaled AR, Durum SK. Death and Baxes: mechanism of lymphotropic cytokines. Immunologic Review 2003; 193 48-57.

[209] Malemud CJ. The discovery of novel experimental therapies for inflammatory arthritis. Mediators of Inflammation doi: 10.1155/2009/698769.

[210] Kim HR, Hwang KA, Park SH, Kang I. IL-7 and IL-15: Biology and roles in T-cell immunity in health and disease. Critical Reviews in Immunology 2008; 28(4) 325-339.

[211] van Roon JA, Hartgring SA, Wenting van Wijk M. Persistence of interleukin-7 activity and levels on tumour necrosis factor α blockade in patients with rheumatoid arthritis. Annals of the Rheumatic Diseases 2007; 66(5) 664-669.

[212] Hartgring SA, van Roon JA, Wenting van Wijk M. Elevated expression of interleukin-7 receptor in inflamed joints mediates interleukin-7-induced immune activation in rheumatoid arthritis. Arthritis & Rheumatism 2009; 60(9) 2595-2605.

[213] Yammani RR, Long D, Loeser RF. Interleukin-7 stimulates secretion of S100A4 by activating the JAK/STAT signaling pathway in human articular chondrocytes. Arthritis & Rheumatism 2009; 60(3) 792-800.

[214] Senolt L, Grigorian M, Lukanidin E et al. S100A4 is expressed at site of invasion in rheumatoid arthritis synovium and modulates production of matrix metalloproteinases. Annals of the Rheumatic Diseases 2006; 65(12) 1645-1648.

[215] Grigorian M, Andresen S, Tulchinsky E et al. Tumor suppressor p53 protein is a new target for the metastasis-associated Mts1/S100A4 protein. Functional consequences of their interaction. Journal of Biological Chemistry 2001; 276(25) 22699-22708.

[216] Senolt L, Grigorian M, Lukanidin E et al. S100A4 (Mts1): Is there any relation to the pathogenesis of rheumatoid arthritis? Autoimmune Reviews 2006; 5(2) 129-131.

[217] Jüngel A, Ospelt C, Lesch M et al. Effect of oral application of a highly selective MMP-13 inhibitor in three different animal models of rheumatoid arthritis. Annals of the Rheumatic Diseases 2010; 69(5) 898-902.

[218] Fleischmann R, Cutolo M, Genovese MC et al. Phase IIB dose-ranging study of the oral JAK inhibitor tofacitinib (CP650,550) or adalimumab monotherapy versus placebo in patients with active rheumatoid arthritis with an inadequate response to DMARDs. Arthritis & Rheumatism 2012; 64(3) 617-629.

[219] Shirakawa T, Kawazoe Y, Tsujikawa T, Jung D, Sato S, Uesugi M. Deactivation of STAT6 through serine 707 phosphorylation by JNK. Journal of Biological Chemistry 2011; 286(5) 4003-4010.

[220] Klinman DM, Tross D, Klaschik S, Shirota H, Sato T. Therapeutic applications and mechanisms underlying the activity of immunosuppressive oligonucleotides. Annals of the New York Academy of Sciences 2009; 1175 80-88.

[221] Lührmann A, Tschernig T, von der Leyen H, Hecker M, Pabst R, Wagner AH. Decoy oligodeoxynucleotides against STAT transcription factors decrease allergic inflammation in a rat asthma model. Experimental Lung Research 2010; 36(2) 85-93.

[222] Hückel M, Schurigt U, Wagner AH et al. Attenuation of murine antigen-induced arthritis by treatment with a decoy oligodeoxynucleotide inhibiting signal transducer and activator of transcription-1 (STAT-1). Arthritis Research & Therapy 2006; 8(1) R17.

[223] Feely MG, Erickson A, O'Dell JR. Therapeutic options for rheumatoid arthritis. Expert Opinion on Pharmacotherapy 2009; 10(13) 2095-2106.

[224] Malemud CJ. Inhibitors of JAK for the treatment of rheumatoid arthritis: rationale and clinical data. Clinical Investigation 2012; 2(1) 39-47.

[225] Malemud CJ. Molecular mechanisms in rheumatic diseases: rationale for novel drug development – Introduction. Anti-Inflammatory & Anti-Allergy Agents in Medicinal Chemistry 2011; 10 73-77.

Chapter 5

The Antibacterial Drug Discovery

Jie Yanling, Liang Xin and Li Zhiyuan

Additional information is available at the end of the chapter

1. Introduction

An antibacterial is a compound or substance that kills or slows down the growth of bacteria. We usually associate the beginning of the modern antibacterial era with the names of Paul Ehrlich and Alexander Fleming. Infectious diseases are the leading causes of human morbidity and mortality for most of human existence. Antibacterials are probably one of the most successful forms of chemotherapy in the history of medicine. They save countless lives and make enormous contribution to the control of infectious diseases since the beginning of antibacterial era. Perhaps most of us born since the Second World War don't know how much enthusiasm, dedication, and hardship have been put in antibacterial drug discovery, and take the success of antibacterial agents too much for granted. Therefore, let's first look back what the human did to combat the infections before antibacterial era and how the outstanding scientists discovered so many efficient antibacterial agents used clinically today and led us enter the antibacterial era.

2. The history of antibacterial discovery

2.1. Pre-antibiotic era

Before the early 20th century, treatments for infections were based primarily on medicinal folklore. Mixtures with antimicrobial properties that were used in treatments of infections were described over 2000 years ago [1]. Even the prehistoric peoples used a number of plants in wound treatment and it seems possible that many plants have the properties of antimicrobial effects [2; 3]. Tetracyclines can be incorporated into the hydroxyapatite mineral portion of bones as well as tooth enamel; once people take it, permanent markers of metabolically active areas will be left. Thus it is much conveniently to trace the exposure of these antibacterials in ancient populations. It was found than the bone sample from Sudanese Nubian (A.D. 350 to 550) was labeled by the antibiotic tetracycline and their dietary regime contained tetracycline-containing materials by X-group cemetery and other advanced technologies [4; 5]. Moreover, another study showed that, bones from the Dakhleh Oasis, Egypt, in a late Roman period, exhibit discrete fluorochromelabelling, exactly like the teeth from patients treated with tetracycline [6]. A large number of customs and anecdotes can also reveal the occurrences of other antibacterials. One popular anecdote is about the antibiotic-like properties of red soil from the Hashemite Kingdom of Jordan. Interestingly, red soil was used for treating skin infections and diaper rash in the past and is still used in some communities today as an inexpensive alternative to antibiotics [7]. In fact, recently, many pharmaceutical antibiotics, such as streptomycin, actinomycin, erythromycin, vancomycin, nystatin and amphotericin, were produced from the soil actinomycetes [8].

The traditional Chinese medicine is the summary of experience about Chinese medical treatment over millennia and may contain a lot of unknown antibiotics [9]. Many traditional Chinese medicines were tested and found effective against four common oral bacteria [10]. Discovery of active components in the ancient herbs could enrich the arsenal of antimicrobials used by the mainstream medicine.

2.2. Foundation of the antibiotic era

Bacteria were first identified in the 1670s by van Leeuwenhoek, following his invention of the microscope. The relationship between bacteria and diseases gradually set up in the nineteenth century. Since then, researchers started to try and find effective antibacterial agents.

Paul Ehrlich is the father of chemotherapy and was honored with the Nobel prize due to the molecular side-chain theory of immunity. His concept of "magic bullet" is that the chemicals selectively target only disease-causing microbes but not the host cells. In 1906, Ehrlich, together with Bertheim, developed hundreds of derivatives of Atoxyl, and finally discovered compound 606, a gold powder [9; 11]. In 1909, he found that Compound 606 could cure syphilis-infected rabbits in experiments; it could also improve terminal patients with dementia and cured early stage patients with infected sores [11]. It was publicly released as salvarsan in 1910. Despite the adverse side effects, salvarsan and it's derivative neosalvarsan kept the status of the most frequently prescribed drug until the introduction of penicillin in the 1940s [12]. Amazingly, the chemical structure of salvarsan hadn't been known until 2005 [13].

The systematic screening approach introduced by Paul Ehrlich became the cornerstone of drug search strategies in the pharmaceutical industry. Sulfonamidochrysoidine (also named prontosil), the first commercially available antibiotic, was first synthesized by Bayer chemists Josef Klarer and Fritz Mietzsch in 1930s by this approach. Then Gerhard Domagk found its effect against Streptococcus pyogenes in mice [14]. Four years later he received the Noble Prize. Eventually prontosil was recognized as a precursor for a new class of antibacterial agents— sulfonamides.

The effect of mould on bacterial colonies hadn't been investigated until 19th century, although the antibacterial properties of mold had been known since ancient times. In 1921, Alexander Fleming observed some substances called lyzosomes which could dissolve bacteria. In 1928, he discovered that a specific mould species inhibited the development of Staphylococcus bacteria. The species was known as Pencilliumnotatum and the filtrate was called penicillin [15]. In 1940, Howard Florey and Ernst Chain worked out how to purify penicillin for clinical testing [16]. All the three researchers were awarded the Nobel Prize in 1945, and since then the era of antibiotics had been initiated. Penicillin became the top therapeutic molecule because of its widespread use and the magnitude of the therapeutic outcomes, and also because of the technologies developed for production of penicillin which became the basis for production of all subsequent antibiotics and other bioproducts in use today [17].

3. Classification

Antibacterials are commonly classified based on their mechanism of action or spectrum of activity. The main classes of antibacterial drugs target only four classical bacterial functions: bacterial-cell-wall biosynthesis (e.g., penicillin and vancomycin); bacterial protein biosynthesis (e.g., aminoglycoside and macrolide); DNA and RNA replication (e.g., ciprofloxacin and rifampin); and folate coenzyme biosynthesis (e.g., sulfamethoxazole) [18]. Antibacterials that target the cell wall or cell membrane or essential bacterial enzymes are more likely to be bactericidal; but generally the bacteriostatic is the antibacterial drugs that inhibits protein synthesis [19]. Another way to distinguish the antibiotics is based on their target specificity. The broad-spectrum antibiotic affects a wide range of disease-causing bacteria, including both Gram-positive and Gram-negative bacteria, in contrast to a narrow-spectrum antibiotic, which acts against specific families of bacteria. For example, ampicillin is a widely used broad-spectrum antibiotic.

4. Antibacterial resistance and its mechanisms

Bacterial resistance to antibacterial drugs increasingly becomes a major health and economic problem, eroding the discovery of antibiotics and their application to clinical medicine. As early as 1946, Alexander Fleming predicted that "There is probably no chemotherapeutic drug to which in suitable circumstances the bacteria cannot react by in some way acquiring 'fastness' (resistance)." Today it is really the truth. Resistance to the antibiotics will emerge only a few years after it is introduced to clinic use [20]. Bacterial resistance is positively correlated with the use of antibacterial agents in clinical practice [21; 22]. Because any use of antibiotics can increase selective pressure in a population of bacteria, allowing survival of the resistant bacteria and death of the susceptible ones. We can find that pathogenic bacteria are resistant to practically all available antibacterial drugs. And many strains, which are informally called superbugs, are even resistant to several different antibiotics. Multidrug resistance has been found in Pseudomonas aeruginosa (P. aeruginosa),

Acinetobacterbaumannii (A. baumannii), E. coli, and Klebsiellapneumoniae (K. pneumoniae), producing extended-spectrum β-lactamases (ESBL), vancomycin-resistant enterococci Enterococcus faecium (E. faecium) (VRE), MRSA, vancomycin-resistant S. aureus VRSA, extensively drug-resistant (XDR) Mycobacterium tuberculosis (M. tuberculosis), Salmonella enterica (S. enterica) serovar Typhimurium, Shigelladysenteriae (S. dysenteriae), Haemophilusinfluenzae (H. influenzae), Stenotrophomonas, and Burkholderia [23; 24].

Great amount of antibiotic is used in nonhuman niches, leading to the spread of resistant bacteria too. Antibiotics have been used for improving the production of livestock and poultry for more than 50 years [25]. The Institute of Food Technologists (IFT), once convened a panel of internationally renowned experts to address the concern that, the emergence of antimicrobial resistance may result from abuse in food production, manufacturing, and elsewhere [26].

Over the past several years, people struggled to search for the mechanisms of resistance. Therefore today there is a large pool of information about how drug resistances come out. Biochemical and genetic aspects of antibiotic resistance mechanisms are shown in Fig. 1.

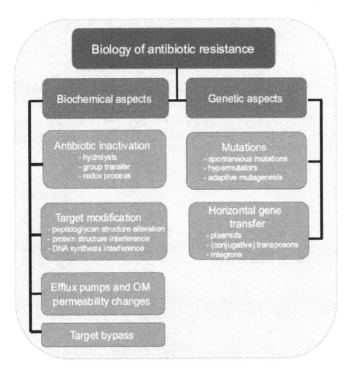

Figure 1. Kinds of antibiotic resistance mechanisms [85].

4.1. Genetics of antibiotic resistance

Resistance can be an intrinsic property of the bacteria themselves or it can be acquired. There are two main ways of acquiring antibiotic resistance: i) chromosomal mutations and ii) horizontal gene transfer. But the question is where the horizontal gene comes from? Some of these genes have an environmental origin and began their evolution before the antibiotic era; most likely, the primary genes originated and diversified within the environmental bacterial communities, then mobilized and penetrated into pathogens. [27; 28]

4.1.1. Mutations

4.1.1.1. Spontaneous mutations

These mutations occur randomly as replication errors or an incorrect repair of a damaged DNA in actively dividing cells, presenting an important mode of generating antibiotic resistance. They are also called the growth dependent mutations. Quinolone resistance in Escherichia coli resulted from the mutations in at least seven positions in the gyrA gene or three positions in the parC gene [29]. There are a large number of biochemical mechanisms of antibiotic resistance related to Spontaneous Mutations. For instance, Mutations in mexR can cause derepression of the mexAB-oprM multidrug efflux operon, causing a multidrug resistance phenotype in Pseudomonas aeruginosa [30].

4.1.1.2. Hypermutators

During a prolonged non-lethal antibiotic selective pressure a small bacterial population enters a transient state of a high mutation rate which is called hypermutable state. Hypermutators are found in many bacteria species such as E. coli, S. enterica, Neisseria meningitides (N. meningitides),H. influenzae, S. aureus, Helicobacter pylori (H. pylori), Streptococcus pneumoniae (S. pneumoniae),and P. aeruginosa [85]. Various studies suggested that hypermutations play an important role in acquisition of antibiotic resistance in pathogens [31; 32; 33].

4.1.1.3. Adaptive mutagenesis

Adaptive mutations arise in non-dividing or slowly dividing cells during the presence of a non-lethal selective pressure that favours them. A great number of antibiotic resistant mutants may come from this mutation process under bacterial natural conditions [85].

4.1.1.4. Horizontal gene transfer

Horizontal transfer of genetic material between bacteria is the most commonly used way to spread antibiotic resistance. In general, this exchange is accomplished mainly through the processes of transduction (via bacteriophages), conjugation (via plasmids and conjugative transposons), and transformation (via incorporation into the chromosome of chromosomal DNA, plasmids, and other DNAs) [34]. This type of genetic transfer not only occurred between closely related bacteria but can also occur between phylogenetically distant bacterial genera, in particular between gram-positive and gram-negative bacteria [35]. Plasmid-encoded antibiotic resistance encompasses most classes of antibiotics in practice, such as aminoglycosides, cephalosporins and fluoroquinolones [36]. Transposons spread quicker than genes in chromosomes and are transferred by conjugation, transformation, or transduction [23; 24]. Integrons acquire and exchange exogenous DNA, known as gene cassettes, by a site-specific recombination mechanism. They can integrate stably into other DNAs where they deliver multiple antibacterial resistant genes in a single exchange. Resistance gene cassettes encoding the metallo-β- lactamases IMP and VIM confer resistance to the potent carbapenem β-lactams imipenem and meropenem [36].

4.1.2. Biochemistry of antibiotic resistance

As so many scientists have been struggling to study the biochemical mechanisms of antibiotic resistance, nowadays there is a large pool of related valuable information left. Biochemical mechanisms may be varied among different bacterial species, but can be mainly classified into four categories (Fig. 2). In fact, each of these four categories also contains an amazing diversity of resistance mechanisms. Sometimes a single bacterial strain may possess several types of resistance mechanisms. Each of the four main categories will be discussed respectively below.

4.1.2.1. Antibiotic inactivation

Biochemical strategies include enzymatic modification and redox mechanisms (which is less important and will not be elaborated in this paper). Enzymes can be divided into two general classes: those such as β-lactamases that degrade antibiotics and others that perform chemical transformations. The antibiotic β-lactam has a four-atom ring known as a beta-lactamin. The β-lactamase enzyme breaks that ring open, destroying the antibacterial properties of the drugs. β-lactamase consists of enzymes with a serine residue at the active site, and metalloenzymes with zinc ion as a cofactor and with a separate heritage [37]. β-lactamase enzymes are the most common and important weapons for Gram-negative bacteria to resist the antibiotics β-lactam [38]. The group transfer approaches are the most diverse and include the modification by acyltransfer, phosphorylation, glycosylation, nucleotidylation, ribosylation, and thiol transfer. They can inactivate antibiotics (aminoglycosides, chloramphenicol, streptogramin, macrolides or rifampicin) by chemical substitution. These modifications reduce the affinity of antibiotics to a target [85]. For example, enzymatic modification is the most prevalent mechanism to destroy aminoglycosides in clinic. Aminoglycoside modifying enzymes can be divided into three classes: acetyltransferases, nucleotidyltranferases, and phosphotransferases; they mainly catalyze the modification at –OH or –NH2 groups of the 2-deoxystreptamine nucleus or the sugar moieties [39]. There are a large number of genes in the chromosomes and other mobile genetic elements coding for these enzymes which let the bacteria resist to more new antibiotics as well as horizontally spread their resistance among bacteria more easily. As a consequence, almost all pathogens are resistant to aminoglycosides through modifying enzymes [39].

4.1.2.2. Target modification

Another important resistance mechanism is the modification of antibiotic targets which makes the antibiotic unable to bind the targets properly. β-lactams target the bacterial enzymes of cell wall biosynthesis (the so-called penicillin-binding proteins, PBPs). Alterations in PBPs can reduce affinity for β-lactams, possibly causing β-lactam resistance in many bacteria strains, such as H. influenzae, N. gonorrhoeae, N. meningitidis, anaerobes, S. dysenteriae [40]. For instance, the mecA resistance gene which encodes PBP2a, a new penicillin binding protein with decreased affinity for oxacillin and most other β-lactam drugs, induces resistance to methicillin and oxacillin in S. aureus [41]. The resistance to antibiotics that interfere with protein synthesis or transcription is achieved by modification of the specific target. rRNAmethylases encoded by a number of genes modificate the 16S rRNA molecule at specific positions critical for aminoglycosides binding [42]. Modification in the 23S rRNA component of the 50S ribosomal subunit also leads to resistance to the macrolide, lincosamide and streptogramin B group of antibiotics in many pathogen strains [43; 44]. Mutations of topoisomerase IV and gyrase genes can sufficiently alter affinity of fluoroquinolones to these enzymes [45].

4.1.2.3. Efflux pumps and outer membrane (OM) permeability

Efflux pumps Membrane proteins that export antibiotics from the cell and maintain their low intracellular concentrations are called efflux pumps. Drug efflux pumps play a key role in drug resistance not just because they can produce multidrug resistance but also because they can elevate level of other resistance mechanisms [46; 47]. Bacterial drug efflux transporters are currently classified into five families: the ATP-binding cassette (ABC) superfamily, the major facilitator superfamily (MFS), the multidrug and toxic compound extrusion (MATE) family, the small multidrug resistance (SMR) family, and the resistance-nodulation-division (RND) superfamily [47]. Efflux transporters can be further classified into single or multicomponent pumps. Tetracycline and macrolide transporters are single component efflux systems that have narrow substrate profiles, while the RND family members have broader substrates and can pump out multiple structurally unrelated compounds [24; 46]. Efflux pumps exist in both Gram-positive and Gram-negative bacteria [48; 49]. MexAB-OprM efflux pumps in Pseudomonas aeruginosa, which belong to RND family, result in higher inhibitory concentration of a large number of antibiotics, such as penicillins, broad-spectrumcephalosporins, chloramphenicol, fluoroquinolones, macrolides, novobiocin, sulfonamides, tetracycline and trimethoprim, dyes and detergents [50; 51].

OM permeability The OM is an asymmetric bilayer: the phospholipid form the inner leaflet and the lipopolysaccharides (LPS) form the outer leaflet. OM of Gram-negative bacteria provides a formidable barrier that must be overcome by drugs. Drug molecules pass the OM by diffusion through porins or the bilayer, or by self-promoted uptake [85]. Small hydrophilic drugs (e.g., β-lactams), enter to the intracellular through the pore-forming porins, while macrolides and other hydrophobic drugs diffuse during their entry [52]. Some resistant clinical strains of Neisseria meningitidis, K. pneumoniae and Enterobacteraerogenes exhibit a noticeable porin variability resulting in decrease of antibacterial uptake [53]. Reduction of

LPS in the outer membrane of Polymyxin-resistant P. aeruginosa strains associates with resistance development [54].

4.1.2.4. Target bypass

This kind of resistance mechanisms is somewhat specific. Bacteria produce two kinds of targets: one is sensitive to antibiotics and the alternative one (usually an enzyme) that is resistant to inhibition of antibiotic. In ampicillin-resistant mutant Enterococcus faecium selected in vitro, bypass of the DD-transpeptidases by a novel class of peptidoglycan polymerases, the LD-transpeptidases, conveyed resistance to all β-lactams, except the carbapenems [55; 56].

5. What should we do?

5.1. Extending the lifespan of existing antibacterials

Although the emergency of antibiotic resistance seems inevitable, measures must be taken to prevent or at least delay this process. As mentioned above, many factors contribute to resistance, so we should adopt a complex approach. The most important way is to strictly control antibiotic misuse and overuse. Interestingly, the EU has implemented a comprehensive ban on the use of all antibiotics for growth promotion since 2006 [25]. And other developed countries also implement similar measures, but in many developing nations antibiotic use is relatively uncontrolled. As hospital-acquired infection is a major cause for antibiotic-resistance, strict antibiotic stewardship and policies should be adopted in the hospitals. For example, we can make some antibiotic policies to optimize the selection, dosing, route of administration, duration of the drug prescribed by the doctor, and limit the unintended consequences of antibiotic utilization [57].

5.2. New antibacterial drug discovery

As serious infectious diseases and multidrug resistance are emerging repeatedly, new antibiotics are needed badly to combat these bacterial pathogens, but the progress of discovery seems relatively slow. Most chemical scaffolds of antibiotics used now were just introduced between the mid-1930s and the early 1960s (fig 2). There are many reasons for this. The first is scientific. We have discovered the easy-to-find antibiotics. Now we have to work harder and think more cleverly to find new drugs. Another reason is commercial. Antibiotics are used much less than other drugs and the new antibiotic are just used to treat serious bacterial infections at most of the time. So antibiotics have a poor return on investment. In 2008 only five major pharmaceutical companies still kept their Enthusiasm in antibacterial discovery. It is most important to delink research and development costs from drug pricing and the return from investment on antibacterial discovery [58]. If the government could establish some subsidies and financial assistance schemes to compensate the cost, more drug companies will be attracted to this area.

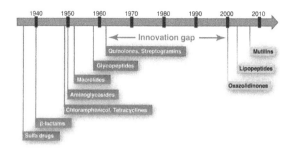

Figure 2. Innovation gap between 1962 and 2000 [59].

Despite the current grim situation in management of resistant bacteria, some new drugs have recently been approved by the FDA or are in late stages of the pipeline (Table 1, 2) [60]. The new drugs belong to the following classes of compounds: oxazolidinones, glycopeptides, ketolides, lycylcyclines, carbapenems and fluoroquinolones.

CLASS OF COMPOUND	PHASE OF DEVELO- PMENT	**ANALOGS**	MECHANISM OF ACTION	RESISTANCE MECHANISM	DRUG COMPANY
Oxazolidinones	FDA Approved 2000	Linezolid, Radezolid, Torezolid, RWJ-416457	Inhibits protein translation (initiation/ elongation)	rRNA mutations	Pfizer, Rib-X, Trius Therapeutics, Johnson & Johnson
Glycopeptides	Phase III	Oritavancin, Dalbavancin, Telavancin	Inhibit peptidoglycan biosysnthesis/ transglycosylation	unidentified	Targanta/The Medicines Co., Pfizer, Theravance
Ketolides	Phase III	Cethromycin	Inhibits protein synthesis	rRNA dimethylation, ribosomal protein mutations	Advanced Life Sciences
Glycylcyclines	FDA Approved 2005	Tigecycline, PTK0796	Inhibits protein synthesis	Efflux pumps	Wyeth, Paratek Pharmaceuticals
Carbapenems	FDA Approved 2007	Doripenem, Razupenem	Inhibits peptidoglycan biosynthesis	Carbapenemases, Efflux pumps, Porin mutations	Johnson & Johnson, Protez Pharmaceuticals
Streptogramins	Phase II	NXL103/XRP2868	Inhibits protein translation	unidentified	Novexel
Fluoroquinolones	Preclinical	JNJ-Q2, finafloxacin	Inhibit type II topoisomerase	gyrA, parC mutations	Johnson & Johnson, MerLion Pharmaceuticals

Table 1. New antibiotics of existing scaffolds

DRUG NAME	TARGET/ MECHANISM OF ACTION	SPECTRUM OF ACTIVITY	PHASE OF DEVELO-PMENT	DRUG COMPANY OR INNOVATOR
Ceftobiprole	Tight binding to PBP2a	Gram-positive, Gram-negative	Phase III	Johnson & Johnson
Ceftaroline	Tight binding to PBP2a	Gram-positive, Gram-negative	Phase III	Forrest Laboratories
Iclaprim	Increased affinity to bacterial DHFR	Gram-positive, Gram-negative	Phase III	Arpida
Sulopenem	Binding to PBPs	Gram-negative	preclinical	Pfizer
BAL30376	Monobactam/β-lactamase inhibitor combination	Multi-drug resistant Gram-negative	preclinical	Basilea
Rx100472	MethionyltRNA synthetase inhibitor	Gram-positive	preclinical	Trius Therapeutics
PC190723	Cell division protein FtsZ	S. aureus	preclinical	Prolysis
MUT7307	Enoyl-ACP FabI reductase (fatty acid biosynthesis)	Gram-positive, Gram-negative	preclinical	Mutabilis
Nitazoxanide	Inhibits vitamin cofactor of pyruvate:ferredoxin oxidoreductase (PFOR)	C. difficile	Phase II	Romark Laboratories
Fidaxomicin (OPT-80)	Inhibits RNA synthesis	C. difficile	Phase II	Optimer Pharmaceuticals
LED209	Quorum sensing	S. typhimurium F. tularensis	preclinical	University of Texas South Western Medical Center,Dallas
BPH652	Virulence factor (antioxidant)	MRSA	preclinical	University of Illinois, Chicago
Omiganan	Antimicrobial peptide; Depolarizes cytoplasmic membrane of bacteria	Gram-positive, fungi	Phase III	MIGENIX, Cadence pharmaceuticals
TMC207	ATP synthase inhibition	M. tuberculosis	Phase II	Johnson & Johnson, Tibotec
CBR2092	Dual pharmacophore	Gram-positive	Phase I	Cumbre
Amikacin	Novel drug delivery: inhaled nanoliposomes	P. aeruginosa biofilm	Phase II	Transave Inc.

Table 2. New antibiotics in development

5.2.1. Tailoring existing scaffolds

It seems that there are many ways to search for new antibacterials, but the key question is: how to search for new antibacterial drugs and where to look for them? The most convenient method is to modify the existing scaffolds to generate their derivates. All antibiotics approved between the early 1960s and 2000 were synthetic derivatives of the old scaffolds except carbapenems. Chemical modifications of old scaffolds may lead to improved bactericidal activities, better resistance profiles, safety, tolerability or superior pharmacokinetic/pharmacodynamic properties. There are four generations of β-Lactam antibiotics, all of which contains a β-lactam nucleus in their molecular structures. The second generation (e.g., cephalexin and cefaclor) and third generation (e.g., cefotaxime, ceftazidime) are not sensitive to plasmid-mediated broad-spectrum β-lactamases and have less allergic reactions, compared with the first generation (penicillins) [61]. The fourth-generation cephalosporins penetrate through the outer membrane of Gram-negative bacteria more easily and have low affinity for clinically important β-lactamases, so they have the advantage of killing many Gram-negative pathogens resistant to most third-generation [86]. Tigecycline is one of glycylcycline antibiotics derived from tetracycline and received approval from the US Food and Drug Administration for the treatment of skin, soft-tissue, and intra abdominal infections in 2005. Tigecycline can overcome the active efflux of drug from inside the bacterial cell and protection of ribosomes, which are two determinants of tetracycline resistance [62; 63]. But this approach is only a good short-term strategy to find new drugs, and but the benefit of these modified drugs will be offset quickly by the resistance to acquired through the horizontal acquisition or molecular evolution [9], which indicates that it is much more attractive to find novel chemical scaffolds.

5.2.2. Novel scaffolds

5.2.2.1. Explore new places

More than two-thirds of clinically used antibiotics come from natural products or their semi synthetic derivatives and most of them came out from soil actinomycetes. But recently researchers have shifted to underexplored ecological niches and bacterial species and found some new scaffolds. Compared to the terrestrial environment, the ocean remains an underexplored habitat with unparalleled biodiversity, leaving it the most promising place to yield new antibacterial metabolites. New antibacterial agents with novelty and/or complexity in chemical structure derived from marine bacteria have been elaborated clearly [64; 65]. Myxobacteria, a untapped bacterial strain, can produce many useful natural products which have great potential to develop into antibacterial drug [66].

5.2.2.2. The genomics

By the mid-1990s, pharmaceutical companies have little enthusiasm for making improvement to the existing antibacterials. Hundreds of bacterial genomes have been completely deciphered since 1995, among which are many important human pathogens, attracting large pharmaceutical companies back into antibacterial discovery [67]. Genomics influence various aspects of the antibiotic development, including new drug target identification, understanding the mechanism of antibiotic action, drug safety and efficacy assessment, bacterial resistance development, and so on [68]. Ecopia Biosciences was very skilled in using genome-scanning approach and discovered the new antibiotic scaffold ECO-0501 which is highly effective against a series of Gram-positive pathogens [59; 69]. GlaxoSmithKline also used a genomics-derived, target-based approach to screen for new drugs. They examined more than 300 genes and employed 70 high-throughput screening campaigns over a period of 7 years, but unfortunately did not create a clinical used antibacterial [70].

5.2.2.3. New targets

It must be admitted that target-based genomic approach has not yielded satisfactory results, nevertheless, retooled target-based strategies can still play an important role in discovery process. Most antibiotic targets are limited to peptidoglycan synthesis, ribosomal protein synthesis, folate synthesis, and nucleic acid synthesis and topoisomerization. In the future we could continue to discover new antibiotics for these old targets through improvement of the existing scaffolds or even finding new scaffolds. For instance, Lipid II is a membrane-anchored cell-wall precursor that is essential for bacterial cell-wall biosynthesis; it is not only classical target for several old antibacterial classes, but is also targeted by the new antibiotics, such as lantibiotics, mannopeptimycins and ramoplanin [71]. Grouping targets by a common inhibitor scaffold rather than by function may lead to new targets; and as mentioned above, insights from outside the antibiotic arena are also important [59].

5.2.2.4. Forward is back

Compared with the fruitless target-based genomic approach, traditional whole-cell assays are more effective in antibiotic discovery. Just because it is not necessary to worry about cell permeability of a novel scaffold in the development process if whole-cell assays are used. As most of the existing libraries have already been used to screen for antibacterial drugs, libraries with new chemical diversity are extremely important in this approach. Sometimes, look for libraries that don't belong to antibacterial development areas may be useful. In fact, most pharmaceutical companies of other therapeutic areas have invested considerable resources in synthesizing small molecule libraries [59]. Candidates with a strong hit in a whole-cell antibacterial assay should be tested in the right animal model early in development, because In vitro experiment results are not always reliable. For example, Antimicrobial drug target type II fatty acid synthesis (FASII) is reported to be essential for their efficacy against infections caused by multiresistant Gram-positive bacteria. But another study showed that Streptococcus agalactiae and S. aureus could take up sufficient unsaturated fatty acids from human serum to obviate the essentiality of FAS II enzymes in vivo [72].

5.2.2.5. Focus on spectrum

Antibacterial spectrum is a major consideration when selecting a target for lead optimization. Permeability and target distribution determine the pectrum [73]. That is to say, the drug candidates should possess two properties at the same time: one is penetrating the cell and evading efflux pump systems, another is retaining potent activity at the molecular targets. However, since almost all targets of the antibacterials in clinical use are present in all bacteria, the antibacterial drug spectra are determined largely by the ability of permeability. Therefore, some compounds are just Gram-positive organism-selective and have no effect against Gram-negative pathogens which have a second membrane acting as a permeability barrier [74; 75]. Efflux pump inhibitors (EPIs) have been explored for broadening the antibacterial spectrum and overcoming bacterial resistance. Although no clinically useful drugs have come out, extensive efforts have been made to test the effectiveness of EPIs across a range of in vitro and in vivo assays, especially the compound MC-207,110 [76].

'Broader is better' is the rule of antibacterial activity spectrum. But developing the agents with a narrower spectrum may be helpful in treating some special antibiotic resistant pathogens or the non-multiplying bacteria. One human squalene synthase inhibitor blocked staphyloxanthin biosynthesis in vitro, resulting in colorless bacteria which became more sensitive to killing by human blood and innate immune clearance [77]. Rifampicin is a standard antibiotic used for clearance of non-multiplying tuberculosis. Monoclonal antibodies (Mabs) have also become potential agents for narrow-spectrum antibacterial therapy. In clinical experiment C. difficile Mab combination MDX-066 and MDX-1388, which targets and neutralizes two main C. difficile toxins, can reduce the recurrence of C. difficile infection [78; 79]. A microbiologic diagnosis should be made before using these kinds of antibiotics for therapy. Such genus-selective agents may have the benefit of leaving more of the endogenous microfloraun unattacked compared with conventional antibiotics.

5.2.2.6. Other new methods

Bacteriophages

Bacteriophages and their fragments could kill the bacteria. They have been developed as antibacterials in humans, poultry and cattle industries, aquaculture and sewage treatment. This approach has novel mechanism of action that is completely different from current antimicrobials, but the problems are that quality control and standardization are difficult. Phage lysins, which are produced late in the viral infection cycle, can bind to cell wall peptidoglycan and rapidly induce Gram-positive bacteria lysis [80]. The sequencing of phages genomes may identify more proteins suitable for novel antibacterials [81; 82].

Other methods to find new drugs could be modulating immunity, developing monoclonal antibody for specific bacteria, designing antibacterial peptides (including antimicrobial peptides and compounds from animals and plants, the natural lipopeptides of bacteria and Fungi [83; 84]), and so on.

6. Conclusion and future issues

While the antibacterial resistance, especially multi-drug resistance continues to rise, what we should do is to investigate the potential mechanisms of drug resistance in bacteria and discover more effective antibacterials to deal with the terrible problems. Luckily there are several promising antibacterial drugs with novel mechanisms of action are in development and new types of targets have emerged. Also we need to be more precise in targeting the pathogens and limit the misuse of antimicrobials and other practices that accelerate the emergence of novel resistance mechanisms. The government must offer robust financial incentives for antibacterial R&D, and build a sustainable model for developing and using antibacterials.

Author details

Jie Yanling, Liang Xin and Li Zhiyuan

Guangzhou Institutes of Biomedicine and Health, Chinese Academy of Sciences, China

References

[1] W.J. Lindblad. Considerations for determining if a natural product is an effective wound-healing agent. Int J Low Extrem Wounds 2008;7(2):75-81.

[2] R.D. Forrest. Early history of wound treatment. J R Soc Med 1982;75(3):198-205.

[3] L.G. Nickell. Antimicrobial activity of vascular plants. Economic Botany 1959;13(4): 281-318.

[4] E.J. Bassett, M.S. Keith, G.J. Armelagos, et al. Tetracycline-labeled human bone from ancient Sudanese Nubia (A.D. 350). Science 1980;209(4464):1532-1534.

[5] M.L. Nelson, A. Dinardo, J. Hochberg, et al. Brief communication: Mass spectroscopic characterization of tetracycline in the skeletal remains of an ancient population from Sudanese Nubia 350-550 CE. Am J PhysAnthropol 2010;143(1):151-154.

[6] M. Cook, E. Molto, C. Anderson. Fluorochromelabelling in Roman period skeletons from Dakhleh Oasis, Egypt. Am J PhysAnthropol 1989;80(2):137-143.

[7] J.O. Falkinham, 3rd, T.E. Wall, J.R. Tanner, et al. Proliferation of antibiotic-producing bacteria and concomitant antibiotic production as the basis for the antibiotic activity of Jordan's red soils. Appl Environ Microbiol 2009;75(9):2735-2741.

[8] J. Clardy. Using genomics to deliver natural products from symbiotic bacteria. Genome Biol 2005;6(9):232.

[9] R.I. Aminov. A brief history of the antibiotic era: lessons learned and challenges for the future. Front Microbiol 2010;1:134.

[10] R.W. Wong, U. Hagg, L. Samaranayake, et al. Antimicrobial activity of Chinese medicine herbs against common bacteria in oral biofilm. A pilot study. Int J Oral MaxilloacSurg 2010;39(6):599-605.

[11] F. Heynick. The original 'magic bullet' is 100 years old - extra. Br J Psychiatry 2009;195(5):456.

[12] J.F. Mahoney, R.C. Arnold, A. Harris. Penicillin Treatment of Early Syphilis-A Preliminary Report. Am J Public Health Nations Health 1943;33(12):1387-1391.

[13] N.C. Lloyd, H.W. Morgan, B.K. Nicholson, et al. The composition of Ehrlich's salvarsan: resolution of a century-old debate. AngewChemInt Ed Engl 2005;44(6):941-944.

[14] J. Kimmig. [Gerhard Domagk, 1895-1964. Contribution to the chemotherapy of bacterial infections]. Internist (Berl) 1969;10(3):116-120.

[15] C. Jesman, A. Mludzik, M. Cybulska. [History of antibiotics and sulphonamides discoveries]. Pol MerkurLekarski 2011;30(179):320-322.

[16] E. Chain, H.W. Florey, A.D. Gardner, et al. THE CLASSIC: penicillin as a chemotherapeutic agent. 1940. ClinOrthopRelat Res 2005;439:23-26.

[17] N. Kardos, A.L. Demain. Penicillin: the medicine with the greatest impact on therapeutic outcomes. ApplMicrobiolBiotechnol 2011;92(4):677-687.

[18] C. Walsh. Where will new antibiotics come from? Nat Rev Microbiol 2003;1(1):65-70.

[19] R.W. Finberg, R.C. Moellering, F.P. Tally, et al. The importance of bactericidal drugs: future directions in infectious disease. Clin Infect Dis 2004;39(9):1314-1320.

[20] S.R. Palumbi. Humans as the world's greatest evolutionary force. Science 2001;293(5536):1786-1790.

[21] S.L. Bronzwaer, O. Cars, U. Buchholz, et al. A European study on the relationship between antimicrobial use and antimicrobial resistance. Emerg Infect Dis 2002;8(3): 278-282.

[22] H. Goossens, M. Ferech, R. Vander Stichele, et al. Outpatient antibiotic use in Europe and association with resistance: a cross-national database study. Lancet 2005;365(9459):579-587.

[23] A. Giedraitiene, A. Vitkauskiene, R. Naginiene, et al. Antibiotic resistance mechanisms of clinically important bacteria. Medicina (Kaunas) 2011;47(3):137-146.

[24] M.N. Alekshun, S.B. Levy. Molecular mechanisms of antibacterial multidrug resistance. Cell 2007;128(6):1037-1050.

[25] 35 years of resistance. Nat Rev Microbiol 2012;10(6):373.

[26] M.P. Doyle, F.F. Busta. Antimicrobial resistance: implications for the food system. Compr. Rev. Food Sci. Food Saf 2006;5:71-137.

[27] J.L. Martinez. Antibiotics and antibiotic resistance genes in natural environments. Science 2008;321(5887):365-367.

[28] R.I. Aminov, R.I. Mackie. Evolution and ecology of antibiotic resistance genes. FEMS MicrobiolLett 2007;271(2):147-161.

[29] D.C. Hooper. Mechanisms of fluoroquinolone resistance. Drug Resist Updat 1999;2(1):38-55.

[30] L. Adewoye, A. Sutherland, R. Srikumar, et al. The mexR repressor of the mexAB-oprM multidrug efflux operon in Pseudomonas aeruginosa: characterization of mutations compromising activity. J Bacteriol 2002;184(15):4308-4312.

[31] J. Blazquez. Hypermutation as a factor contributing to the acquisition of antimicrobi-
      al resistance. Clin Infect Dis 2003;37(9):1201-1209.

[32] A. Oliver, R. Canton, P. Campo, et al. High frequency of hypermutable Pseudomonas
      aeruginosa in cystic fibrosis lung infection. Science 2000;288(5469):1251-1254.

[33] I. Chopra, A.J. O'Neill, K. Miller. The role of mutators in the emergence of antibiotic-
      resistant bacteria. Drug Resist Updat 2003;6(3):137-145.

[34] S.B. Levy, B. Marshall. Antibacterial resistance worldwide: causes, challenges and re-
      sponses. Nat Med 2004;10(12 Suppl):S122-129.

[35] P. Courvalin. Transfer of antibiotic resistance genes between gram-positive and
      gram-negative bacteria. Antimicrob Agents Chemother 1994;38(7):1447-1451.

[36] P. Nordmann, L. Poirel. Emerging carbapenemases in Gram-negative aerobes. Clin-
      Microbiol Infect 2002;8(6):321-331.

[37] G.A. Jacoby, L.S. Munoz-Price. The new beta-lactamases. N Engl J Med 2005;352(4):
      380-391.

[38] S.M. Drawz, R.A. Bonomo. Three decades of beta-lactamase inhibitors. ClinMicrobiol
      Rev 2010;23(1):160-201.

[39] M.S. Ramirez, M.E. Tolmasky. Aminoglycoside modifying enzymes. Drug Resist Up-
      dat 2010;13(6):151-171.

[40] K. Poole. Resistance to beta-lactam antibiotics. Cell Mol Life Sci 2004;61(17):
      2200-2223.

[41] F.C. Tenover. Mechanisms of antimicrobial resistance in bacteria. Am J Med
      2006;119(6 Suppl 1):S3-10; discussion S62-70.

[42] S. Jana, J.K. Deb. Molecular understanding of aminoglycoside action and resistance.
      ApplMicrobiolBiotechnol 2006;70(2):140-150.

[43] G. Ackermann, A. Degner, S.H. Cohen, et al. Prevalence and association of macro-
      lide-lincosamide-streptogramin B (MLS(B)) resistance with resistance to moxifloxacin
      in Clostridium difficile. J AntimicrobChemother 2003;51(3):599-603.

[44] B. Weisblum. Erythromycin resistance by ribosome modification. Antimicrob Agents
      Chemother 1995;39(3):577-585.

[45] D. Ince, X. Zhang, L.C. Silver, et al. Dual targeting of DNA gyrase and topoisomerase
      IV: target interactions of garenoxacin (BMS-284756, T-3811ME), a new desfluoroqui-
      nolone. Antimicrob Agents Chemother 2002;46(11):3370-3380.

[46] X.Z. Li, H. Nikaido. Efflux-mediated drug resistance in bacteria. Drugs 2004;64(2):
      159-204.

[47] X.Z. Li, H. Nikaido. Efflux-mediated drug resistance in bacteria: an update. Drugs
      2009;69(12):1555-1623.

[48] K.P. Langton, P.J. Henderson, R.B. Herbert. Antibiotic resistance: multidrug efflux proteins, a common transport mechanism? Nat Prod Rep 2005;22(4):439-451.

[49] M. Putman, H.W. van Veen, W.N. Konings. Molecular properties of bacterial multi-drug transporters. MicrobiolMolBiol Rev 2000;64(4):672-693.

[50] J.M. Thomson, R.A. Bonomo. The threat of antibiotic resistance in Gram-negative pathogenic bacteria: beta-lactams in peril! CurrOpinMicrobiol 2005;8(5):518-524.

[51] D.M. Livermore. Multiple mechanisms of antimicrobial resistance in Pseudomonas aeruginosa: our worst nightmare? Clin Infect Dis 2002;34(5):634-640.

[52] A.H. Delcour. Outer membrane permeability and antibiotic resistance. BiochimBio-physActa 2009;1794(5):808-816.

[53] W. Achouak, T. Heulin, J.M. Pages. Multiple facets of bacterial porins. FEMS Micro-biolLett 2001;199(1):1-7.

[54] M.E. Falagas, S.K. Kasiakou. Colistin: the revival of polymyxins for the management of multidrug-resistant gram-negative bacterial infections. Clin Infect Dis 2005;40(9): 1333-1341.

[55] J.L. Mainardi, R. Legrand, M. Arthur, et al. Novel mechanism of beta-lactam resist-ance due to bypass of DD-transpeptidation in Enterococcus faecium. J BiolChem 2000;275(22):16490-16496.

[56] S. Triboulet, M. Arthur, J.L. Mainardi, et al. Inactivation kinetics of a new target of beta-lactam antibiotics. J BiolChem 2011;286(26):22777-22784.

[57] I.C. Gyssens. Antibiotic policy. Int J Antimicrob Ag 2011;38:11-20.

[58] T. Braine. Race against time to develop new antibiotics. Bull World Health Organ 2011;89(2):88-89.

[59] M.A. Fischbach, C.T. Walsh. Antibiotics for emerging pathogens. Science 2009;325(5944):1089-1093.

[60] G. Devasahayam, W.M. Scheld, P.S. Hoffman. Newer antibacterial drugs for a new century. Expert OpinInvestig Drugs 2010;19(2):215-234.

[61] H.C. Neu, K.P. Fu. Cefaclor: in vitro spectrum of activity and beta-lactamase stabili-ty. Antimicrob Agents Chemother 1978;13(4):584-588.

[62] G.A. Noskin. Tigecycline: a new glycylcycline for treatment of serious infections. Clin Infect Dis 2005;41Suppl 5:S303-314.

[63] P.J. Petersen, N.V. Jacobus, W.J. Weiss, et al. In vitro and in vivo antibacterial activi-ties of a novel glycylcycline, the 9-t-butylglycylamido derivative of minocycline (GAR-936). Antimicrob Agents Chemother 1999;43(4):738-744.

[64] H. Rahman, B. Austin, W.J. Mitchell, et al. Novel anti-infective compounds from ma-rine bacteria. Mar Drugs 2010;8(3):498-518.

[65] C.C. Hughes, W. Fenical. Antibacterials from the sea. Chemistry 2010;16(42): 12512-12525.

[66] S.C. Wenzel, R. Muller. The biosynthetic potential of myxobacteria and their impact in drug discovery. CurrOpin Drug DiscovDevel 2009;12(2):220-230.

[67] C. Freiberg, H. Brotz-Oesterhelt. Functional genomics in antibacterial drug discovery. Drug Discov Today 2005;10(13):927-935.

[68] S. Amini, S. Tavazoie. Antibiotics and the post-genome revolution. CurrOpinMicrobiol 2011;14(5):513-518.

[69] A.H. Banskota, J.B. McAlpine, D. Sorensen, et al. Genomic analyses lead to novel secondary metabolites. Part 3. ECO-0501, a novel antibacterial of a new class. J Antibiot (Tokyo) 2006;59(9):533-542.

[70] D.J. Payne, M.N. Gwynn, D.J. Holmes, et al. Drugs for bad bugs: confronting the challenges of antibacterial discovery. Nat Rev Drug Discov 2007;6(1):29-40.

[71] E. Breukink, B. de Kruijff. Lipid II as a target for antibiotics. Nat Rev Drug Discov 2006;5(4):321-332.

[72] S. Brinster, G. Lamberet, B. Staels, et al. Type II fatty acid synthesis is not a suitable antibiotic target for Gram-positive pathogens. Nature 2009;458(7234):83-86.

[73] L.L. Silver. Challenges of antibacterial discovery. ClinMicrobiol Rev 2011;24(1): 71-109.

[74] E. Andre, L. Bastide, S. Michaux-Charachon, et al. Novel synthetic molecules targeting the bacterial RNA polymerase assembly. J AntimicrobChemother 2006;57(2): 245-251.

[75] J. Wang, S. Kodali, S.H. Lee, et al. Discovery of platencin, a dual FabF and FabH inhibitor with in vivo antibiotic properties. ProcNatlAcadSci U S A 2007;104(18): 7612-7616.

[76] O. Lomovskaya, K.A. Bostian. Practical applications and feasibility of efflux pump inhibitors in the clinic--a vision for applied use. Biochemical pharmacology 2006;71(7):910-918.

[77] C.I. Liu, G.Y. Liu, Y. Song, et al. A cholesterol biosynthesis inhibitor blocks Staphylococcus aureus virulence. Science 2008;319(5868):1391-1394.

[78] I. Lowy, D.C. Molrine, B.A. Leav, et al. Treatment with monoclonal antibodies against Clostridium difficile toxins. N Engl J Med 2010;362(3):197-205.

[79] M.N. Gwynn, A. Portnoy, S.F. Rittenhouse, et al. Challenges of antibacterial discovery revisited. Ann N Y AcadSci 2010;1213:5-19.

[80] V.A. Fischetti, D. Nelson, R. Schuch. Reinventing phage therapy: are the parts greater than the sum? Nat Biotechnol 2006;24(12):1508-1511.

[81] T.D. Bugg, A.J. Lloyd, D.I. Roper. Phospho-MurNAc-pentapeptidetranslocase (MraY) as a target for antibacterial agents and antibacterial proteins. Infect Disord Drug Targets 2006;6(2):85-106.

[82] J. Liu, M. Dehbi, G. Moeck, et al. Antimicrobial drug discovery through bacterio-phage genomics. Nat Biotechnol 2004;22(2):185-191.

[83] R.E. Hancock, H.G. Sahl. Antimicrobial and host-defense peptides as new anti-infective therapeutic strategies. Nat Biotechnol 2006;24(12):1551-1557.

[84] A. Makovitzki, D. Avrahami, Y. Shai. Ultrashort antibacterial and antifungal lipopeptides. ProcNatlAcadSci U S A 2006;103(43):15997-16002.

[85] S.Dzidic, J.Suskovic, B. Kos. Antibiotic resistance mechanisms in bacteria: biochemical and genetic aspects. FoodTechnolBiotechnol2008;46(1), 11-21.

[86] J.Garau, W. Wilson, M, Wood, J,Carlet. Fourth-generation cephalosporins: a review of in vitro activity, pharmacokinetics, pharmacodynamics and clinical utility.ClinMicrobiol Infect 1997;3 (Suppl 3): S87 -S101.

Chapter 6

Transition State Analogues of Enzymatic Reaction as Potential Drugs

Karolina Gluza and Pawel Kafarski

Additional information is available at the end of the chapter

1. Introduction

All chemical transformations pass through an unstable structure called the transition state, which is poised between the chemical structures of the substrates and products. The transition states for chemical reactions are proposed to have lifetimes near 10^{-13} sec, the time for a single bond vibration. Thus, the transition state is the critical configuration of a reaction system situated at the highest point of the most favorable reaction path on the potential-energy surface, with its characteristics governing the dynamic behavior of reacting systems decisively. It is used primarily to understand qualitatively how chemical reactions take place.

Yet transition state structure is crucial to understanding enzymatic catalysis, because enzymes function by lowering activation energy. Linus Pauling coiled an accepted view, that incredible catalytic rate enhancements caused by enzyme is governed by tight binding to the unstable transition state structure in 1948. Because reaction rate is proportional to the fraction of the reactant in the transition state complex, the enzyme was proposed to increase the concentration of these reactive species. This proposal was further formalized by Wolfenden (1972) and coworkers, who hypothesized that the rate increase imposed by enzymes is proportional to the affinity of the enzyme to the transition state structure relative to the Michaelis complex.

Transition state structures of enzymatic targets for cancer, autoimmunity, malaria and bacterial antibiotics have been explored by the systematic application of kinetic isotope effects and computational chemistry. Today the combination of experimental and computational access to transition-state information permits the design of transition-state analogs as powerful enzymatic inhibitors and exploration of protein features linked to transition-state structure.

Molecular electrostatic potential maps of transition states serve as blueprints to guide synthesis of transition state analogue inhibitors of chosen enzymes. Substances, that ideally mimic geometric and electrostatic features of a transition state (or other intermediates of high energy) are considered as excellent enzyme inhibitors (Fig.1). They bind up to 10^8 times tighter than substrate. Thus, the goal of transition-state analogs design is to create stable chemical structures with van der Waals geometry and molecular electrostatic potential surfaces as close as possible to those of the transition state.

Although some reviews on the subject have been published, this concept has not been reviewed in detail [Wolfenden, 1999; Robertson, 2005; Schramm, 2005; Schramm, 2007; Dyba-ła-Defratyka et al. 2008; Schramm, 2011]. In this review the current trends, alongside with appropriate case studies in designing of such inhibitors will be presented.

2. Choice of the target enzyme

The sequencing of the human genome has promised a revolution in medicine. The genome encodes 20,000- 25,000 human genes, and thousands more proteins as a result of alternative gene splicing. Many of these hold the keys to treating disease, especially numerous enzymes of undefined so far physiologic functions [Gonzaga-Jagureui et al., 2012]. Out of 1200 registered drugs over 300 act as enzyme inhibitors. Most of them are simple analogs of substrates of certain enzymatic reaction. Analogy to transition state as a mean to obtain effective inhibitors emerged in 1970s [Lienhard, 1973]. Through the 1970s and 1980s, most of the known examples were natural products [Wolfenden, 1976]. The situation has changed in 1990s when synthetic inhibitors became the predominate examples of transition-state inhibitors. In 1995, there were transition-state analogues for at least 130 enzymes [Radzicka & Wolfenden, 1995].

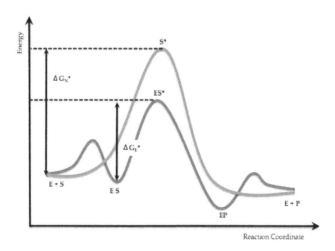

Figure 1. Progress of the enzymatic reaction versus uncatalyzed one.

The design of transition-state inhibitors is likely to become more frequent in the future, alongside with the development of theory and technology for understanding enzyme transition states. Today the sequence of information required to obtain transition state analog of enzymatic reaction considers: choice of the suitable enzyme (most likely suited to kinetic isotope effect measurement), selection of presumable mechanism(s) of catalyzed reaction, measurement of kinetic isotope effects (KIE), computer-aided calculations matching the intrinsic KIEs, construction of steric and electronic map of transition state and synthesis of stable compound(s) matching this map [Schramm, 2007]. This procedure has been developed gradually in parallel with the advances in KIE enzymology, computational chemistry, and synthetic organic chemistry.

3. Determination of transition state architecture

At present, the most reliable method to determine three-dimensional architecture of transition state is through the use of computational methods in conjunction with experimentally measured kinetic isotope effect (KIE).

Isotopic substitution is a useful technique for probing reaction mechanisms. The change of an isotope may affect the reaction rate in a number of ways, providing clues to the pathway of the reaction. The advantage of isotopic substitution is that this is the least disturbing structural change that can be effected in a molecule. Replacement of one isotope of the substrate by another at vicinity where bonds are being or re-hybridizing typically leads to a change in the rate of the reaction. Thus, kinetic isotope effects measurements compare k_{cat}/K_M values between isotope-labeled and natural abundance reactants. This provides information about which bonds are broken or formed, and identifies changes in hybridization that occur during the rate limiting step of a reaction. It is reached by conversion of atom-by-atom KIE values to a specific static model with fixed bond angles and lengths by computational matching to a quantum chemical model of the reaction of interest. Substrate, intermediate and product geometries are located as the global minima. Transition-state structures are located with a single imaginary frequency, characteristic of true potential energy saddle points.

Such an analysis was performed recently for human thymidine phosphorylase, an enzyme responsible for thymidine homeostasis, action of which promotes angiogenesis. Thus, inhibitors of this enzyme might be considered as promising anticancer agents. Its transition state was characterized using multiple kinetic isotope effect measurements applying isotopically (^{3}H, ^{14}C and ^{15}N) enriched thymidines, which were synthesized enzymatically [Schwartz et al, 2010]. A transition state constrained to match the intrinsic KIEs was found using density functional theory. In the proposed mechanism (Fig.2), departure of the thymine results in a discrete ribocation intermediate. Thymine likely leaves deprotonated at N1 and undergoes enzyme-catalyzed protonation before the next step. In the following step, the intermediate undergoes nucleophilic attack from an activated water molecule to form the products. The latter step is a reaction rate limiting step as determined by energetics of its transition state.

The transition state model predicts that deoxyribose adopts a mild 3'-*endo* conformation during nucleophilic capture (Fig. 2).

Such studies, although cumbersome and difficult, are being recently more and more popular, as demonstrated by representative studies on *Escherichia coli* t-RNA-specific adenosine deaminase [Luo & Schramm, 2008], glucoside hydrolases [Lee et al, 2004], human purine nucleoside phosphorylase [Murkin et al., 2007], *Trypasnosoma cruzi trans*-sialidase [Pierdominici-Sottile et al., 2011], L-dopa decarboxylase [Lin & Gao, 2011] or *cis*-prenyltransferase [Hu et al., 2010].

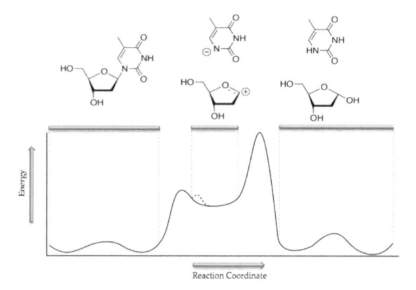

Figure 2. Mechanism of human thymidine phosphorylase catalyzed depirymidation of thymidine. The dash line represents protonation step.

Computational chemistry provides techniques for the generation and exploration of the multi-dimensional energy surfaces that govern chemical reactivity. Therefore, energy minima and saddle points can be located and characterized. The pathways that interconnect them can be determined. Thus, computational methods are increasingly at the forefront of elucidating mechanisms of enzyme-catalyzed reactions, and shedding light on the determinants of specificity and efficiency of catalysis [Kollman et al., 2002; Parks et al., 2010; Williams, 2010; Lonsdake et al., 2012].

At the beginning of a molecular modeling study choice upon the specific catalytic process to model has to be undertaken. This decision may sound simple, but it includes the nontrivial task of exhaustively searching the literature to determine what is already known about the selected enzymatic system, either from experiments or from previous computational studies. Reaction mechanisms may have already been proposed in the literature, and thus provide a logical starting point for modeling studies. The three-dimensional structure of the enzyme, preferably with a bound substrate analog, reaction product or inhibitor, is among the most critical sources of information. In practice, this usually means that a high-resolution X-ray crystal structure of a reacting enzyme complex is required.

Molecular mechanics methods are important in simulations of enzymes, even though these methods cannot model chemical reactions. For that molecular dynamics simulations, or combination of molecular mechanics with quantum mechanical methods are commonly used [Senn & Thiel, 2007; Hou & Cui, 2011; Kosugi & Hayashi, 2012; Londsdale et al., 2012]. Enzymes are large molecules consisting of thousands of atoms whereas the active site may comprise only around 100 atoms. Since quantum chemical calculations are nowadays affordable only for up to a few hundred atoms (depending on the level of accuracy) the system is split into two regions: a small region encapsulating the reaction at the active site is modeled with a quantum mechanical methods, while the rest of the enzyme alongside with surrounding water is modeled using molecular mechanics (Fig. 3.)

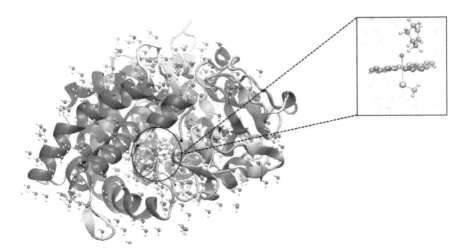

Figure 3. Quantum mechanics/molecular mechanics calculation of an enzymatic reaction illustrated by cytochrome P450 with bound cyclohexene [Lonsdake et al., 2010].

These calculations do not take in the consideration such an important factor as protein dynamic. There is an agreement that fast (at nano- or picosecond scale) protein motions couple directly to transition state formation in enzymatically catalyzed reactions and are an integral part of the reaction coordinate. Slower protein dynamic motions also influence the heights of barriers in enzymatic reactions, however detailed description of these effects require elaboration of new computational methods [Saen-oon et al., 2008].

4. Inhibitors of proteinases

First inhibitors being transition state analogs were designed for proteolytic enzymes. The design was based on the resemblance of transition state of phosphonamidates and phosphonic, phosphinic (Fig. 4) acids to the sp^3 intermediate of the hydrolysis of peptide bond. Because the lengths of oxygen-to-phosphorus and carbon-to-phosphorus bonds are significantly longer than the corresponding carbon-to-carbon and carbon-to-oxygen bonds, organophosphorus fragment of the molecule might be considered as "swollen" tetrahedral intermediate and thus can be treated similar to the transition state of this reaction.

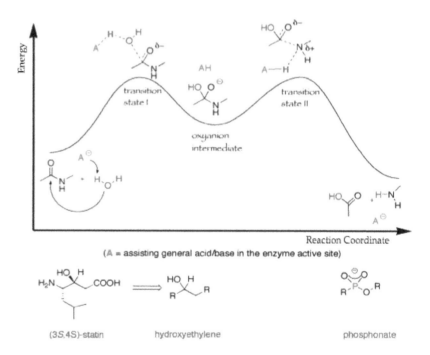

Figure 4. Organophosphoprus compounds as transition state analog inhibitors of hydrolysis of peptide bonds.

Crystallography of enzyme-inhibitor complexes and molecular modeling studies had shown that their potent inhibitory activities result from both: resemblance to the transition state and strong electrostatic interactions between positively charged active-site metal ions (predominantly zinc ions) and negatively charged phosphonic acid (or related) group [Mucha et al., 2010; Mucha et al., 2011]. Although the phosphonate/phosphinate group is a rather weak zinc complexing moiety, it offers other advantageous structural and electronic features [Collinsova & Jiráček, 2000].

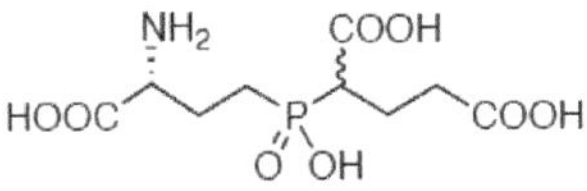

inhibitor of human glutamate
carboxypeptidase II
(Barinka et. a., 2008)

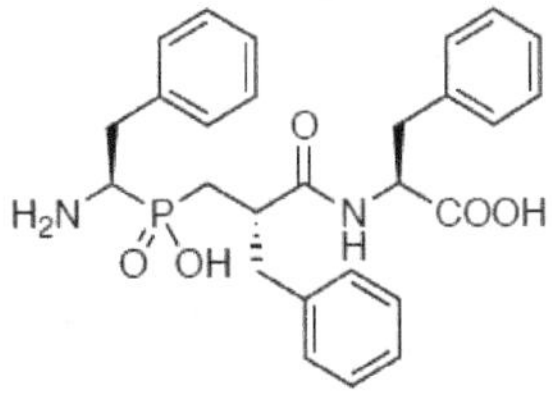

inhibitor of aminopeptidase from
Escherichia coli
(Fournie-Zaluski et al., 2009)

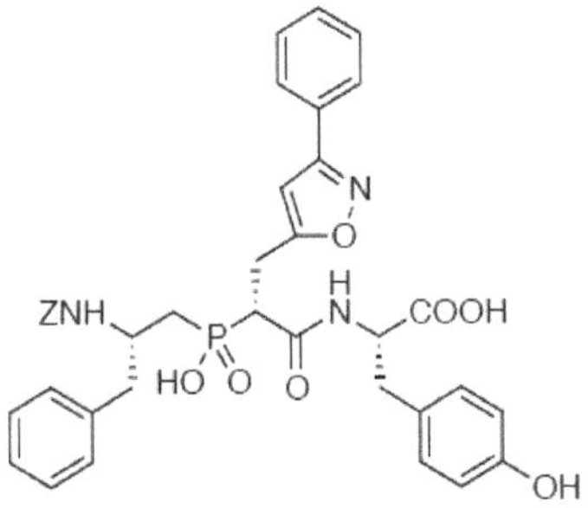

inhibitor of angiotensin converting enzyme
(Ákif et al., 2011)

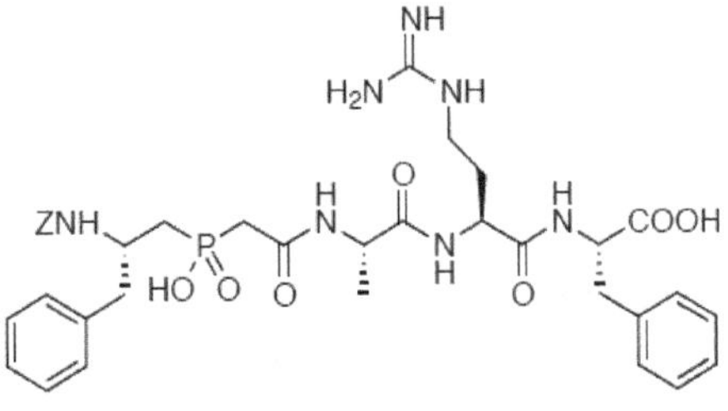

inhibitor of bradykinin hydrolyzing protease
(Chaerkady & Sharma, 2004)

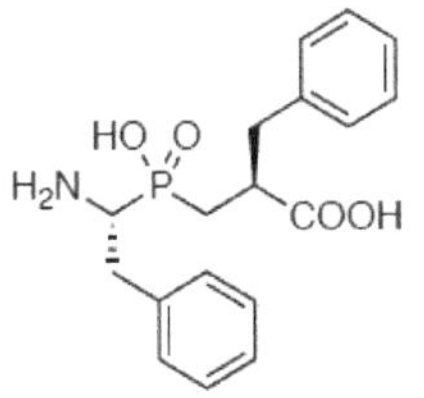

inhibitor od leucine aminopeptidases
from porcine kidney (Mucha et al, 2008)
from *Plasmodium falciparum* (Stack et al., 2007)

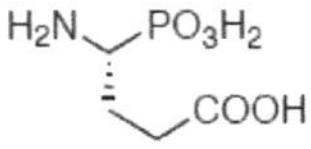

inhibitor od aspartyl aminopeptidase
(Teuscher et al., 2007)

Figure 5. Representative organophosphorus inhibitors of metalloproteinases.

Simple phosphonic acid analogs of amino acids and pseudopeptides, containing phosphinate moiety replacing scissile peptide bond, are acting via this mechanism and rank amongst most potent inhibitors of metalloproteinases (Fig. 5). Inhibitors of neutral alanyl (M1) and leucine (M17) aminopeptidases are among the most recognized and most intensively studied representatives of metal-containing exopeptidases of biomedical significance [Lowther & Matthews, 2002; Grembecka et al., 2003; Vassiliou et. al. 2007]. Functions related to tumorigenesis and invasion makes these enzymes molecular targets for the development of potential anticancer drugs [Grembecka & Kafarski, 2001; Zhang & Xu, 2008; Fournié-Zaluski et al., 2009; Grzywa et al., 2010]. The recognized role of neutral aminopeptidase in the pathogenesis of hypertension provides also an opportunity for regulating arterial blood pressure by their inhibitors [Banegas et al., 2006; Bodineau et al., 2008]. Additionally, two of these pseudodipeptides appear to be excellent inhibitors when applied to *Plasmodium falciparum* M1 and M17 aminopeptidases (Fig. 5), the protozoan counterparts of neutral and leucine aminopeptidases [Stack et al., 2007; Cunningham et al, 2008; McGowan et al., 2009; McGowan et al., 2010]. They efficiently controlled the growth of *P. falciparium* in cultures, including those of malaria cells lines resistant to chloroquine, and significantly reduced malaria infections in murine model (*Plasmodium chabaudi*) [Skinner-Adams et al., 2007]. These findings positively validated *P. falciparum* M1 and M17 aminopeptidases as promising targets for a novel treatment of malaria and identify new leads with anti-parasite potential [Skinner-Adams et al., 2010; Thivierge et al., 2012].

The design and development of pseudopeptidic inhibitors of aminopeptidases are greatly facilitated by two factors. First, the results of extensive structure-activity relationship studies, available for a wide collection of fluorogenic substrates, have defined the requirements of the S1 binding pockets of these enzymes [Drag & Salvesen, 2009; Drag et al., 2010; Gajda et al., 2012; Poręba et al., 2011; Poręba 2012]. Second, computer-aided analysis of numerous crystal structures available for leucine aminopeptidase has pointed to this enzyme as a primary molecular target for extending and optimizing interactions within the S1' pocket [Grembecka et al., 2001; Jørgensen et al., 2002; Evdokimov et al., 2007; Khandelwal et al., 2005; Khaliullin et al. 2010; Li et al., 2010].

Phosphinic pseudopeptides have also clearly revealed their potential for the regulation of matrix metalloproteinases (MMPs, matrixins), zinc-dependent endopeptidases implicated in the breakdown of the extracellular matrix [Yiotakis at al., 2004; Fisher & Mobashery, 2006]. Cleavage of the matrix component (collagen, lamanin, elastin, gelatin, etc.) is physiologically essential for tissue remodeling processes such as morphogenesis, embryogenesis and reproduction [Overall & Kleifield, 2006; Sang et. al., 2006]. Overexpression or inadequate level of matrix metalloproteinases leads to pathological states such as osteoarthritis, rheumatoid arthritis and inflammation, but it is most associated with tumor growth, invasion, and metastasis. Angiogenetic process favored by these enzymes is essential for vascoularization and growth of tumors. Thus, they were the first proteinase targets seriously considered for combating cancer. Despite that preliminary clinical/preclinical studies on MMP inhibition in tumor models brought positive results the outcome in the drug market has been so far unsatisfactory. The spectacular failure of the last-step clinical trials is mainly due to a lack of selectivity and serious side effects [Fisher & Mobashery, 2006]. The field is now resurging with careful reinvestigation of the precise roles of each particular MMP member and a focus on the development of selective inhibitors that fully discriminate between different members of the MMP family [Reiter et al., 2003; Matziari et al., 2007; Zucker & Cao, 2009; Devel et al., 2010; Johnson et al., 2011]. Such selectivity had been reached by variation of peptide scaffold by means of combinatorial pseudopeptide synthesis [Buchardt et al, 2000; Dive et al., 2004] or by application of molecular modeling based on crystallographic studies of these enzymes [Rao, 2005; Pirard, 2007; Verma & Hansch, 2007; Anzellotti & Farrell, 2008; Kalva et al., 2012]. Representative selective inhibitors of this class are shown in Figure 6.

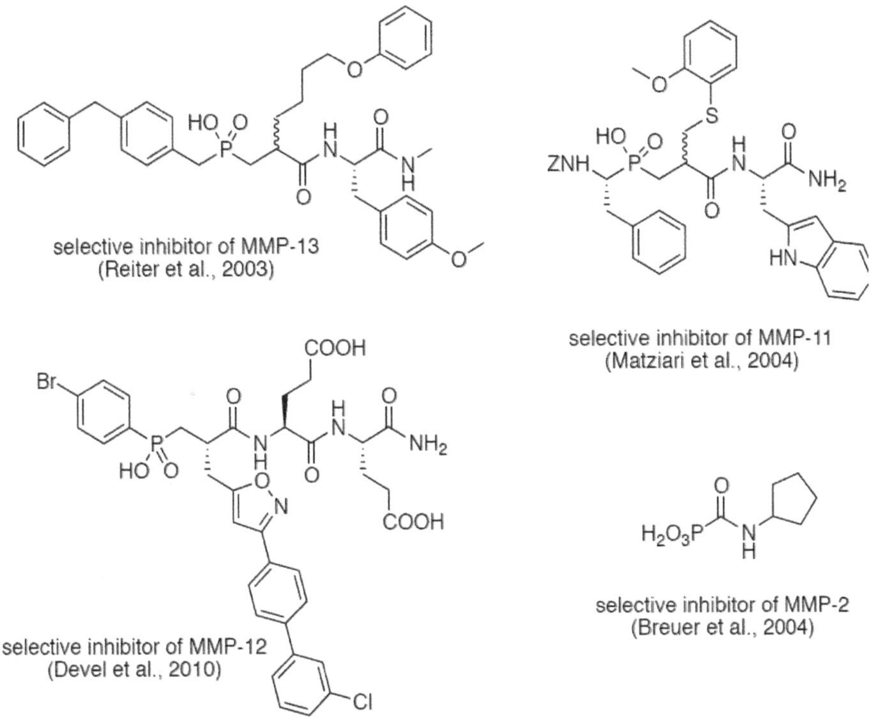

Figure 6. Representative inhibitors selective against chosen matrix metalloproteinases.

Quite interesting approach is preparation of hybrid systems as this composed of a phosphinate transition state analogue that has been incorporated within a triple-helical peptide template. The template sequence was based on the $\alpha 1(V)436$-450 collagen region, which is hydrolyzed at the Gly_{439}-Val_{440} bond selectively by MMP-2 and MMP-9. In that manner highly selective inhibitor towards these two gelatinases was found [Lauer-Fields et al., 2007; Lauer-Fields et al., 2008].

Phosphinic transition state analog approach has been also recently applied for the design and synthesis of novel potent inhibitors of other proteinases of medicinal importance. Thus, inhibitors of angiotensin converting enzyme [Mores et al., 2008; Julien et al. 2010; Akif et al., 2011] are potential drugs against hypertension, aspartyl aminopeptidase as antimalarial agent [Teuscher et al., 2007], inhibitors of cathepsin C and renal dipeptidase may be considered as potential anticancer agents [Gurulingappa et al., 2003: Mucha et al., 2004], inhibitors of sortase, which is bacterial virulence protein [Kruger et al., 2004], whereas inhibition of pyroglutamyl peptidase II enhances the analeptic effect of thyrotropin [Matziari et al., 2008; Lazcano et al. 2012].

It is worth mentioning that *Monopril®*, the sodium salt of fosinopril [Fig. 7], the ester prodrug of an angiotensin-converting enzyme (ACE) inhibitor fosinoprilat, is perhaps one of the most effective implementation of transition state analogy in medicine [Powell et al., 1984].

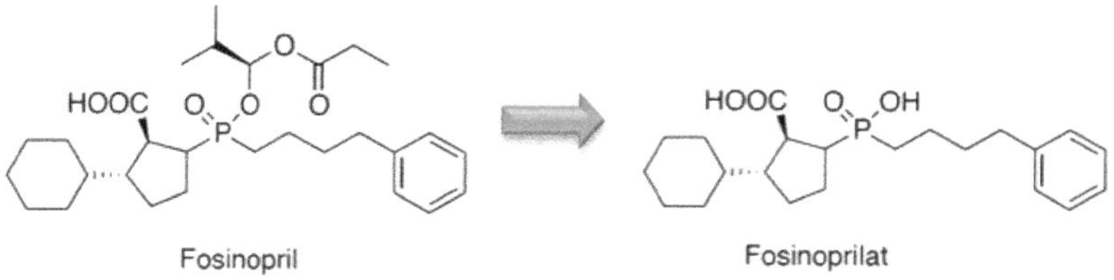

Fosinopril   Fosinoprilat

Figure 7. Fosinopril and fosinoprilat.

Sulfonamides also mimic both shape and electronic environment of the transition state of peptide bond hydrolysis. This approach was used for introduction of transition state inhibitors of HIV-protease, thermolysin and thrombine as well as haptens for generation of catalytic antibodies (Fig. 8) [Moree, et al., 1993; Moree, et al., 1995; Löwik et al., 2000; Liskamp & Kruijzer, 2004; Turcotte et al., 2012]. Unfortunately most of them appeared to be ineffective. This might be explained by non-typical bonding of potent inhibitor of this class with HIV protease (Fig. 9). It appeared that sulfonamide moiety displaces water molecule from active site and forms hydrogen bonds with two isoleucines, not as expected with catalytic aspartic acids [Meanwell, 2011]. Thus, sulfonamide group does not act as transition state analogue.

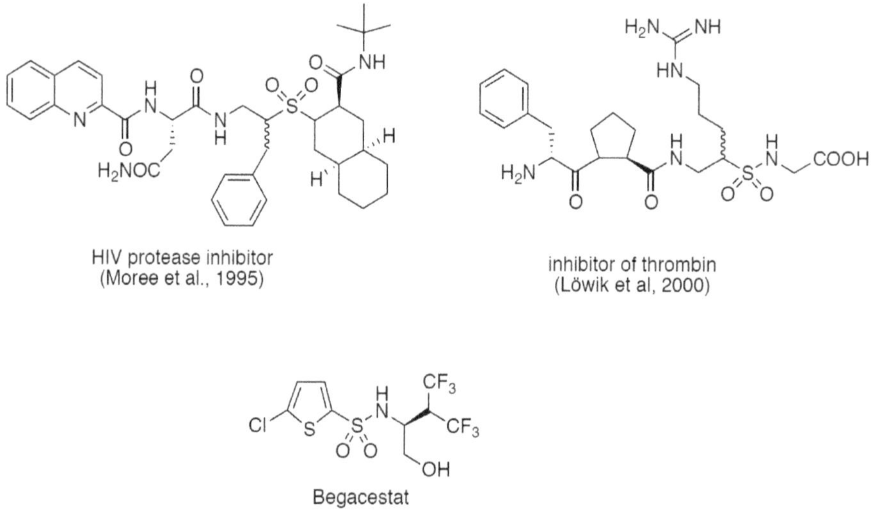

HIV protease inhibitor
(Moree et al., 1995)

inhibitor of thrombin
(Löwik et al, 2000)

Begacestat

Figure 8. Sufonamides as inhibitors of proteases.

Begacestat (Fig. 8), an effective and potent inhibitor of γ-secretase is an exception here [Mayer et al., 2008; Martone et al., 2009]. γ-Secretase catalyzes the final step in the generation of amyloid β peptides from amyloid precursor protein. Amyloid β-peptides aggregate to form neurotoxic oligomers, senile plaques, and congophilic angiopathy, some of the cardinal pathologies associated with Alzheimer's disease. Begacestat appeared to be well tolerated in mouse and dog toxicity studies and has been advanced to human clinical trials for the treatment of this neurological disease.

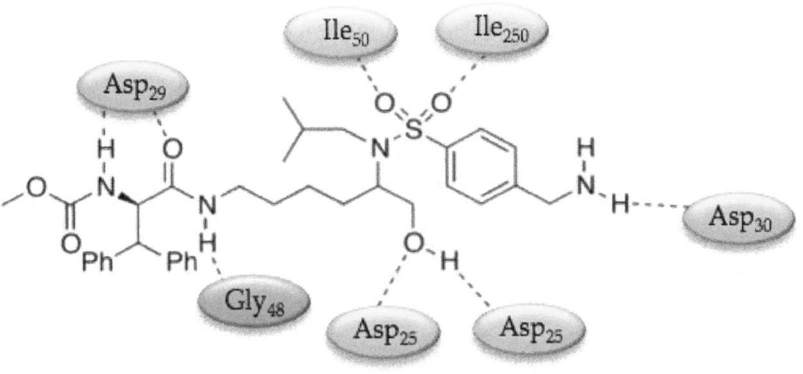

Figure 9. Mode of binding of sulfonamide HIV protease inhibitor.

inhibitor of angiotensin converting enzyme
(Mutahi et al., 2002)

HIV protease inhibitors
(Chen et al., 2001)

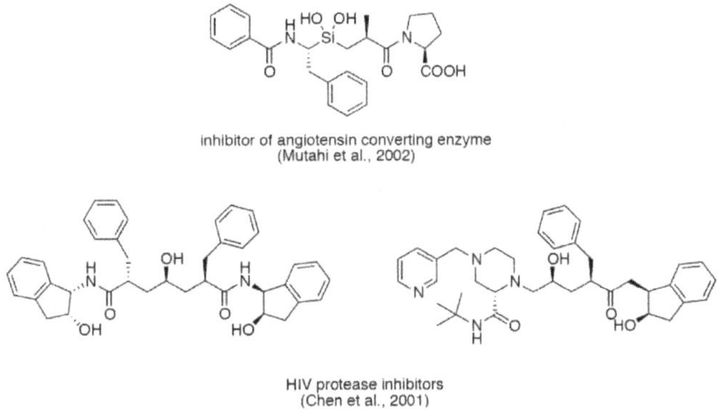

Figure 10. Silenediols as proteinase inhibitors.

Dialkylsilanediols are tetrahedral functional groups that can mimic hydrated carbonyls and thus might be also considered as „swollen" intermediates of peptide bond hydrolysis. When silanediols are embedded in a peptide-like structure, they are recognized by proteinases and act as hydrolytically stable entities. Thus, dialkylsilanol is an effective functional group for the design of active site-directed protease inhibitors. This concept has been successfully tested by replacing the presumed tetrahedral carbon of thermolysin, HIV-protease and angiotensin converting enzyme substrates with silanediol groups (Fig. 10), which resulted in potent inhibitors of these enzymes [Juers et al., 2005; Sieburth & Chen, 2006; Bo et al., 2011; Meanwell, 2011].

5. Hydroxyethylene intermediate analogs as inhibitors of proteases

Aspartic proteases generally bind 6-10 amino acid regions of their polypeptide substrates, which are typically processed with the aid of two catalytic aspartic acid residues in the active site. Thus, there is usually considerable scope for building inhibitor specificity for a particular aspartic protease by taking advantage of the collective interactions between a putative inhibitor on both sides of its scissile amide bond, and a substantial portion of the substrate-binding groove of the enzyme [Eder et al., 2007]. A very effective group of their inhibitors are simple hydroxyethylene analogs of tetrahedral oxyanion intermediates of the hydrolysis of peptide bonds. This approach is based on the structure of bestatin, a general inhibitor of aminopeptidases and aspartyl proteinases isolated in 1976 from *Streptomyces olivoreticuli* [Umezawa et al., 1976].

Today, HIV protease inhibitors constitute around 40% of available drugs against HIV. Nearly all of them contain hydroxyethylene unit as transition state analog mimic, to mention only Darunavir, Atazanavir, Fosamprenavir, Lopinavir (or Ritonavir) or the oldest one Saquinavir (Fig. 11) [Brik & Wong, 2003; Pokorna et. al, 2009].

Availability of anti-HIV drugs enabled to introduce highly active antiretroviral therapy (HAART), which resulted in dramatic decrease of the mortality and morbidity for a wide variety of opportunistic viral, bacterial, fungal and parasitic infections among HIV-infected individuals in economically developed countries [Andreoni & Perno, 2012]. Thus, the design, development and clinical success of HIV protease inhibitors represent one of the most remarkable achievements of molecular medicine. However, both the academias, as well as, the industry need to continue in their effort to develop novel, more potent compounds. This is mainly connected with HIV drug resistance, which in turn results from the high mutation rate, caused by the lack of proofreading activity of the viral reverse transcriptase. The pattern of mutations associated with the viral resistance is extremely complex as shown in Figure 12 [Pokorna et al., 2009]. Taken together, in spite of the indisputable success of the HAART and benefit to patients, new approaches to the antiviral treatment are highly desirable [Clarke, 2007; Adachi et al., 2009; Pokorna et al., 2009; Alfonso & Mozote, 2011].

Quite interestingly, small modifications of core structure of the inhibitor results in minute changes in inhibitor affinity to HIV protease as demonstrated in Figure 13 [Wu et al., 2008; Mahalingham et al., 2010].

Studies conducted in order to evaluate the influence of these antiviral drugs on the development of parasites, which are known to co-infect HIV-positive individuals, surprisingly

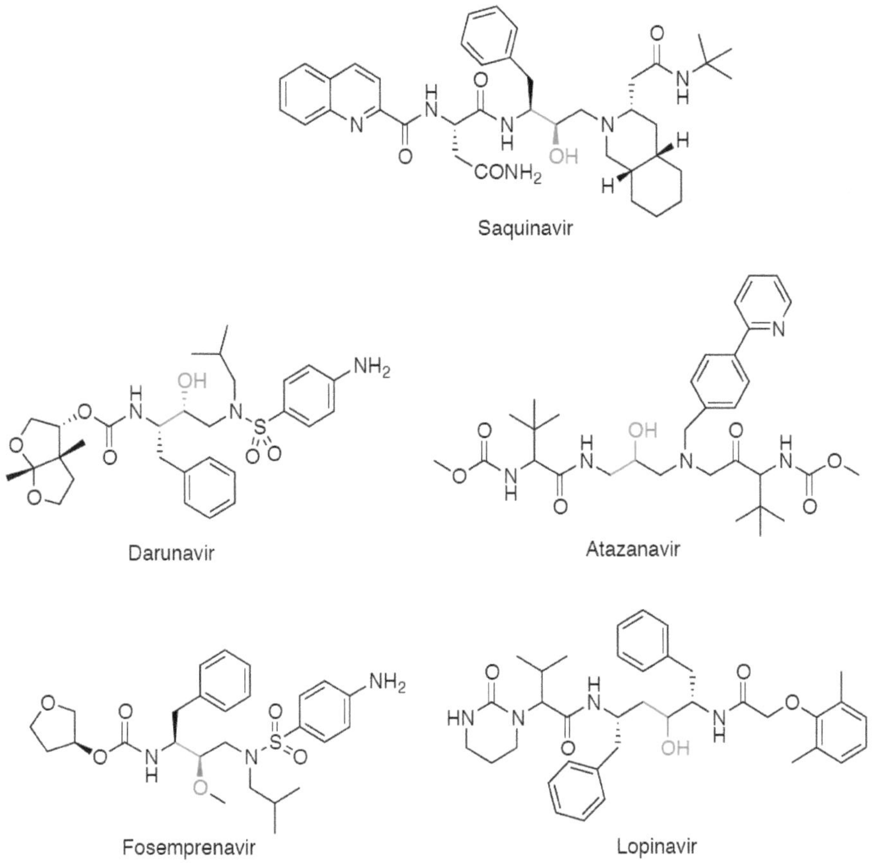

Saquinavir

Darunavir

Atazanavir

Fosemprenavir

Lopinavir

Figure 11. Representative examples of clinical HIV protease drugs.

shown, that these drugs exhibit marked antiprotozoal activity. For example Saquinavir, Lopinavir, Indinavir directly inhibited the grown of *Plasmodium falciparum* in vitro at clinically relevant concentrations. This findings suggest that some inhibitors of HIV protease are active against the most virulent human malaria parasite *P. falciparum* that is known to express number of aspartic proteases (plasmepsins) [Skinner-Adams, et al., 2004; Alfonso & Mozote, 2011].

More than 25 million people are suffering from dementia, and the annual socioeconomic worldwide costs have been estimated to exceed U.S. $200 billion. γ-Secretase, along with β-secretase produces the amyloid β-protein of Alzheimer's disease. Because of its key role in the pathogenesis γ-secretase has been a prime target for drug discovery, and many inhibitors of this protease have been developed. These enzymes are also effectively inhibited by

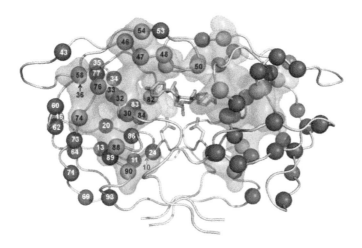

Figure 12. Three-dimensional structure of HIV protease complexed with Darunavir. Mutations associated with resistance to clinically used inhibitors are depicted as balls.

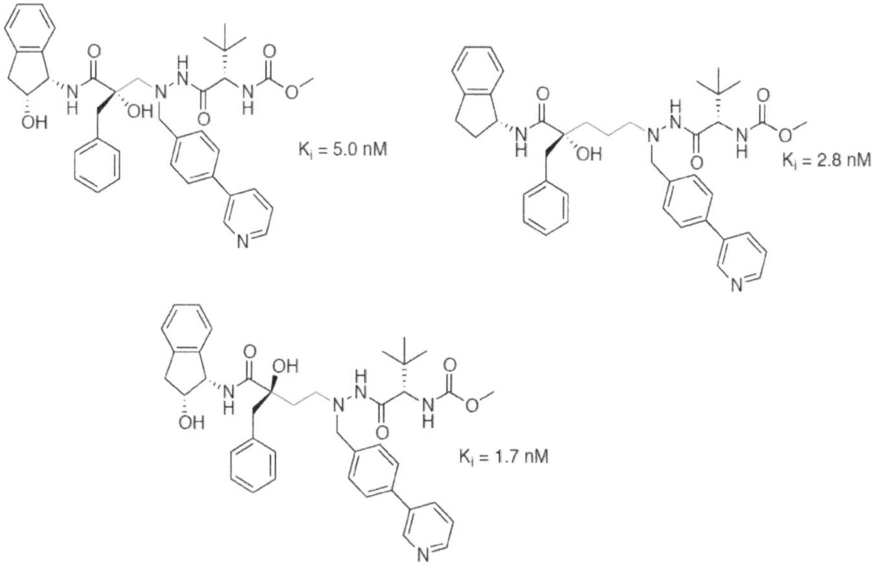

$K_i = 5.0$ nM

$K_i = 2.8$ nM

$K_i = 1.7$ nM

Figure 13. Influence of linker length on activity of HIV protease inhibitors.

peptidomimetics containing hydroxyethylene fragment replacing hydrolyzed peptide bond. Only one drug (Semagacestat, Fig. 14) reached phase III clinical studies so far, however, uncovered evidence of cognitive worsening in treated patients compared with placebo led to suspension of the trials in 2010. Anyway, design, synthesis and evaluation of new low-molecular, nanomolar inhibitors of secretases, structure of which significantly drifted away from peptidic transition state analogs (Fig. 14), is still challenging and brought new promising results [Osterman et al., 2006; Wolfe, 2012]. Due to rapid technological progress in chemistry, bioinformatics, structural biology and computer technology, computer-aided drug design plays more and more important role in this respect [Avram et al., 2006; Fujimoto et al., 2008; Xu et al., 2009; Al-Tel et al. 2011; Hamada et al., 2012].

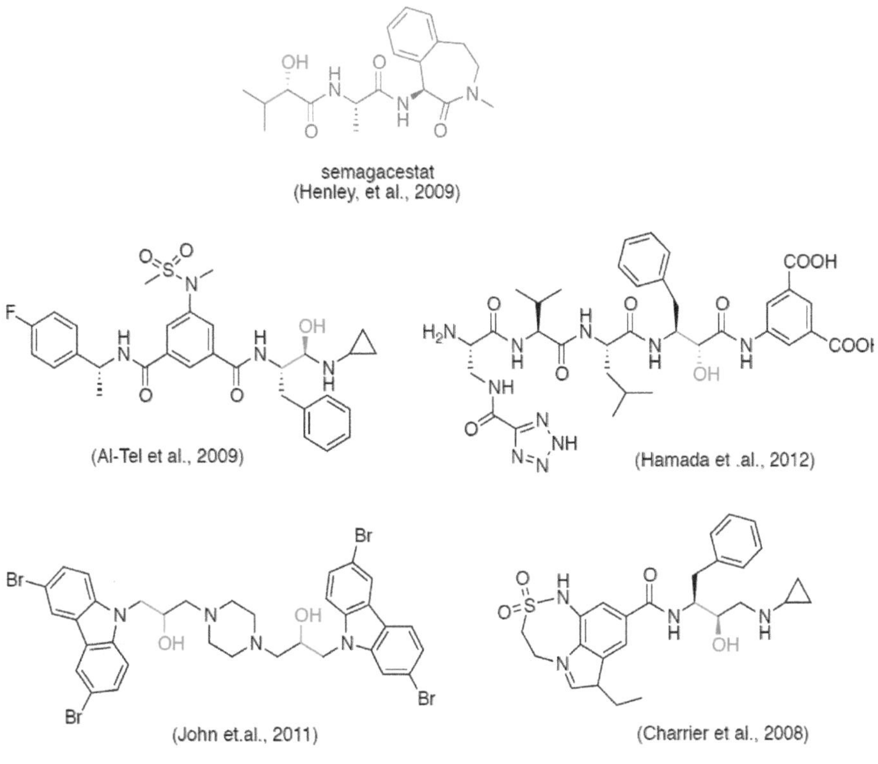

semagacestat
(Henley, et al., 2009)

(Al-Tel et al., 2009)

(Hamada et .al., 2012)

(John et.al., 2011)

(Charrier et al., 2008)

Figure 14. Inhibitors of secretases.

Hypertension is a major risk factor for cardiovascular diseases such as stroke, myocardial infarction, and heart failure, the leading causes of death in the Western world. Inhibitors of the renin–angiotensin system have proven to be successful treatments for hypertension. As renin specifically catalyses the rate limiting step of this system, it represents the optimal target for antihypertensive drugs. Aliskiren (Fig. 15), a promising drug lowering blood pressure in sodium-depleted marmosets and hypertensive human patients, was developed using a combination of crystal structure analysis of renin–inhibitor complexes and computational methods [Wood et al., 2003]. The therapy was introduced under the names Takturna and Rasilez.

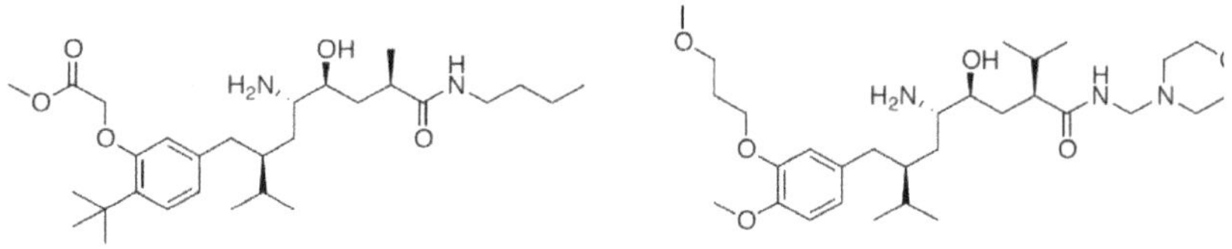

Figure 15. Aliskiren (left hand side) and its more potent analog.

Another possibility arose from use of fluoroketone derivatives. α-monofluoroketones are approximately 50% hydrated, whereas the α,α-difluoroketones are 100% hydrated in aqueous solutions (Fig. 16). The latter ones are obviously of choice because of their striking similarity to phosphinic inhibitors (two hydroxyls placed at terahedral atom). This approach is applied very rarely but gave good inhibitors of fungal endothiapepsin [Tuan et al., 2007] and matrix metalloprotease [Reiter et al., 2000] (Fig. 16).

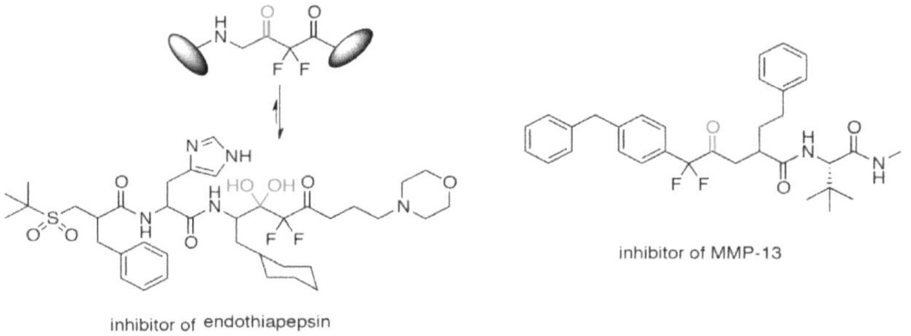

inhibitor of endothiapepsin

inhibitor of MMP-13

Figure 16. Difluoroketones as transition state inhibitor.

6. Suicide substrates yielding transition state analogues

Peptide aldehydes and boronic acids are inhibitors of serine and threonine enzymes forming both, hydrogen and covalent bonds in the enzyme active site. Tetrahedral adduct generated from these compounds upon their action on enzymes bear a closer relationship to the structure of the true intermediate and they may be considered as suicidal substrates. There is, however, an important difference between these two types of inhibitors. The boronic acid derivative possesses a negative charge, whereas the hemiacetal adduct is neutral (Fig 17).

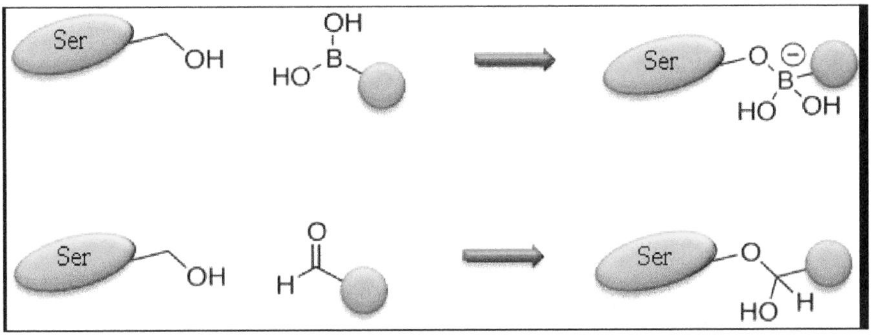

Figure 17. Suicidal substrates yielding transition state analogs

Hence, the peptidyl boronic acid adduct is a better transition state analog than the hemiacetal formed from peptidic aldehyde [Polgár, 2005]. Aldehydes typically have a low prevalence in drugs and drug candidates because of their potential chemical reactivity and susceptibility to be engaged in a reduction/oxidation pathways in vivo. Therefore peptidyl boronic acids are considered as far better drug candidates. Additionally slight changes in pH can result in release of the inhibitor from the active site, which is profitous.

In 2003, bortezomib (Fig. 18), a first-in-class therapeutic, gained approval from the US Federal Drug Administration for the treatment of relapsed multiple myeloma and mantle cell lymphoma. Approval in the UK, for multiple myeloma, followed in 2006. It possesses a unique mode of action. Bortezomib acts as inhibitor of the 26S proteasome, the key regulator of intracellular protein degradation, found in the nucleus and cytosol of all eukaryotic cells, and forming part of the critical ubiquitin-proteasome system. This inhibition results in disruption of homeostatic mechanisms within the cell that can lead to cell death.

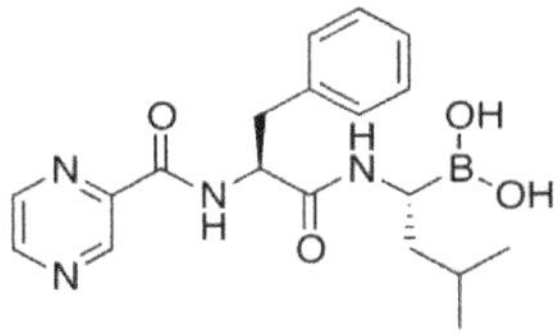

Figure 18. Structure of bortezomib.

This finding initiated intensive researches on boronic inhibitors of serine and threonine proteases [Trippier & McGuigan, 2010]. For, example recently inhibitors of Lon proteases (bacterial ATP-dependent protease conferring bacterial virulence) afforded interesting antibacterial agents [Frase and Lee, 2007], inhibitors of prostate-specific antigen for prostate cancer imaging and therapy [LeBeau et al., 2008], antifungal inhibitors of kexin (regulatory proteins from *Candida*) [Holyoak et al., 2004; Wheatley & Holyoak, 2007], inhibitor of HCV NS3 protease as potential drug against hepatitis [Zhang et al., 2003; Venkatraman et al., 2009], and anticancer and antibacterial inhibitors of proteasome [Hu et al., 2006]. Representative examples of these inhibitors are shown in Figure 19.

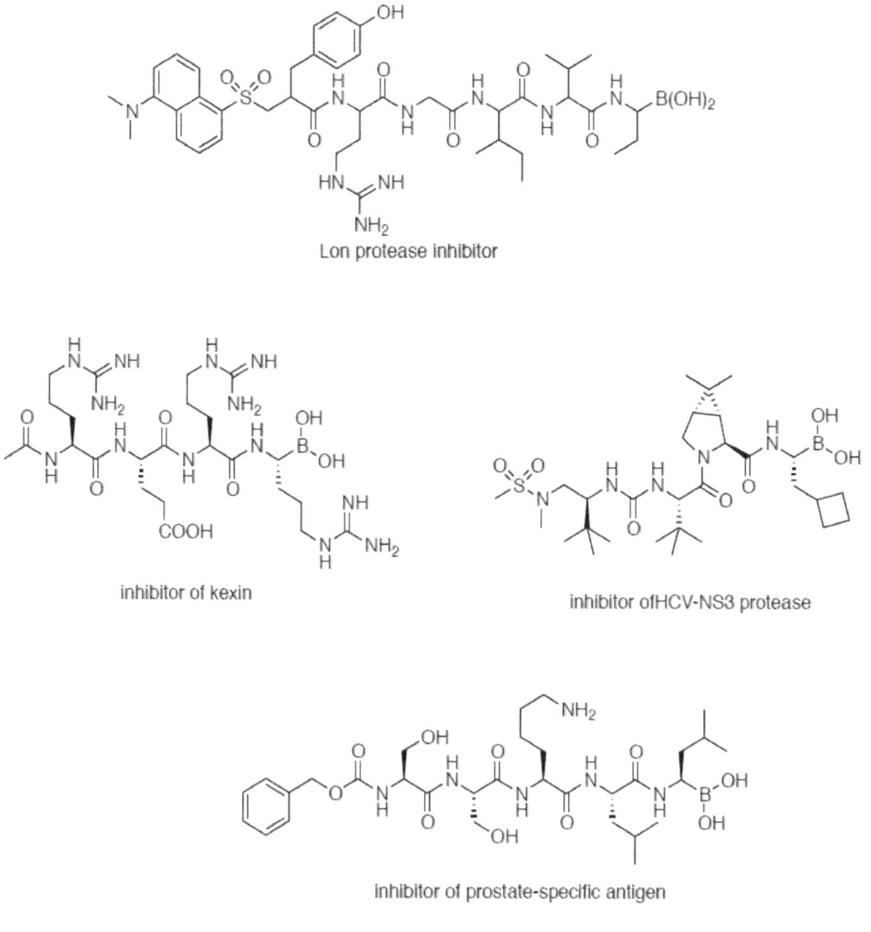

Lon protease inhibitor

inhibitor of kexin

inhibitor ofHCV-NS3 protease

inhibitor of prostate-specific antigen

Figure 19. Boronic acid based inhibitors.

7. Other hydrolases

The data considering transition state analogue inhibitors of other hydrolases are practically limited to inhibitors of β–lactamases, arginase and urease.

Antibiotic resistance, especially to widely prescribed β-lactam antibiotics, is a serious threat to public health and is responsible for the increase in morbidity, mortality, and health care costs related to the treatment of bacterial infections. In most cases emergence of antibiotic-resistant bacteria is primarily driven by overuse of β-lactam antibiotics in food and agricultural products. The most prominent resistance mechanism is related to the expression of β-lactamases, which hydrolyze β–lactam fragment of the drug molecule. In nature, four classes of these enzymes exist. Three of them are serine-based, whereas fourth is zinc-dependent-hydrolase. To counteract β-lactamases, mechanism-based inhibitors were developed to be administered in concert with β-lactam antibiotics. Presently, there are three commercially available β-lactamase inhibitors (clavulanate, sulbactam, and tazobactam). The new approach to obtain such inhibitors is combination of structure of potent β-lactam antibiotics with a boronic [Thomson, et al., 2007; Eidam et al., 2010: Ke, et al., 2011; Chan, et al., 2012] or phosphonic [Nukaga, et al., 2004] acid moieties with the goal of mimicking the transition state and creating a high-affinity, reversible inhibitor that cannot be inactivated by β-lactamases since they do not bear hydrolyzable β-lactam ring.

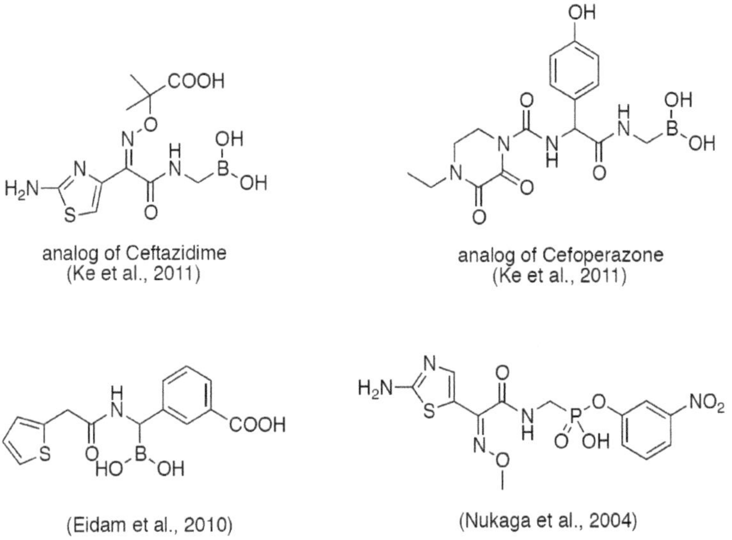

analog of Ceftazidime
(Ke et al., 2011)

analog of Cefoperazone
(Ke et al., 2011)

(Eidam et al., 2010)

(Nukaga et al., 2004)

Figure 20. Transition state inhibitors of lactamases.

Arginase is a binuclear manganese metalloenzyme that serves as a therapeutic target for the treatment of asthma, erectile dysfunction, and atherosclerosis. The hydrolysis of L-arginine to *L*-ornithine and urea (Fig. 21) is also the final cytosolic step of the urea cycle in mammalian liver. *S*-(2-Boronoethyl)-*L*-cysteine is one of the most effective inhibitor of the enzyme (Fig 21). The specificity determinants of amino acid recognition by arginase were identified by X-Ray structure of human arginase I enzyme complexed with this inhibitor. These studies undoubtedly shown that boronate adopts tetrahedral configuration [Cama et al., 2003 & 2003a; Shishova, et al., 2009]. Also aldehydes and sulfonamides similar to boronic acids appeared to be promising inhibitors of arginases [Shin et al., 2004].

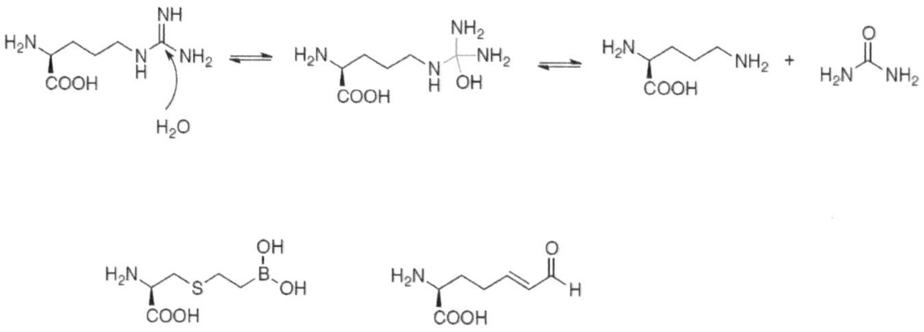

(Shishova et al., 200(9))   (Shin et al., 2004)

Figure 21. Arginase catalyzed reaction and representative inhibitors of the enzyme.

Urease catalyzes hydrolysis of urea in the last step of organic nitrogen mineralization to give ammonia and carbamate, which decomposes to give a second molecule of ammonia and bicarbonate (Fig. 22). The hydrolysis of the reaction products induces an overall pH increase that has negative implications both in human and animal health as well as in the ecosphere. Urease is a virulence factor in infections of urinary (*Proteus mirabilis*, *Ureaplasma urealyticum*) and gastrointestinal tracts (*Helicobacter pylori*), causing severe diseases such as peptic ulcers, stomach cancer, and formation of urinary stones. The efficiency of soil nitrogen fertilization with urea (the most used fertilizer worldwide) decreases due to ammonia volatilization and root damage caused by soil pH increase. Thus, control of the activity of urease through the use of inhibitors could counteract these negative effects [Kosikowska & Berlicki, 2011; Zambelli et al., 2011]. Di- and triamides of phosphoric acid represent a group of urease inhibitors with the highest activity. It is the direct consequence of their similarity to the tetrahedral transition state of the enzymatic reaction of urea hydrolysis. Takeda Chemicals have patented a large group of N-acyltriamido phosphates and found over 90 examples with nanomolar activity against *H. pylori* urease, with flurofamide being the most effective (Fig. 22) [Kosikowska & Berlicki, 2011].

Recently design, synthesis, and evaluation of novel ogranophosphonate inhibitors of bacterial urease have been described as an attractive alternative to known phosphoramidates. On the basis of the crystal structure of *Bacillus pasteurii* urease, several phosphinic acids and their short peptides have been designed by using the computer-aided techniques. The step-wise scheme of inhibitor design, shown in Figure 21, led to the synthesis of compounds with low structural complexity, high hydrolytic stability and satisfactory biological activity against various ureases, including cytoplasmic urease from pathogenic *Proteus* species [Vassiliou et al., 2008; Berlicki et al., 2012; Vassiliou et al., 2012].

8. Peptide bond formation by ribosome

Ribosomes are molecular machines that synthesize proteins in the cell. Recent biochemical analyses and high-resolution crystal structures of the bacterial ribosome have shown that the active site for the formation of peptide bonds – the peptidyl-transferase center – is composed solely of rRNA. Thus, the ribosome is the largest known RNA catalyst and the only natural ribozyme that has a synthetic activity. Peptide bond formation during ribosomal protein synthesis involves an aminolysis reaction between the aminoacyl α-amino group and the carbonyl ester of the growing peptide via a transition state with a developing negative charge - the oxyanion. Therefore the observed intermediates and transition states are similar to those observed in proteinases (Fig. 23). Structural and molecular dynamic studies have suggested that the ribosome may stabilize the oxyanion in the transition state of peptide bond formation via a highly ordered water molecule [Rodnina et al., 2006; Carrasco et al., 2011].

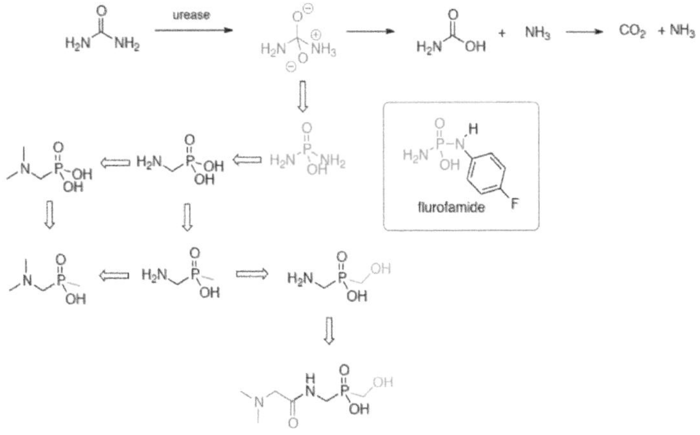

Figure 22. Urease hydrolysed reaction and evolution of the structure of its inhibitors.

To biochemically elucidate how the ribosome stabilizes the developing negative charge in the transition state of peptide bond formation, a series of tetrahedral transition state mimics were synthesized. Their relative binding affinities for the ribosomes also were measured (Fig. 23). The obtained results confirmed high affinity of predicted mechanism of ribosome action [Green & Lorsch, 2002; Weinger et al., 2004; Carrasco, et al., 2011].

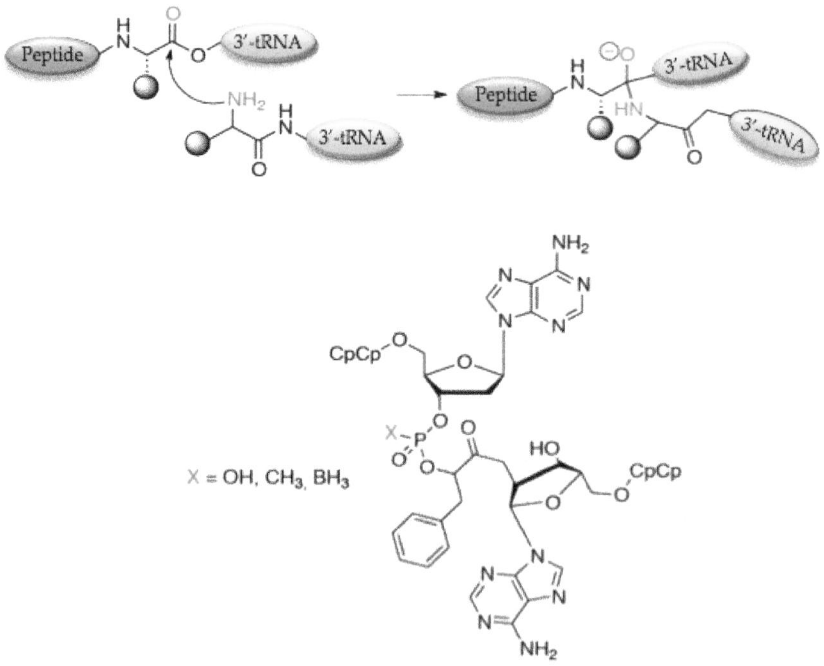

Figure 23. Transition state analog inhibitor of peptidyl transferase.

9. Enzymes forming amide and ester bonds via carboxylic-phosphate anhydride

Activation of carboxylic group of amino acid by ATP-phosphorylation yielding mixed carboxylic-phosphate anhydride is quite popular mechanism of synthesis of amide and ester bonds.

D-Alanyl-D-alanine ligase is one of the key enzymes in peptidoglycan biosynthesis and is an important target for antibacterial drugs. The enzyme catalyzes the condensation of two alanine molecules using ATP to produce D-Ala-D-Ala (Fig. 24), which is the terminal peptide of a peptidoglycan monomer. Analogs of D-Ala-D-Ala, in which phosphonate or phosphinate moiety replaces peptide bond appear to be potent inhibitors. As determined by kinetic [Ellsworth et al., 1996], X-Ray [Wu et al., 2008], and molecular modeling studies the inhibitor behaves as substrate and reacts with ATP to produce ADP and a tight-binding phosphorylated transition state analogue, which exerts inhibitory action against the enzyme (Fig. 24). Thus, these compounds might be rather considered as suicide substrates.

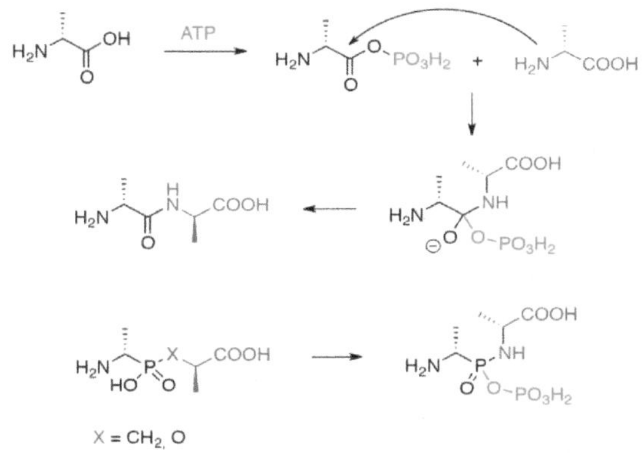

Figure 24. Mechanism of condensation of two molecules of D-Ala catalyzed by *D*-alanine-*D*-alanine ligase.

Similarly acting inhibitors have been found for glutamine synthetase (phosphinothricin and methionine sulfoximine and their analogs) [Berlicki et al., 2005; Berlicki & Kafarski 2006; Berlicki, 2008], γ-glutamylcysteine synthetase [Hibi et al., 2004], or penicillin binding proteins [Dzekieva et al., 2010; Dzekieva et al., 2012] (Fig. 25).

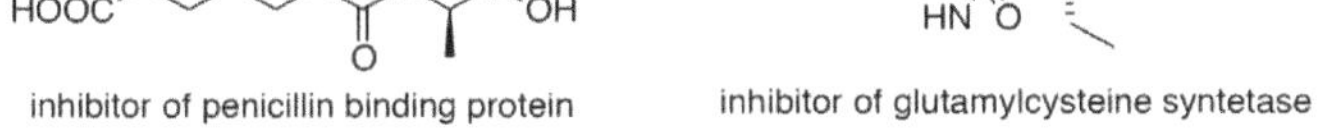

phosphinothricin

methionine sulfoximine

inhibitor of penicillin binding protein

inhibitor of glutamylcysteine syntetase

Figure 25. Inhibitors activated by ATP.

10. Nucleotide deaminases

Enzymes of the deaminase superfamily catalyze deamination of bases in nucleotides and nucleic acids across in diverse biological contexts. Representatives that act on free nucleotides or bases are primarily involved in the salvage of pyrimidines and purines, or in their catabolism in bacteria, eukaryotes and phages. Other members of the deaminase superfamily catalyze the *in situ* deamination of bases in both RNA and DNA. Such modifications play a central role in RNA editing, which is critical for generating the appropriate anti-codon sequences for decoding the genetic code, modification of the sequences of microRNA and other transcripts and alteration of the reading frames in mRNAs, defense against viruses via hypermutation-based inactivation, and somatic hypermutation or class switching of antigen receptor genes in vertebrates [Iyer et al., 2011].

Adenosine deaminase (ADA) is an enzyme present in all organisms and catalyzes the irreversible deamination of adenosine and deoxyadenosine to inosine and deoxyinosine (Fig. 26). Both adenosine and deoxyadenosine are biologically active purines that can have a deep impact on cellular physiology. For example it plays a vital role in regulating T-cell coactivation. Deficiency of this enzyme in humans causes severe combined immunodeficiency. Increased serum activity of this enzyme have been found in many infectious diseases caused by microorganisms infecting the macrophages, in leprosy, brucellosis, HIV infections, viral hepatitis, infectious mononucleosis, liver cirrhosis and tuberculosis. Its extended transition state inhibitor – conformycin was isolated from *Nocardia interforma* and *Streptomyces kaniharaensis*. Analogs of conformycin (Fig. 26) are proposed as an antineoplastic synergists and immunosuppressants [Wolfenden, 2003].

The wide potential of these inhibitors may be illustrated by the fact that deaminoformycin was recently applied to evaluate mechanisms responsible for lethality caused by genetic and herbicide-based activity of adenosine deaminase [Sabina et al., 2007], as well as identification of highly selective inhibitor of purine salvage pathway in malaria parasites [Tyler et al., 2007]. This is because of a unique feature of *Plasmodium falciparum* enzyme that catalyzes the deamination of both adenosine and 5'-methylthioadenosine.

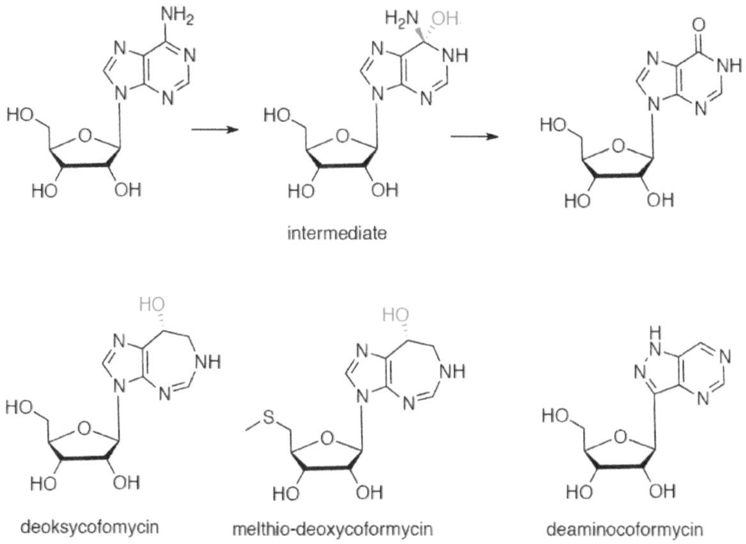

intermediate

deoksycofomycin   melthio-deoxycoformycin   deaminocoformycin

Figure 26. Inhibitors of adenosine deaminase.

Guanine deaminase is an enzyme that hydrolyzes guanine to form xanthine that is unsuitable for DNA/RNA buildup. This enzyme has been found in normal or transformed human organs and sera. One of the approaches for antiviral/anticancer therapy is to design structural mimics of natural guanine as nucleic acid building blocks, with an anticipation that such analogs would be incorporated into DNA/RNA of virus for cancer cells, interrupting their normal replicative processes. Unfortunately these potent anticancer mimics are believed to be substrates for the enzyme guanine deaminase, which converts them into their respective inactive forms. A potent inhibitor would restore the original potency of these anticancer compounds. Such an activity was determined for azepinomycin [Isshiki et al., 1987] and its analog designed as transition state of this reaction (Fig. 27) [Chakraborty et al., 2011].

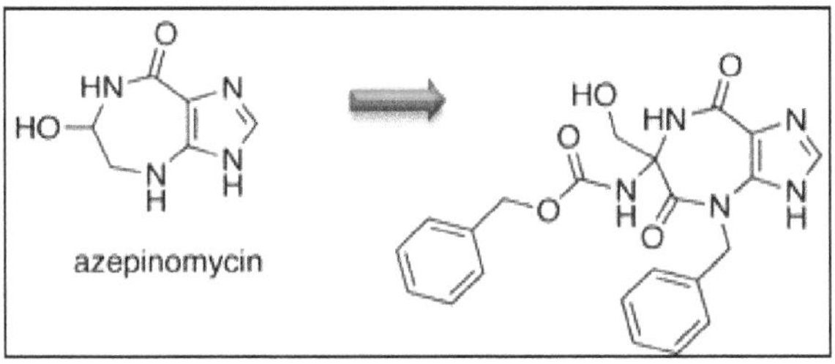

Figure 27. Apizenomycin as a template for guanine deaminase inhibitor.

11. Glycosidases and related enzymes

Glycoside hydrolases, the enzymes catalyzing hydrolysis of the glycosidic bond in di-, oligo- and polysaccharides, and glycoconjugates, are ubiquitous in Nature and fundamental to existence. The extreme stability of the glycosidic bond caused that they have evolved into highly proficient catalysts, with an estimated 10^{17} fold rate enhancement over the uncatalysed reaction. Such rate enhancements mean that enzymes bind the substrate at the transition state with extraordinary affinity [Gloster & Davies, 2010].

In the most cases of glycoside hydrolysis, the short-lived transition state possesses substantial oxocarbenium character (Fig. 27) resembling classical S_N1 reaction intermediate. Under these conditions the anomeric carbon possesses trigonal character, which causes sp^2 hybridisation predominantly along the bond between the anomeric carbon and endocyclic oxygen and significant relative positive charge accumulation on the pyranose ring [Lee et al., 2004; Biarnés et al., 2011; Davies at al., 2012].

The quest for potent and selective inhibitors of glycosidases is extremely active at present. This results from the involvement of glycosidases in lysosomal storage disorders, cancer, viral infections, diabetes and many others. Consequently a plethora of glycosidase inhibitors have been already synthesized and evaluated. The number of them is continually growing. It is outside the scope of this chapter to mention all of them in detail. One of the most appealing ways to design a transition state analog would be to incorporate both the features of geometry and charge present at the transition state. Distortion of the ring to generate compounds which may resemble the geometry of the transition state can be done by introducing a double bond in the pseudo-glycoside ring itself, whereas introduction of the charge might be done by application of sulfonium or ammonium ions [Rempel & Withers, 2008; Gloster & Davies, 2010; Sumida et al., 2012].

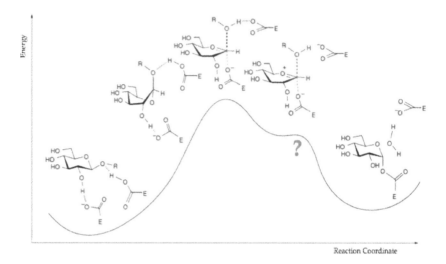

Figure 28. Mechanism of β-glucosidase action [after Vasella et al., 2002].

Some representatives, which fulfills these requirements are: salicinol, one of the active principles in the aqueous extracts of *Salacia reticulata* that is traditionally used in Sri Lanka and India for the treatment of diabetes [Ghavami et al., 2001] and its structurally variable analogues [Liu et al., 2006; Bhat et al., 2007; Mohan & Pinto, 2008].

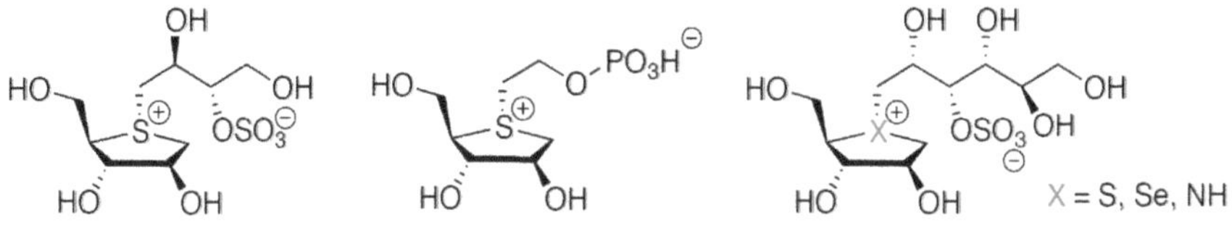

Figure 29. Salicinol and its analogs.

Sialic acids play an important role in a variety of biological processes. They are usually attached to the terminal positions of glycoproteins, glycolipids and oligosaccharides. From more than 100 different sialic acids, *N*-acetylneuraminic acid (NeuAc) is the most abundant one. Sialidases or neuraminidases are a family of exo-glycoside hydrolases that catalyze the cleavage of terminal sialic acid residues from sialylated oligosaccharides, glycoproteins, and glycolipids. Aberrant expression of different human sialidases was found to associate with various pathological conditions, including lysosomal storage diseases such as sialidosis and galactosialidosis. Non-specific transition-state analog of sialidase, 2-deoxy-2,3-dehydro-N - acetylneuraminic acid (DANA, Fig. 30) is a good starting point for the synthesis of specific inhibitors of human enzymes [Streicher & Busse, 2006; Li et al., 2011].

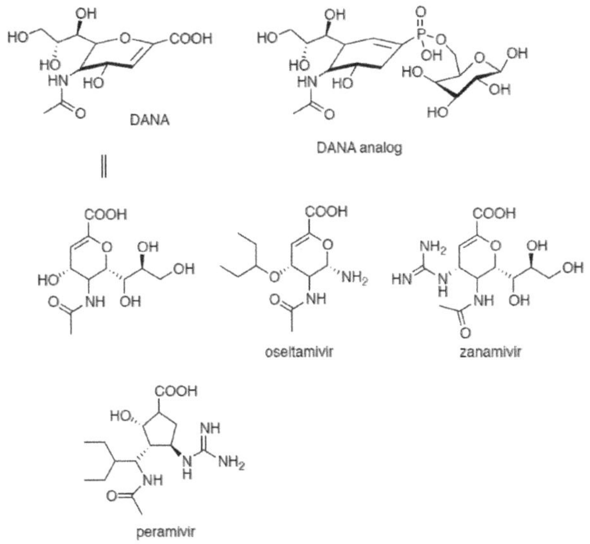

Figure 30. Chemical structures of neuraminidaze inhibitors.

Influenza viruses, in particular those of type A that can infect animals and humans, continue to represent a major threat to public health and animal health worldwide. The social and economic burden associated with a pandemic is substantial. Two viral surface glycoproteins, the sialoside-hydrolysing neuraminidase and the sialic acid-binding hemagglutinin, have become important targets for such approach. Most likely, the function of flu virus neuraminidase is to remove sialic acid receptors for the virus from the host cells, and also, perhaps more importantly, from the newly formed virus particles themselves [Nelson & Holmes, 2007; Medina & Garcia-Sastre, 2011]. Three inhibitors of neuraminidase have been successfully introduced as anti-influenza drugs, all of them being transition state analog inhibitors. They were designed by systematic reduction of DANA structure using crystallographic data and computer-aided methods [Wei, et al., 2006]. Relenza (zanamivir) was the first inhibitor to be synthesized which specifically inhibited neuraminidases of both Type A and Type B influenza viruses and is effective in controlling influenza infections. In people is given as a powder by oral inhalation [Palese et al., 1974]. Interestingly, it is weaker inhibitor of neuramidase than DANA, however, DANA inhibited influenza virus replication in tissue culture but failed to prevent disease in flu-infected animals. In order to produce a neuraminidase inhibitor, which was orally bioavailable and which was taken orally in capsules or as a suspension, Tamiflu (oseltavimir) was developed in 1997 [Kim et al.]. Third drug, which has been authorized for the emergency use of treatment of certain hospitalized patients with known or suspected 2009 H1N1 influenza, is permavir [Chand, et al., 2005]. Structures of these drugs are presented in Figure 30.

All three drugs soon became lead structures for the design and preparation of new, presumably more effective ones. Syntheses and eveluation of phosphinic analogs and significantly simplified analogs of permavir (Fig. 31) have been recently described [Kati et al., 2001; Bianco et al., 2005; Shie et al., 2007; Udommaneethanakit et al., 2009].

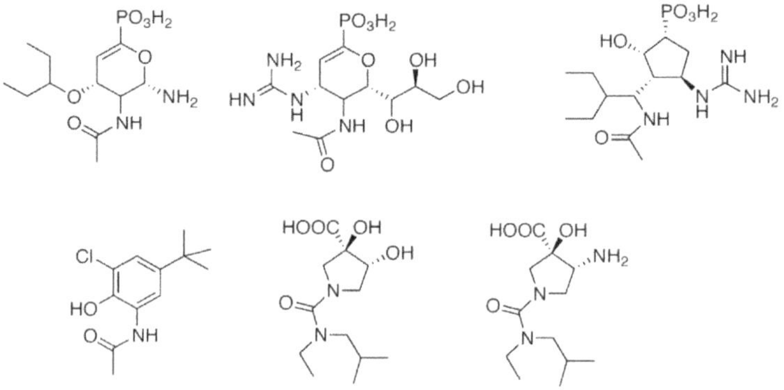

Figure 31. Second generation of influenza neuraminidase inhibitors.

Modified phosphonic analogs of oseltamivir were used to functionalize gold nanoparticles and were found to bind strongly and selectively to all seasonal and pandemic influenza virus strains, and thus could serve as prototypes for novel virus sensors. This may be helpul in fast influenza diagnosis [Stanley et al., 2012].

12. Transition state analogues of nucleic acids metabolism

N-Ribosyltransferases are a general class of enzymes that catalyze nucleophilic displacement reactions by migration of the cationic ribooxacarbenium carbon from the fixed purine to phosphate and water nucleophiles, respectively. Two major classes of these enzymes are hydrolases and phosphorylases. Hydrolases, which release the heterocycle to generate a free sugar ribosyl unit, include enzymes for DNA repair, RNA depurinations by plant toxins, and purine and pyrimidine nucleoside and nucleotide metabolism. Phosphorylases, which transfer ribosyl groups to phosphate, are also involved in the pathway for nucleoside salvage. Genetic defects in this pathway prevent normal purine catabolism in humans.

The focus on transition states for a family of N-ribosyltransferases roots from physiologic importance of these enzymes. Similarly as in the case of glycosidases, most sugar transferases form transition states with cationic charge at the anomeric carbon. The geometry is altered at this center from sp^3 (tetrahedral geometry) in the reactant sugar to sp^2 (trigonal planargeometry) at the transition state (Fig. 32) [Schramm, 2002; Murkin et al., 2007; Silva et al., 2011].

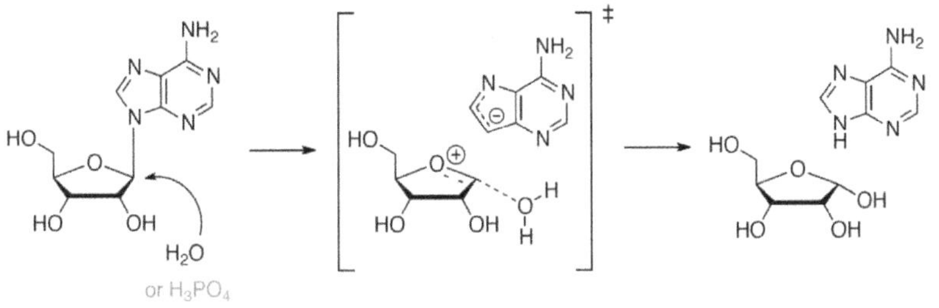

Figure 32. Course of reaction catalyzed by N-ribosyltransferases.

Newborns with a genetic deficiency of purine nucleoside phosphorylase are normal, but exhibit a specific T-cell immunodeficiency during the first years of development. All other cell and organ systems remain functional. Human purine nucleoside phosphorylase degrades deoxyguanosine, and apoptosis of T-cells occurs as a consequence of the accumulation of deoxyguanosine in the circulation. Thus, control of T-cell proliferation is desirable in T-cell cancers, autoimmune diseases, and tissue transplant rejection. The search for powerful inhibitors of these enzymes as anti-T-cell agents has culminated in the discovery of immucillins. The atomic replacements between inosine and immunocilin H make an insignificant change in atomic size, but a dramatic change in the molecular electrostatic potential surface (Fig. 33). Thus, analysis of the molecular electrostatic potential surface similarity between transition state and immucilin confirmed utility of this simple approach in helping to design effective inhibitor [Schramm, 2002; Schramm, 2007].

Evolution of immucilin structure, performed using standard structural analogy techniques, enabled to obtain new inhibitors of purine nucleotide phosphorylase of nano- to picomolar affinities to the enzyme (Fig. 34) [Evans et al., 2008; Edwards et al., 2009; Ho et al. 2010; Rejman et al., 2012].

Plasmodium parasites (causative agents of malaria) are purine auxotrophs and require preformed purine bases for synthesis of nucleotides, cofactors, and nucleic acids. The purine phosphoribosyltransferases catalyze transfer the 5-phosphoribosyl group from 5-phospho-α-D-ribofuranosyl-1-pyrophosphate to salvage hypoxanthine, guanine, or xanthine to form intracellular nucleosides. Purine salvage in *Plasmodium falciparum* uses hypoxanthine formed in erythrocytes or in parasites by the sequential actions of adenosine deaminase and purine nucleoside phosphorylase

inosine
immucilin H

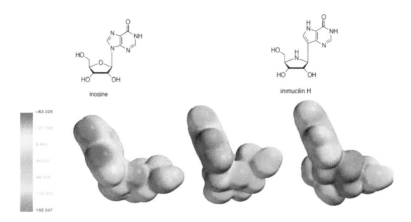

Figure 33. Molecular electrostatic potential surfaces for inosine, the transition state of purine nucleoside phosphorylase and immucilin H.

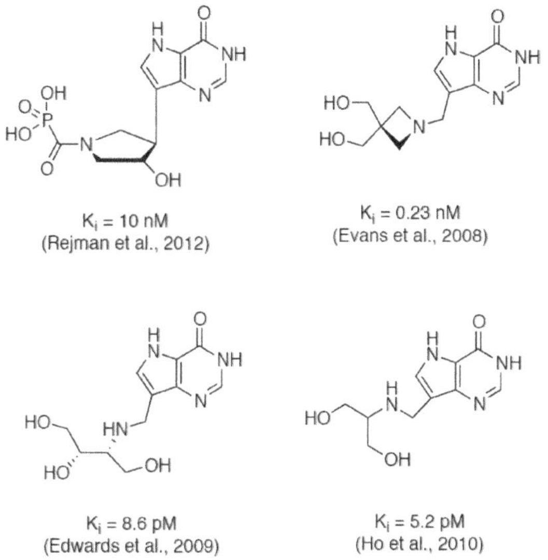

K$_i$ = 10 nM
(Rejman et al., 2012)
K$_i$ = 0.23 nM
(Evans et al., 2008)
K$_i$ = 8.6 pM
(Edwards et al., 2009)
K$_i$ = 5.2 pM
(Ho et al., 2010)

Figure 34. Effective inhibitors of purine nucleotide phosphorylase.

Therefore, effective inhibitors of both enzymes influence the life cycle of P. falciparum and these pathways have been targets for antimalarials since the discovery that *Plasmodium* parasites are purine auxotrophs.

Immunocillins HP and GP [Shi et al., 1999] and BCX4945 [Cassera et al., 2011] (Fig. 35) appear to be effective inhibitors of phosphoribosyltransferases and are also able to influence purine nucleoside phosphorylase, being dual inhibitor of the process. Especially the efficacy, oral availability, chemical stability, unique mechanism of action and low toxicity of BCX4945 demonstrate potential for combination therapies with this novel antimalarial agent. Similar studies have been also carried out for acyclic nucleoside phosphonates [Keough et al., 2009].

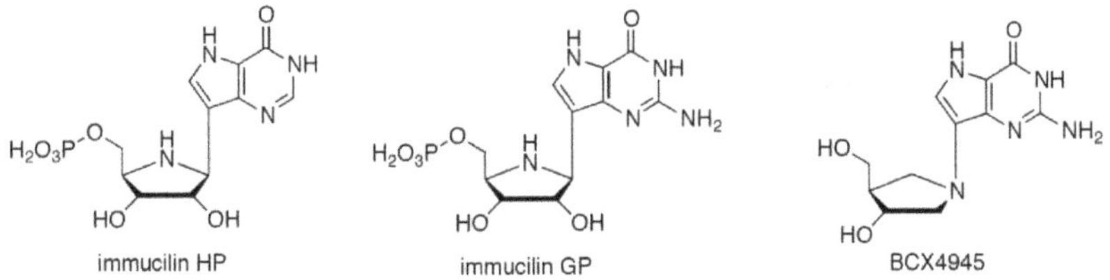

Figure 35. Antimalarial agents of dual inhibitory action.

Acknowledgements

This work is dedicated to Professor Henri-Jean Cristau from Ecole Nationale Superieure de Chimie in Mointpellier on the occasion of his 70th birthday.

Authors thank Polish Ministry of Science and Higher Education for financial support.

Author details

Karolina Gluza and Pawel Kafarski

Department of Bioorganic Chemistry, Faculty of Chemistry, Wroclaw University of Technology, Wybrzeze Wyspianskiego, Wroclaw, Poland

References

[1] Abbenante, G.; Fairlie, D. P. (2005) Protease Inhibitors in the Clinic. Medicinal Chemistry Vol. 1 (No. 1): 71-104

[2] Adachi, M.; Ohhara, T.; Kurihara, K.; Tamada, T.; Honjo, E.; Okazaki, N.; Arai, S.; Shoyama, Y.; Kimura, K.; Matsumura, H.; Sugiyama, S.; Adachi, H.; Takano, K.; Mori, Y.; Hidaka, K.; Kimura, T.; Hayashi, Y.; Kiso, Y. & Kuroki, R. (2009) Structure of HIV-1 Protease in Complex with Potent Inhibitor KNI-272 Determined by High-Resolution X-ray and Neutron Crystallography. *Proc. Natl. Acad. Sci. U.S.A.* Vol. 106 (No. 12): 4641-4646

[3] Akif, M.; Schwarger, S. L.; Anthony, C. S., Czrny, B.; Beau, F.; Dive, V.; Sturrock, E. D. & Acharya, D. L. (2011) Novel Mechanism of Inhibition of Human Angiotensin-I-Converting Enzyme (ACE) by a Highly Specific Phosphinic Tripeptide. *Biochem. J.* Vol. 436 (No. 1): 53-59

[4] Alfonso, Y. & Monzotte, L. (2011) HIV Protease Inhibitors: Effect on the Opportunistic Protozoan Parasites. *Open Med. Chem. J.* Vol. 5 (March 2011): 40-50

[5] Al-Tel, T. H.; Al-Qawasmeh, R. A.; Schmidt, M. F.; Al-Aboudi, A.; Rao, S. N.; Sabri, S. S. & Voelter, W. (2009) Rational Design and Synthesis of Potent Dibenzazepine Motifs as -Secretase Inhibitors. *J. Med. Chem.* Vol. 52 (No. 20): 6484-6488

[6] Al-Tel, T. H.; Samreen, M. H.; Al-Quawasmeh, R. A.; Schmidt, M. F.; El-Awadi, R.; Ardah, M.; Zaarour, R.; Rao, S. N. & El-Agnaf, O. (2011) Design, Synthesis, and Qualitative Structure-Activity Evaluations of Novel -Secretase Inhibitors as Potential Alzheimer's Drug Leads. *J. Med. Chem.* Vol. 54 (No. 24): 8373-8385

[7] Andreoni, M. & Perno, C. F. (2012) Positioning of HIV-Protease Inhibitors in Clinical Practice. *Eur. Rev. Med. Pharmacol. Sci.* Vol. 16 (No. 1): 10-18

[8] Anzellotti, A. I., & Farrell, N. P. (2008) Zinc Metalloproteins as Medicinal Targets. *Chem. Soc. Rev.* Vol. 37 (No. 8): 1629-1651

[9] Avram, S.; Milac, A. L.; Mihailescu, D. L.; Dabu, A. & Flonta M. L. (2006) Computer-Aided Drug Design Applied to Beta and Gamma Secretase Inhibitors-Perspectives for New Alzheimer Disease Therapy. *Curr. Enzyme Inhib.* Vol. 2 (No. 4): 311-328

[10] Banegas, I.; Prieto, I; Vives, F.; Alba, F.; deGAsparo, M.; Segarra, A. B.; Hermoso, F.; Durán, R. & Ramirez, M. (2006) Brain Aminopeptidases and Hypertension. *J. Renin Angiotensin Aldosterone Syst.* Vol. 7 (No.3): 129-134

[11] Barinka, C.; Hlouchova, K.; Rovenska, M.; Majer, P.; Dauter, M.; Hin, N.; Ko, Y.-S.; Tsukamoto, T.; Slusher, B. S.; Konvalinka, J. & Lubkowski, J. (2008) Structural Basis of Interactions between Human Glutamate Carboxypeptidase II and Its Substrate Analogs. *J. Mol. Biol.* Vol. 376 (No. 5): 1438-1350

[12] Berlicki, L.; Obojska, A.; Forlani, G. & Kafarski, P. (2005) Design, Synthesis, and Activity of Analogues of Phosphinothricin as Inhibitors of Glutamine Synthetase. *J. Med. Chem.* Vol. 48 (No. 20): 6340-6349

[13] Berlicki, L. & Kafarski P. (2006) Computer-aided Analysis of the Interactions of Glutamine Synthetase with its Inhibitors. *Bioorg. Med. Chem.* Vol. 14 (No. 13): 4578 - 4585

[14] Berlicki, L. (2008) Inhibitors of Glutamine Synthetase and Their Potential Application in Medicine. *Mini-reviews Med. Chem.*Vol. 8 (No. 9): 869 - 878

[15] Berlicki, L.; Bochno, M.; Grabowiecka, A.; Białas, A.; Kosikowska, P. & Kafarski P. (2012) N-Substituted Aminomethanephosphonic and Aminomethane-P-methylphosphinic Acids as Inhibitors of Ureases. *Amino Acids* Vol. 42 (No. 5): 1937-1942

[16] Bhat, R. G.; Kumar, N. G. & Pinto, B. M. (2007) Synthesis of Phosphate Derivatives Related to the Glycosidase Inhibitor Salacinol. *Glycomimetics* Vol. 342 (No. 12-13): 1934-1942

[17] Bianco, A.; Brufani, M.; Dri, D. A.; Melchioni, C. & Filocamo, L. (2005) Design and Synthesis of a New Furanosic Sialylmimetic as a Potential Influenza Neuraminidase Viral Inhibitor. *Lett. Org. Chem.* Vol. 2 (No. 1): 83-89

[18] Biarnés, X.; Ardèvol. A.; Iglesias-Fernández, J.; Planas, A. & Rovira, C. (2011) Catalytic Itinerary in 1,3-1,4--Glucanase Unraveled by QM/MM Metadynamics. Charge Is Not Yet Fully Developed at the Oxocarbenium Ion-like Transition State. *J. Am.Chem. Soc.* Vol. 133 (No. 50): 20301-20309

[19] Bo, Y.; Singh, S.; Duong, H. Q.; Cao, C. & Sieburtf, S. McN. (2011) Efficient, Enantio-selective Assembly of Silanediol Protease Inhibitors. *Org. Lett.* Vol. 13 (No.7): 1387-1389

[20] Bodineau, L.; Fugière, A.; Marc, Y.; Inguimbert, N.; Fassot, C.; Balavoine, F.; Roques, B. & Llorens-Cortes, C. (2008) Orally Active Aminopeptidase A Inhibitors Reduce Blood Pressure A New Strategy for Treating Hypertension. *Hypertension* Vol. 51 (No. 5): 1318-1325

[21] Breuer, E.; Salomon, C. J.; Katz, Y.; Chen, W.; Lu, S.; Röschenthaler, G.-V.; Hander, R. & Reich, R. (2004) Carbamoylphosphonates, a New Class of *In vivo* Active Matrix Metalloproteinase Inhibitors. 1. Alkyl- and Cycloalkylcarbamoylphosphonic Acids. *J. Med. Chem.* Vol. 47 (No. 11): 2826-2832

[22] Brik, A. & Wong, C.-H. (2003) HIV-1 Protease: Mechanism and Drug Discovery. *Org. Biomol. Chem.* Vol. 1 (No.)1: 5-14

[23] Buchardt, J; Bruun Schiødt, K.; Krsog-Jensen, K.; Dellaise, J.-M.; Tækker Foged, N. & Meldal, M. (2000) Solid Phase Combinatorial Library of Phosphinic Peptides for Discovery of Matrix Metalloproteinase Inhibitors. *J. Comb. Chem.* Vol. 2 (No. 6): 624-6238

[24] Cama, E.; Colleluori, D. M.; Emig, F. A.; Shin, H.; Kim, S. W.; Kim, N. N.; Traish, A. M.; Ash, D. E. & Christianson, D. W. (2003) Human Arginase II: Crystal Structure and Physiological Role in Male and Female Sexual Arousal. *Biochemistry* Vol. 43 (No. 28): 8445-8451

[25] Cama, E.; Shin, H. & Christianson, D. W. (2003a) Design of Amino Acid Sulfonamides as Transition-State Analogue Inhibitors of Arginase. *J. Am. Chem. Soc.* Vol. 125 (No. 43): 13052-13057

[26] Carrasco, N.; Hiller, D. A. & Strobel S. A. (2011) Minimal Transition State Charge Stabilization of the Oxyanion During Peptide Bond Formation by the Ribosome. *Biochemistry* Vol. 50 (No. 48): 10491-10498

[27] Cassera, M. B.; Hazleton, K. Z.; Merino, E. F.; Obladia III, N.; Ho, M.-C.; Murkin, A. S.; DePinto, R.; Gutierrez, J. A.; Almo, S. C.; Evans, G. B.; Babu, Y. S. & Schramm, V.

L. (2011) Plasmodium falciparum Parasites Are Killed by a Transition State Analogue of Purine Nucleoside Phosphorylase in a Primate Animal Model, *PloS ONE* Vol. 6 (No. 11): e26916

[28] Chaerkady, R. & Sharma, K. K. (2004) Characterization of a Bradykinin-Hydrolyzing Protease from the Bovine Lens. *Invest. Ophthalmol. Vis. Sci.* Vol. 45 (No. 4): 1214-1223

[29] Chakraborty, S.; Shah, N. K.; Fishbein, J. C. & Hoschamne R. S. (2011) A Novel Transition State Analog Inhibitor of Guanase Based on Azepinomycin Ring Structure: Synthesis and Biochemical Assessment of Enzyme Inhibition. *Bioorg. Med. Chem. Lett.* Vol. 21 (No. 2): 756-759

[30] Chan, F. Y.; Neves, M. A. C.; Sun, N.; Tsang, M. W.; Leung, Y. C.; Chan. T.-H.; Abagyan, R. & Wong, K. Y. (2012) Validation of the AmpC -Lactamase Binding Site and Identificationof Inhibitors with Novel Scaffolds. *J. Chem. Inf. Model.* Vol. 52 (No. 5): 1367-1375

[31] Chand, P.; Bantia, S.; Kotian, P.; El-Kattan, Y.; Lin, T. & Babu, Y. S. (2005) Comparison of the Anti-influenza Virus Activity of Cyclopentanederivatives with Oseltamivir and Zanamivir In Vivo. *Bioorg. Med. Chem.* Vol. 13 (No. 12): 4071–4077.

[32] Charrier, N.; Clarke, B.; Cutler, L.; Demont, E.; Dingwall, C.; Dunsdon, R.; East, P.; Hawkins, J,.; Howes, C.; Hussain, I.; Jeffrey, P.; Maile, G.; Matico, R.; Mosley, J.; Naylor, A.; O'Brien, A.; Redsahw, S.; Rowland, P.; Soleil, V.; Smith, K.; Sweitzer, S.; Theobald, P,; Vesey, D.; Walter, D. S. & Wayne, G. (2008) Second Generation of Hydroxyethylamine BACE-1 Inhibitors: Optimizing Potency and Oral Bioavailability. *J. Med. Chem.* Vol 51 (no.11): 3313-3317

[33] Chen, S. A.; Sieburth S. McN.; Glekas, A.; Hewitt, G. W.; Trainor, G. L.; Erickson-Viitanen, S.; Garbor, S. S.; Cordova, B.; Jeffrey, S. & Klabe, R. M. (2001) Drug Design with a New Transition State Analog of the Hydrated Carbonyl: Silicon-based Inhibitors of the HIV Protease. *Chem. Biol.* Vol. 8 (No.12): 1161-1166

[34] Clarke, S. G. (2007) HIV Protease Inhibitors and Nuclear Lamin Processing: Getting the Right Bells and Whistles. *Proc. Natl. Acad. Sci. U.S.A.* Vol. 104 (No. 35): 13857-13858

[35] Collinsova, M. & Jiráček, J. (2000) Phosphinic Acid Compounds in Biochemistry, Biology and Medicine. *Curr. Med. Chem.* Vol. 7 (No. 6): 629-647

[36] Cunningham, E.; Drąg, M.; Kafarski, P. & Bell, A. (2008) Chemical Target Validation Studies of Aminopeptidase in Malaria Parasites Using alpha-Aminoalkylphosphonate and Phosphonopeptide Inhibitors. *Antimirob. Agnets Chemother.* Vol. 52 (No. 9): 3221 – 3228

[37] Davies, G. J.; Planas, A. P. & Rovira C. (2012) Conformational Analyses of the Reaction Coordinate of Glycosidases. *Acc. Chem. Res.* Vol. 45 (No.2): 308-316

[38] Devel, L.; Garcia, S.; Czarny B.; Beau, F.; Lajeunesse, E.; Vera, L.; Georgiadis, D.; Sture , E. & Dive, V. (2010) Insights from Selective Non-phosphinic Inhibitors of

MMP-12 Tailored to Fit with an S_1' Loop Canonical Conformation. *J. Biol. Chem.* Vol. 285 (No. 46): 35900-35909

[39] Dive, V.; Georgiadis, D.; Matziari, M.; Beau, F.; Cuniasse, P. & Yiotakis, A. (2004) Phosphinic Peptides as Zinc Metalloproteinase Inhibitors. *Cell. Mol. Life Sci.* Vol. 61 (No. 16): 2010-2019

[40] Drag, M. & Salvesen, G. S. (2010) Emerging Principles in Protease-based Drug Discovery. *Nature Rev. Drug. Discov.* Vol. 9 (September 2010): 690-701

[41] Drag, M.; Bogya, M.; Ellman, J. A. & Salvesen, G. S. (2010) Aminopeptidase Fingerprints, an Integrated Approach for Identification of Good Substrates and Optimal Inhibitors. *J. Biol. Chem.* Vol. 285 (No. 5): 3310-3318

[42] Dybala-Defratyka, A.; Rostkowski, M. & Paneth, P. (2008) Enzyme Mechanisms from Molecular Modeling and Isotope Effects. *Archiv. Biochem. Biophys.* Vol. 474 (No. 2): 274-282

[43] Dzekieva, L.; Rocaboy, M.; Kerff, F.; Charlier, P.; Sauvage, E. & Pratt, R. F (2010) Crystal Structure of a Complex between the *Actinomadura* R39 DD-Peptidase and a Peptidoglycan-mimetic Boronate Inhibitor: Interpretation of a Transition State Analogue in Terms of Catalytic Mechanism. *Biochemistry* Vol. 49 (No. 30): 6411-6419

[44] Dzekieva, L.; Kumar, I. & Pratt, R. F. (2012) Inhibition of Bacterial DD-Peptidases (Penicillin-Binding Proteins) in Membranes and in Vivo by Peptidoglycan-Mimetic Boronic Acid, *Biochemistry* Vol. 58 (No. 13): 2804-2811

[45] Eder, J.; Hommel, U.; Cumin, F.; Martoglio, B. & Gerthartz, B. (2007) Aspartic Proteases in Drug Discovery. *Curr. Pharm. Des.* Vol. 13 (No. 3): 271-285

[46] Edwards, A. A.; Mason, J. M.; Clinch, K.; Tyler, P. C.; Evans, G. B. & Schramm V. L. (2009) Altered Enthalpy-Entropy Compensation in Picomolar Transition State Analogues of Human Purine Nucleoside Phosphorylase. *Biochemistry* Vol. 48 (No. 23): 5226-5238

[47] Eidam, Oliv.; Romagnoli, C.; Caselli, E.; Babaoglu, K.; Teotico Pohlhaus, D.; Karpiak, J.; Bonnet, R.; Stoichet, B. K. & Prati, F. (2010) Design, Synthesis, Crystal Structures, and Antimicrobial Activity of Sulfonamide Boronic Acids as -Lactamase Inhibitors. *J. Med. Chem.* Vol. 53 (No.21): 7852-7863

[48] Ellsworth, B. A.; Tom, N. J. & Bartlett, P. A. (1996) Synthesis and Evaluation of Inhibitors of Bacterial D-Alanine:D-Alanine Ligases. *Chem.Biol.* Vol. 3, (No. 1): 37–44

[49] Evans, G. B.; Furneaux, R. H.; Greatrex, B.; Murkin, A. S.; Schramm, V. L. & Tyler, P. C. (2008) Azetidine Based Transition State Analogue Inhibitors of N-Ribosyl Hydrolases and Phosphorylases. *J. Med.Chem.* Vol. 51 (No. 4): 948-956

[50] Evdokimov, A. G.; Pokross, M.; Walter, R. M.; Mekel, M.; Barnett, B. L.; Amburger, J.; Seibel, W. L.; Soper, S.J.; Djung, J, F.; Fairweather, N.; Diven, C.; Rastogi, V.; Grinius, L.; Klanke, C.; Siehner, R.; Twinem, T. & Andrews, R. (2007) Serendipitous Discovery

of Novel Bacterial Methionine Aminopeptidase Inhibitors. *Proteins* Vol. 66 (No. 3): 538-546

[51] Fisher, J. F. & Mobashery S. (2006) Recent Advances in Recent MMP Inhibitor Design. *Cancer Matastasis Rev.* Vol. 25 (No. 1): 115-136

[52] Fournié-Zaluski, M.-C.; Poras, H.; Roques, B.P.; Nakajima, Y.; Ito, K. & Yoshimoto, T. (2009) Structure of Aminopeptidase N from *Escherichia coli* Complexed with the Transition-state Analogue Aminophosphinic Inhibitor PL250. *Acta Crystallogr. D* Vol. 65 (No. 8): 814-822

[53] Frase, H. F. & Lee, I. (2007) Peptidyl Boronates Inhibit *Salmonella enterica* Serovar Typhimurium Lon Protease by a Competitive ATP-Dependent Mechanism, *Biochemistry* Vol. 46 (No.22): 6647-6657

[54] Fujimoto, T.; Matsushita, Y.; Gouda, H.; Yamaotsu, N. & Hirono, S. (2008) In Silico Multi-filter Screening Approaches for Developing Novel -Secretase Inhibitors. *Bioorg. Med. Chem. Lett.* Vol. 18 (No. 9): 2771-2775

[55] Gajda, A.; Pawelczak, M. & Drag, M. (2012) Substrate Specificity Screening of Oat (*Avena sativa*) Seeds Aminopeptidase Demonstrate Unusually Broad Tolerance in S1 Pocket. *Plant Physiol. Biochem.* Vol. 54 (May 2012): 6-9

[56] Ghavami, A.; Johnston, B. D. & Pinto, B. M. (2001) A New Class of Glycosidase Inhibitor: Synthesis of Salacinol and Its Stereoisomers. *J. Org. Chem.,* Vol. 66 (No .7): 2312-2317

[57] Gloster, T. M. & Davies, G. J. (2010) Glycosidase Inhibition: Assessing Mimicry of the Transition State. *Org. Biomol. Chem.* Vol. 8 (No.): 305-320

[58] Gonzaga-Jagureui, C.; Lupski, J. R. & Gibbs, R. A. (2012) Human Genome Sequencing in Health and Disease. *Annu. Rev. Med.* Vol. 63: 35-61

[59] Green, R. & Lorsch, J. R. (2002) The Path to Perdition Is Paved with Protons. *Cell* Vol. 110 (No. 6): 665-668

[60] Grembecka, J. & Kafarski, P. (2001) Leucine Aminopeptidase as a Target for Inhibitor Design. *Mini Rev. Med. Chem.* Vol. 1 (No. 2): 133 - 144.

[61] Grembecka, J.; Mucha, A.; Cierpicki, T. & Kafarski, P. (2003) The Most Potent Organophosphorus Inhibitors of Leucine Aminopeptidase. Structure-based Design, Chemistry, and Activity. *J. Med. Chem.* Vol. 46 (No. 13): 2641 – 2655

[62] Grzywa, R.; Oleksyszyn, J.; Salvesen, G. S. & Drag, M. (2010) Identification of Very Potent Inhibitor of Human Aminopeptidase N (CD13). *Bioorg. Med. Chem. Lett.* Vol. 20 (No.8): 2497-2499

[63] Gurulingappa, H.; Buckhaults, P.; Kumar, S. K.; Kinzler K. W.; Vogelstein, B. & Khazn, S. R. (2003) Design, Synthesis and Evaluation of New RDP Inhibitors. *Tetrahedron Lett.* Vol. 44 (No. 9): 1871-1873

[64] Hamada, Y.; Tagad, H. D.; Nishimura, Y.; Ishiura, S. & Kiso, Y. (2012) Tripeptidic BACE1 Inhibitors Devised by *In-silico* Conformational Structure-based Design. *Bioorg. Med. Chem.* Vol. 22 (No. 2): 1130-1135

[65] Henley, D. B.; May, P. C.; Dean, R.A. & Siemers, R. E. (2009) Development of Semagacestat (LY450139), a Functional Gamma-secretase Inhibitor, for the Treatment of Alzheimer's Disease. *Expert Opinion Pharmacoother.* Vol. 10 (No. 10): 1657-1654

[66] Hibi, T.; Nii, H.; Nakatsu, T.; Kimura, A.; Kato, H.; Hiratake, J. & Oda, J. (2004) Crystal Structure of γ -Glutamylcysteine Synthetase: Insights Into the Mechanism of Catalysis by a Key Enzyme for Glutathione Homeostasis. *Proc. Natl. Acad. Sci. U.S.A.* Vol. 101 (No. 42): 15052-15057

[67] Holyoak, T.; Kettner, C. A.; Petsko, G. A; Fuller, R. S. & Ringe, D. (2004) Structural Basis for Differences in Substrate Selectivity in Kex2 and Furin Protein Convertases. *Biochemistry* Vol. 43 (No. 9): 2412-2421

[68] Hou, G. & Cui, Q. (2011) QM/MM Analysis Suggests that Alkaline Phosphatase (AP) and Nucleotide Pyrophosphatase/Phosphodiesterase Slightly Tighten the Transition State for Phosphate Diester Hydrolysis Relative to Solution: Implication for Catalytic Promiscuity in the AP Superfamily. *J. Am. Chem. Soc.* Vol. 134 (No. 1): 229-246

[69] Hu, G.; Lin, G.; Wang, M.; Dick, L.; Xu, R. M.; Nathan, C. & Li, H. (2006) Structure of the Mycobacterium tuberculosis Proteasome and Mechanism of Inhibition by a Peptidyl Boronate. *Mol. Microbiol.* Vol. 59 (No. 5): 1417-1428

[70] Hu, Y. P; Liu, H. G.; Teng, K. H. & Liang, P. H. (2010) Mechanism of cis-Prenyltransferase Reaction Probed by Substrate Analogues. *Biochem. Biophys. Res. Commun.* Vol. 400 (No. 4): 758-762

[71] Iyer, L. M.; Zhang, D. P. ; Rogozhin, I. B. & Aravind, L. (2011) Evolution of the Deaminase Fold and Multiple Origins of Eukaryotic Editing and Mutagenic Nucleic Acid Deaminases from Bacterial Toxin Systems. *Nucl. Acid. Res.* Vol. 39 (No. 22): 9473-9497

[72] Jeurs, D. H.; Kim, J.; Matthews, B. W. & Sieburth, S. McN. (2005) Structural Analysis of Silanediols as Transition-State-Analogue Inhibitors of the Benchmark Metalloprotease Thermolysin. *Biochemistry* Vol. 44 (No. 50): 16524-16528

[73] John, S.; Thangapandian, S.; Sakkiah, S. & Lee, K. W. (2011) Potent Bace-1 Inhibitor Design Using Pharmacophore Modeling, In Silico Screening and Molecular Docking Studies. *BMC Bioinformatics* Vol. 12 (Suppl. 1): S28

[74] Johnson, J. L.; Devel, L.; Czarny, B.; George, S. J.; Jackson, C. L.; Rogakos, V.; Beau, F.; Yiokatis, A.; Newby, A. C. & Dive, V. (2011) A Selective Matrix Metalloproteinase-12 Inhibitor Retards Atherosclerotic Plaque Development in Apolipoprotein E-knockout Mice. *Arterioscl. Tromb. Vasc. Biol.* Vol. 31 (No. 3): 528-535

[75] Jørgensen, A. T.; Norrby, P. O. & Liljefors, T. (2002) Investigation of the Metal Binding Site in Methionine Aminopeptidase by Density Functional Theory. *J. Comput. Aided Mol. Des.* Vol. 16 (No. 3): 167-179

[76] Julien, N.; Makritis, A; Georgiadis, D.; Beau, F.; Yiotakis, A. & Dive, V. (2010) Phosphinic Tripeptides as Dual Angiotensin-Converting Enzyme C-Domain and Endothelin-Converting Enzyme-1 Inhibitors. *J. Med. Chem,. Vol.* 53 (No. 1): 208-220

[77] Kalva, S.; Vadivelan, S.; Sanam, R.; Jagarlapudi, S. A. R. P. & Saleena, L. M. (2012) Lead Identification and Optimization of Novel Collagenase Inhibitors; Pharmacophore and Structure Based Studies. *Bioinformation* Vol. 8 (No. 7): 301-308

[78] Kati, W. M.; Montgomery, D.; Maring, C.; Stoll, V. S.; Giranda, V.; Chen, X.; Laver, W. G.; Kohlbrenner, W. & Norbeck, D. W. (2001) Novel - and -Amino Acid Inhibitors of Influenza Virus Neuraminidase. *Antimicrob. Agents Chemither.* Vol. 45 (No. 9): 2563-2570

[79] Ke, W.; Sampson, J. M.; Ori, C.; Prato, F.; Drawz, S. E.; Bethel, C. R.; Bonomo, R. A.; & van den Akken, F. (2011) Novel Insights into the Mode of Inhibition of Class A SHV-1 -Lactamases Revealed by Boronic Acid Transition State Inhibitors. *Antimicrob. Agents Chemother.* Vol. 55 (No. 1): 174-183

[80] Keough, D. T.; Hoćkova, D.; Holy, A.; Naesenes, L. M. J.; Skinner-Adams, T. S.; de Jersey, J.; & Guddat, L. W. (2009) Inhibition of Hypoxanthine - Guanine Phosphoribosyltransferase by Acyclic Nucleoside Phosphonates:A New Class of Antimalarial Therapeutics. *J. Med. Chem.* Vol. 52 (No.): 4391-4399

[81] Khaliullin, I. G.; Suplatov, D. A.; Dalaeva, D. L.; Otsuka, M.; Asano, Y. & Švedas, V. K. (2010) Bioinformatic Analysis, Molecular Modeling of Role of Lys65 Residue in Catalytic Triad of D-aminopeptidase from Ochrobactrum anthropi. Acta Naturae Vol. 2 (No. 2): 66-71

[82] Khandelwal, A.; Lukacova, V.; Comez, D.; Kroll, D. M.; Raha, S. & Balaz, S. (2005) A Combination of Docking, QM/MM Methods, and MD Simulation for Binding Affinity Estimation of Metalloprotein Ligands. *J. Med. Chem.* Vol. 48 (No. 17): 5437-5447

[83] Kim, C. U.; Williams, M. A.; Lui, H.; Zhang, L.; Swaminathan, S.; Bischofberger, N.; Chen, M. S.; Mendel, D.B.; Tai, C. Y.; Laver, W. G. & Stevens, R. C. (1997). Influenza Neuraminidase Inhibitors Possessing a Novel Hydrophobic Interaction in the Enzyme Active Site: Design, Synthesis and Structural Analysis of Carbocyclic Sialic Acid Analogues with PotentAanti-influenza Activity. *J. Am. Chem. Soc.* Vol. 119 (No. 4) 681–690.

[84] Kollman, P. A.; Kuhn, B. & Peräkylä, M. (2002) Computational Studies of Enzyme-Catalyzed Reactions: Where Are We in Predicting Mechanisms and in Understanding the Nature of Enzyme Catalysis? *J. Phys. Chem. B* Vol. 106 (No. 7): 1537-1542

[85] Kosikowska, P. & Berlicki, L. (2011) Urease Inhibitors as Potential Drugs for Gastric and Urinary Tract Infections: a Patent Review. *Expert Opin. Ther. Patents* Vol. 21 (No. 6): 945-957

[86] Kotsugi, T. & Hayashi, S. (2012) Crucial Role of Protein Flexibility in Formation of a Stable Reaction Transition State in an -Amylase Catalysis. *J. Am. Chem. Soc.* Vol. 134 (No. 16): 7045-7055

[87] Kruger, R. G.; Barkallah, S.; Frankel, B. A. & Mc Cafferty, B. G. (2004) Inhibition of the *Staphylococcus aureus* Sortase Transpeptidase SrtA by Phosphinic Peptidomimetics. *Bioorg. Med. Chem.* Vol. 12 (No.13): 3723-3729

[88] Lauer-Fields, J. L.; Brew, K.; Whitehead, J. K.; Li, S.; Hammer, R. P. & Fields, G.B. (2007) Triple-Helical Transition State Analogues: A New Class of Selective Matrix Metalloproteinase Inhibitors. *J. Am. Chem. Soc.* Vol. 129 (No. 30): 10408-10417

[89] Lauer-Fields, J. L.; Whitehead, J. K.; Li, S.; Hammer, R. P. ; Brew, K. & Fields, G.B. (2008) Selective Modulation of Matrix Metalloproteinase 9 (MMP-9) Functions via Exosite Inhibition. *J. Biol. Chem.* Vol. 283 (No.29): 20087-20095

[90] Lazcano, I.; Uribe, R. M.; Martinez-Cháves, E.; Vargas, M. A.; Matziari, M.; Joseph-Bravo P. & Charli, J. M. (2012) Pyroglutamyl Peptidase II Inhibition Enhances the Analeptic Effect of Thyrotropin-Releasing Hormone in the Rat Medial Septum. *J. Pharmacol. Exp. Ther.* Vol. 342 (No. 1): 222-231

[91] Lebeau, A.; Singh, P.; Isaacs, J, & Denmeade, S. R. (2008) Potent and Selective Peptidyl Boronic Acid Inhibitors of the Serine Protease Prostate-Specific Antigen. *Chem. Biol.* Vol. 15 (No. 7): 665-674

[92] Lee, J. K.; Bain, A. D. & Berti, P. J. (2004) Probing the Transition States of Four Glucoside Hydrolyses with ^{13}C Kinetic Isotope Effects Measured at Natural Abundance by NMR Spectroscopy. *J. Am. Chem. Soc.* Vol. 126 (No. 12): 3769-3776

[93] Li, X.; Hayik, S. A. & Merz Jr, K. M. (2010) QM/MM X-Ray Refinement of Zinc Metalloenzymes. *J. Inorg. Biochem.* Vol. 104 (No. 5): 512-522

[94] Li, Y.; Cao, H.; Hai, Y.; Chen, Y.; Lau, K.; Qu, J.; Thon, V.; Sugirato, G. & Chen, X. (2011) Identifying Selective Inhibitors Against Human Cytosolic Sialidase NEU2 by Substrate Specificity Studies. *Mol. Biosyst.* Vol. 7 (No. 4): 1060-1072

[95] Lienhard, G. E. (1973) Enzymatic Catalysis and Transition-state Theory, *Science* Vol. 180 (No. 4082): 149-154

[96] Lin, Y.-L & Gao, J. (2011) Kinetic Isotope Effects of *L*-Dopa Decarboxylase, *J. Am. Chem. Soc.* Vol,. 133 (No. 12): 4398-4403

[97] Lipscamp, R. M. J. & Kruijtzer J. A. W. (2004) Peptide Transformation Leading to Peptide-peptidosulfonamide Hybrids and Oligo Peptidosulfonamides. *Mol. Divers.* Vol. 8 (No. 2): 787-97

[98] Liu, H.; Sim. L.; Rose, D. L. & Pinto, B. M. (2006) A New Class of Glucosidase Inhibitor: Analogues of the Naturally Occurring Glucosidase Inhibitor Salacinol with Different Ring Heteroatom Substituents and Acyclic Chain Extension. *J. Org. Chem.* Vol. 71 (No. 8): 3007-3013

[99] Lonsdale, R.; Harvey, J. N. & Mulholland, A. J. (2010) Compound I Reactivity Defines Alkene Oxidation Selectivity in Cytochrome P450cam. *J. Phys. Chem. B* Vol.114, (No. 2): 1156–1162

[100] Lonsdale, R.; Harvey, J. N. & Mulholland, A. J. (2012) A Practical Guide to Modelling Enzyme-Catalysed Reactions. *Chem. Soc. Rev.* Vol. 41 (No. 8): 3025–3038

[101] Löwik, D. W. P. M. and Liskamp, R. M. J. (2000) Synthesis of - and -Substituted Aminoethane Sulfonamide Arginine-Glycine Mimics. *Eur. J.Org. Chem.*, Vol. 2000 (No. 7): 1219-1228

[102] Lowther, W. T. & Matthews, B. W. (2002) Metalloaminopeptidases: Common Functional Themes in Disparate Structural Surroundings. *Chem. Rev.* Vol. 102 (No.12): 4581-4607

[103] Mahalingham, A. K.; Axelsson, L.; Ekegren, J. K.; Wanneberg, B.; Kihlström, J.; Unge, T,; Wallberg, H.; Samuelsson, B.; Larhed, M. & Hallberg, A (2010) HIV-1 Protease Inhibitors with a Transition-State Mimic Comprising a Tertiary Alcohol: Improved Antiviral Activity in Cells. *J. Med. Chem.* Vol. 53 (No. 2): 607-615

[104] Martone, R. L.; Zhou, H.; Atchison, K.; Comery, T.; Xu, J. Z.; Huang, X.; Gong, X.; Jin, M.; Kreft, A.; Harrison, B.; Mayer, S. C.; Aschmies, S.; Gonzales, C.; Zaleska, M. M.; Riddel, D. R.; Wagner, E.; Lu, P.; Sun, S.-C.; Sonnenberg-Reines, J.; Oganesian, A.; Adkins, K.; Leach, M.W.; Clarke, D. W.; Huryn, D.; Abou-Gharbia, M.; Magolda, R.; Bard, J.; Frick, G.; Raje, S.; Forlow, S. B.; Balliet, C.; Burczynski R. E.; Reinhart, P. H.; Wan, H. I.; Pangalos, M. N. & Jacobsen, J. S. (2009) Begacestat (GSI-953): A Novel, Selective Thiophene Sulfonamide Inhibitor of Amyloid Precursor Protein -Secretase for the Treatment of Alzheimer's Disease. *J. Parmacol. Exp. Ther.* Vol. 331 (No. 2): 598-608

[105] Matziari, M.; Beau, F.; Cuniasse, P.; Dive, V. & Yiotakis, A. (2004) Evaluationof P1'-Diversified Phosphinic Peptides Leads to the Development Ofhighly Selective Inhibitors of MMP-11. *J. Med. Chem.* Vol. 47 (No. 2): 325-336

[106] Matziari, M.; Dive, V. & Yiotakis, A. (2007) Matrix Metalloproteinase 11 (MMP-11; Stromelysin-3) and Synthetic Inhibitors. *Med. Res. Rev.* Vol. 27 (No. 4): 528-552

[107] Matziari, M.; Bauer, K.; Dive, V. & Yiotakis, A. (2008) Synthesis of the Phosphinic Analogue of Thyrotropin Releasing Hormone. *J. Org. Chem.* Vol. 73 (No. 21): 8591-8693

[108] Mayer, S. C.; Kreft, A. S.; Harrison, B.; Abou-Gharbia, M.; Antane, M.; Aschmies, S.; Atchison, K.; Chlenov, M.; Cole, D. C.; Comery, T.; Diamantis, G.; Ellingboe, J.; Fan, K.; Gallante, R.; Gonzales, K.; Ho, D. M.; Hoke, M. E.; Hu, Y.; Huryn, D.; Jain, U.; Jin, M.; Kremer, K.; Kubrak, D.; Lin, M.; Lu, P.; Magolda, R.; Martone, R.; Moore, W.; Oganesian, A.; Pangalos, M. N.; Porte, A.; Reinhart, P.; Resnick, L.; Riddel, D. R.; Sonnenberg-Reines, J.; Stock, J. R.; Sun, S.-C.; Wagner, E.; Wang, T.; Woller, K.; Xu, Z.; Zaleska, M. M.; Zeldis, J.; Zhang, M.; Zhou, H. & Jacobsen J. S. (2008) Discovery of Begacestat, a Notch-1-Sparing -Secretase Inhibitor for the Treatment of Alzheimer's Disease. *J. Med. Chem.* Vol. 51 (No. 23): 7348-7351

[109] McGowan, S.; Oellig, C. A.; Birru, W. A.; Caradoc-Davies, T. T.; Stack, C. M.; Lowther, J.; Skinner-Adams, T.; Mucha, A.; Kafarski, P.; Grembecka, J.; Trenholme, K. R.; Buckle, A. M.; Gardiner, D. L.; Dalton, J. P. & Whisstock, J. C. (2010) Structure of the *Plasmodium falciparum* M17 Aminopeptidase and Significance for the Design of Drugs Targeting the Neutral Exopeptidases. *Proc. Natl. Acad. Sci. U.S.A.* Vol. 107, (No. 6), 2449 – 2454

[110] McGowan, S.; Porter, C. J.; Lowther. J.; Stack, C. M.; Golding, S. J.; Skinner-Adams, T. S.; Trenholme, K. R.; Teuscher, F.; Donnelly, S. M.; Grembecka, J.; Mucha, A.; Kafarski, P.; Degori, R.; Buckle, A. M.; Gardiner, D. L.; Whisstock, J. C. & Dalton, J. P. (2009) Structural Basis for the Inhibition of the Essential Plasmodium falciparum M1 Neutral Aminopeptidase. *Proc. Natl. Acad. Sci. U.S.A.* Vol. 106 (No. 8): 2537 – 2542

[111] Medina, R. A. & Garcia-Sastre, A. (2011) Influenza A Viruses: New Research Developments. *Nat. Rev. Microbiol.* Vol. 9 (August 2011): 590-603

[112] Meanwell, N. A. (2011) Synopsis of Some Recent Tactical Application of Bioisosteres in Drug Design. *J. Med. Chem.* Vol. 54 (No. 8): 2529-2591

[113] Mohan, S. & Pinto, B. M. (2008) Zwitterionic Glycosidase Inhibitors: Salacinol and Related Analogues. *Carbohydr. Res.* Vol. 342 (No. 12-13): 1551-1580

[114] Moree, W. J.; Van Gent, L. C.; Van Der Marel, G. A. & Liskamp,R. M. J., (1993) Synthesis of Peptides Containing a Sulfinamide or a Sulfonamidetransition State Isostere. *Tetrahedron* Vol. 49 (No.5): 1133-1150

[115] Moree, W. J.; Van Der Marel, G. A. & Liskamp, R. M. J. (1995) Synthesis of Peptidosulfinamides and Peptidosulfonamides Containing the Sulfinamide or Sulfonamide Transition-state Isostere. *J. Org. Chem.*, Vol. 60 (No. 16): 5157-5169

[116] Mores, A.; Matziari, M.; Beau, F.; Cuniasse, P.; Yiotakis, A. & Dive, V,.(2008) Development of Potent and Selective Phosphinic Peptide Inhibitors of Angiotensin-Converting Enzyme 2. *J. Med. Chem.* Vol. 51 (No.7): 2216-2226

[117] Mucha, A.; Pawelczak, M.; Hurek, J. & Kafarski, P. (2004) Synthesis and Activity of Phosphinic Tripeptide Inhibitors of Cathepsin C. *Bioorg. Med. Chem. Lett.* Vol. 14 (No. 12) 3113 – 3116

[118] Mucha, A.; Lämmerhoffer, M.; Lindner, W.; Pawelczak, M. & Kafarski, P. (2008) Individual Stereoisomers of Phosphinic Dipeptide Inhibitor of Leucine Aminopeptidase. *Bioorg. Med. Chem. Lett.* Vol. 18 (No. 5): 1550-1554

[119] Mucha, A.; Drag, M.; Dalton, J. P. & Kafarski, P. (2010) Metallo-Aminopeptidase Inhibitors. *Biochimie* Vol. 92 (No. 11): 1509 - 1529.

[120] Mucha, A.; Kafarski, P. & Berlicki, L. (2011) Remarkable Potential of the -Aminophosphonate/Phosphinate Structural Motif in Medicinal Chemistry. *J. Med. Chem.* Vol. 54 (No. 17): 5955-5980

[121] Muo, L. & Schramm, V. L. (2008) Transition State Structure of E. coli tRNA-Specific Adenosine Deaminase. *J. Am. Chem. Soc.* Vol. 130 (No. 8): 2649-2655

[122] Murkin, A. S.; Birck, M. R.; Rinaldo-Matthis, A.; Shi, W.; Taylor, E. A.; Almo, S. C. & Schramm, V. L. (2007) Neighboring Group Participation in the Transition State of Human Purine Nucleoside Phosphorylase. *Biochemistry* Vol. 26 (No. 17): 5038-5049

[123] Mutahi, M.; Nittoli, T.; Guo, L.; Sieburth, S. McN. (2002) Silicon-based Metalloprotease Inhibitors: Synthesis and Evaluation of Silanol and Silanediol Peptide Analogues as Inhibitors of Angiotensin-converting Enzyme. *J. Am. Chem. Soc.* Vol. 124 (No. 25): 7363-7365

[124] Nelson, M. I. & Holmes, E. C. (2007) The Evolution of Epidemic Influenza, *Nat. Rev, Genet.* Vol. 8 (March 2007): 196-205

[125] Neuhaus, F. C. (2010) Role of Arg301 in Substrate Orientation and Catalysis in Subsite 2 of D-Alanine:D-alanine (D-Lactate) Ligase from Leuconostoc mesenteroides: A Molecular Docking Study. J. *Mol. Graphics Model.* Vol. 28 (No. 8): 728–734

[126] Nukaga, M.; Kumar, S.; Nukaga, K.; Pratt, R. F. & Knox, J. R. (2004) Hydrolysis of Third-generation Cephalosporins by Class C -Lactamases. *J. Biol. Chem.* Vol. 10 (No. 5): 9344-9352

[127] Osterman, N.; Eder, J.; Eidhoff, U.; Zink, F.; Hassiepen, U.; Worpenberg, S.; Mainbaum, J. Simic, O.; Hommel, U. & Gerhartz, B. (2006) Crystal Structure of Human BACE2 in Complex with a Hydroxyethylamine Transition-state Inhibitor. *J. Mol. Biol.* Vol. 355 (No.)2: 249-261

[128] Overall, C. M. & Kleifield O. (2006) Validating Matrix Metalloproteinases as Drug Targets and Anti-targets for Cancer Therapy *Nat. Rev. Cancer* Vol. 6 (No. 3): 227-239

[129] Palese, P.; Schulman, J. N.; Bodo, G. &Meindl, P. (1974). Inhibition of Influenza and Parainfluenza Virus Replication in Tissue culture by 2-Deoxy-2,3-dehydro-N-trifluoroacetylneuraminic Acid (FANA). *Virology* Vol. 59 (No. 2) 490–498.

[130] Parks, J. M., Imhof, P. & Smith, J. C. (2010) Understanding Enzyme Catalysis Using Computer Simulation. *Encyclopedia of Catalysis 2nd Ed.* John Wiley & Sons 2010

[131] Pauling, L. (1949) Achievement and Hope for the Future. *Am. Sci.* Vol. 36: 50-58

[132] Pierdominici-Sottile, G.; Horenstein, N. A. & Roitberg A. E. (2011) Free Energy Study of the Catalytic Mechanism of *Trypanosoma cruzi trans*-Sialidase. From the Michaelis Complex to the Covalent Intermediate. *Biochemistry* Vol. 22 (No. 46): 10150-10158

[133] Pirard, B. (2007) Insight Into the Structural Determinants for Selective Inhibition of Matrix Metalloproteinases. *Drug Discovery Today* Vol. 12 (No.15/16): 640-646

[134] Pokorná, J.; Machala, L.; Řezáčova, P. & Konvalinka, J. (2009) Current and Novel Inhibitors of HIV Protease. *Viruses* Vol. 1 (No. 3): 1209-1239

[135] Polgár, L. (2005) The catalytic triad of serine peptidases. *Cell. Mol. Life Sci.* Vol. 62 (No. 19-20): 2161-2172

[136] Poreba, M.; Gajda, A.; Picha, J.; Jiráček, J.; Marschner, A.; Klein, C. D., Salvesen, G. S. & Drag, M. (2011) S1 Pocket Fingerprints of Human and Bacterial Methionine Aminopeptidases Determined Using Fluorogenic Libraries of Substrates and Phosphorus Based Inhibitors. *Biochimie* Vol. 94 (No. 3): 704-710

[137] Poreba M.; McGowan, S.; Skinner-Adams, T. S.; Trenholme, K. S.; Gardiner, D. L.; Whisstock, J. C.; To, J.; Salvesen, G. S.; Dalton, J. P. & Drag, M. (2012) Fingerprinting the Substrate Specificity of M1 and M17 Aminopeptidases of Human Malaria, *Plasmodium falciparum. PLOS One* Vol. 7 (No. 2): e31938

[138] Powell, J. R.; DeForrest, J. M.; Cushman, D. W.; Rubin, B. & Petrillo, E. W. (1984) Antihypertensive Effects of a New ACE Inhibitor, SQ. 28555. *Fed. Proc.* Vol. 43 (No. 3): 733

[139] Radzicka, A., and Wolfenden, R. (1995) Transition State and Multisubstrate Analog Inhibitors, *Methods Enzymol.* Vol. 249: 284-312

[140] Reiter, L. A.; Martinelli, G. J.; Reeves, L. A. & Mitchell, P. G. (2000) Difluoroketones as Inhibitors of Matrix Metalloprotease-13. *Bioorg. Med. Chem. Lett.* Vol. 10 (No.14): 1581-1584

[141] Reiter, L. A.; Mitchell, P. G.; Martinelli, G. J.; Lopresti-Morrow, L. L.; Yocum, S. A. & Escra, J. D. (2003) Phosphinic Acid-Based MMP-13 Inhibitors That Spare MMP-1 and MMP-3. *Bioorg. Med. Chem. Lett.* Vol. 13 (No. 14): 2331-2336

[142] Rejman, D.; Panova, N.; Klener, P.; Maswabi, B.; Pohl, R. & Rosenberg, I. (2012) N-Phosphonocarbonylpyrrolidine Derivatives of Guanine: A NewClass of Bi-Substrate Inhibitors of Human Purine Nucleoside Phosphorylase. *J. Med. Chem.* Vol. 55 (No. 4): 1612-1621

[143] Rempel, B. R. & Withers, S. G. (2008) Covalent Inhibitors of Glycosidases and Their Applications in Biochemistry and Biology. *Glycobiology* Vol. 18 (No 8): 570-586

[144] Robertson, J. G. (2005) Mechanistic Basis of Enzyme-Targeted Drugs. *Biochemistry* Vol. 44 (No. 15): 5561-5571

[145] Rodnina, M. V.; Beringer, L. & Wintermeyer, W. (2006) How Ribosomes Make Peptide Bonds. *Trends Biochem. Sci.* Vol 31 (No.1): 20-26

[146] Sabina, R. L.; Paul, A.-L.; Ferl, R. J.; Laber, B. & Lindell, S. D. (2007) Adenine Nucleotide Pool Perturbation Is a Metabolic Trigger for AMP Deaminase Inhibitor-Based Herbicide Toxicity. *Plant Physiol.* Vol. 143 (No. 4): 1752-1760

[147] Saen-oon, S.; Quaytman-Machleder, S.; Schramm, V. L. & Schwartz, S. D. (2008) Atomic Detail of Chemical Transformation at the Transition State of an Enzymatic Reaction. *PNAS* Vol. 105 (No. 43): 16543-16545

[148] Sang, Q.-X. A.; Jin, Y.; Newcomer, R. G.; Monroe, S. C.; Fang, X.; Hurst, D. R.; Lee, S.; Cao, Q. & Schwartz, M. A. (2006) Matrix Metalloproteinase Inhibitors as Prospective Agents for the Prevention and Treatment of Cardiovascular and Neoplastic Diseases. *Curr. Top. Med. Chem.* Vol. 6 (No. 4): 289-316

[149] Schramm, V. L. (2002) Development of Transition State Analogues of Purine Nucleoside Phosphorylase as Anti-T-cell Agents. *Biochim. Biophys. Acta* Vol. 1587 (No. 2-3): 107-117

[150] Schramm, V. L. (2005) Enzymatic Transition States and Transition State Analogues. *Curr. Opin. Struct. Biol.* Vol. 15 (No. 7): 604-613

[151] Schramm, V. L. (2007) Enzymatic Transition State Theory and Transition State Analogue Design. *J. Biol. Chem.* Vol. 282 (No. 39): 28297-28300

[152] Schramm, V. L. (2011) Enzymatic Transition States, Transition-State Analogs, Dynamics, Thermodynamics, and Lifetimes. *Annu. Rev. Biochem.* Vol. 80: 703-732

[153] Schwartz, P. A.; Vetticatt, J. & Schramm V. L. (2010) Transition State Analysis of Thymidine Hydrolysis by Human Thymidine Phosphorylase. *J. Am. Chem. Soc.* Vol. 132 (No. 38): 13425-13433

[154] Senn, H. M. & Thiel, W. (2007) QM/MM Studies of Enzymes. *Curr. Opin. Chem. Biol.* Vol. 11 (No. 2): 182-187

[155] Shi, W.; Wu, C. M.; Tyler, P.C.; Furmeaux, R. H.; Cahill, S. M.; Girvin, M. E.; Grubmeyer, C.; Schramm, V. L & Almo, S.C. (1999) The 2.0 Å Structure of Malarial Purine Phosphoribosyltransferase in Complex with a Transition-State Analogue Inhibitor. *Biochemistry* Vol. 38 (No. 31): 9872-9880

[156] Shie, J. J.; Fang, J. M.; Wang, S. Y.; Tsai, K. C.; Chemg, Y.-S. E.; Yang, A. S.; Hsiao, S. C.; Su, C. Y. & Wong C. H. (2007) Synthesis of Tamiflu and its Phosphonate Congeners Possessing Potent Anti-Influenza Activity. *J. Am. Chem. Soc.* Vol. 129 (No. 39): 11892-11893

[157] Shin, H.; Cama, E. & Christianson, D. W. (2004) Design of Amino Acid Aldehydes as Transition-State Analogue Inhibitors of Arginase. *J. Am. Chem. Soc.* Vol. 126 (No. 33): 10278-10284

[158] Shishova, E. Y.; Di Costanzo, L.; Emig, S. A.; Ash, D. E. & Christianson, D. W. (2009) Probing the Specificity Determinants of Amino Acid Recognition by Arginase. *Biochemistry* Vol. 48 (No. 1): 121-131

[159] Sieburth, S. McN. & Chen, C.-A. (2006) Silanediol Protease Inhibitors: From Conception to Validation. *Eur. J. Org. Chem.* Vol. 2006 (No. 2): 311-322

[160] Skinner-Adams, T.; McCarthy, J. S.; Gardiner, D. L.; Hilton, P. M.& Andrews, K. T. (2004) Antiretrovirals as Antimalarial Agents. *J. Infect. Dis.* Vol. 190 (No. 11); 1998-2000

[161] Skinner-Adams, T. S.; Lowther, J.; Teuscher, F.; Stack, C. M.; Grembecka, J.; Mucha, A.; Kafarski, P.; Trenholme, K. R.; Dalton, J. P.; & Gardiner, D. L.(2007) Identification of Phosphinate Dipeptide Analog Inhibitors Directed Against the *Plasmodium falciparum* M17 Leucine Aminopeptidase as Lead Antimalarial Compounds. *J. Med. Chem.* Vol. 50 (No. 24): 6024 - 6031.

[162] Skinner-Adams, T. S.; Stack, C. M.; Trenholme, K. R.; Brown, C. L.; Grembecka, J.; Lowther, J.; Mucha, A.; Drag, M.; Kafarski, P.; McGowan, S.; Whisstock, J. C.; Gardiner, D. L. & Dalton, J. P. (2010) *Plasmodium falciparum* Neutral Aminopeptidases: New Targets for Anti-malarials. *Trends Biochem. Sci.* Vol. 35 (No. 1): 53 – 61

[163] Silva, R. G.; Hirschi, J. S.; Ghanem, M.; Murkin, A. S.; & Schramm, V. L. (2011) Arsenate and Phosphate as Nucleophiles at the Transition States of Human Purine Nucleoside Phosphorylase. Biochemistry, Vol. 50 (No.): 2701-2709

[164] Stack, C. M.; Lowther, J.; Cunningham, E.; Donnelly, S.; Gardiner, D. L.; Trenholme, K. R.; Skinner-Adams, T. S.; Teuscher, F.; Grembecka, J.; Mucha, A.; Kafarski, P.; Lua, L.; Bell, A. & Dalton, J. P. (2007) Characterization of the *Plasmodium falciparum* M17 Leucyl Aminopeptidase. A Protease Involved in Amino Acid Regulation with Potential for Antimalarial Drug Development. *J. Biol. Chem.* Vol. 282 (No. 3): 2069 – 2080

[165] Stanley, M.; Cattle, N.; McCauley, J.; Martin, S. R.; Rashid, A.; Field, R. A.; Carbain, B. & Streicher, H. (2012) 'TamiGold': Phospha-oseltamivir-Stabilised Gold Nanoparticles as the Basis for Influenza Therapeutics and Diagnostics Targeting the Neuraminidase (Instead of the Hemagglutinin). *MedChemComm* doi: 10.1039/c2md20034a

[166] Streicher, H. & Busse, H. (2006) Building a Successful Structural Motif into Sialylmimetics - Cyclohexenephosphonate Monoesters as Pseudo-sialosides with Promising Inhibitory properties. *Bioorg. Med. Chem.* Vol. 14 (No. 4): 1047-1057

[167] Sumida, T.; Stubbs, K. A.; Ito, M. & Yokohama, S. (2012) Gaining Insight into the Inhibition of Glycoside Hydrolase Family 20 exo--N-Acetylhexosaminidases Using a Structural Approach. *Org. Biomol. Chem.*Vol. 10 (No. 13): 2607-2612

[168] Teuscher, F.; Lowther, J.; Skinner-Adams, T.S.; Spielmann, T.; Dixon, M.W.A.; Stack, C.M.; Donnelly, S.; Mucha, A.; Kafarski, P.; Vassiliou, S.; Gardiner, D.L.; Dalton, J.P.; Trenholme, K. (2007) The M18 Aspartyl Aminopeptidase of the Human Malaria Parasite *Plasmodium falciparum*. *J. Biol. Chem.* Vol. 282 (No. 42): 30817 – 30826

[169] Thivierge, K.; Mathew, R. T.; Nsangou, D. N. N.; Da Silva, F.; Cotton, S. Skinner-Adams, T. S.; Trenholme, K. R.; Brown, C. L.; Stack, C. M.; Gardiner D. M. & Dalton, J. P. (2012) Anti-malaria Drug Development Targeting the M1 Alanyl and M17 Leucyl Aminopeptidases. ARKIVOC 2012 (No. 4): 330-346

[170] Thomson, J. M.; Prati, F.; Bethel, C. R. & Bonomo, R. A. (2007) Use of Novel Boronic Acid Transition State Inhibitors To Probe SubstrateAffinity in SHV-Type Extended-Spectrum -Lactamase. *Antimicrob. Agents Chemother.* Vol. 51 (No. 4): 1577-1579

[171] Trippier P. C. & McGuigan, C. (2010) Boronic Acids in Medicinal Chemistry: Anticancer, Antibacterial and Antiviral Applications. *Med. Chem. Commun.* Vol. 1 (No. 3): 183-198

[172] Tuan, H. F.; Erskin, P.; Langan, P. Cooper, J. & Coates, L. (2007) Preliminary neutron and ultrahigh-resolution X-ray diffraction studies of the aspartic proteinase endothiapepsin cocrystallized with a gem-diol inhibitor. *Acta Crystallogr.* Vol. 63 (No. 12): 1080-1083

[173] Turcotte, S.; Bouayad-Gervais, H. & Lubell, W. (2012) N-Aminosulfamide PeptideMimic Synthesis by Alkylation of Aza-sulfurylglycinyl Peptides. *Org. Lett.* Vol. 14 (No. 5): 1318-1321

[174] Tyler, P. C.; Taylor, E. A.; Fröhlich, F. R. G. & Schramm, V. L. (2007) Synthesis of 5'-Methylthio Coformycins: Specific Inhibitors for Malarial Adenosine Deaminase. *J. Am. Chem. Soc.* Vol. 129 (No. 21): 6872-6879

[175] Udommaneethanakit, T. Rungrotmongkol, T.; Bren, U.; Frecer, V. & Miertus, S. (2009) Dynamic Behavior of Avian Influenza A Virus Neuraminidase Subtype H5N1 in Complex with Oseltamivir, Zanamivir, Peramivir, and Their Phosphonate Analogues. *J. Chem. Inf.Model.* Vol. 49 (No.10): 2323-2332

[176] Umezawa, H.; Aoyagi, T.; Suda, H.; Hamada, M. & Takeuchi, T. (1976) Bestatin, an Inhibitor of Aminopeptidase B, Produced by Actinomycetes. Journal of Antibiotics (Tokyo) Vol. 29 (No. 1): 97-99

[177] Vasella, A.; Davies, G. J. & Böhm, M (2002) Glycosidase Mechanisms. *Curr. Opin. Chem. Biol.* Vol. 5 (No. 6): 619-629

[178] Vassiliou, S.; Xeilari, M.; Yiotakis, A.; Grembecka, J.; Pawelczak, M.; Kafarski, P. & Mucha, A. (2007) A Synthetic Method for Diversification of the P1' Substituent in Phosphinic Dipeptides as a Tool for Exploration of the Specificity of the S1' Binding Pockets of Leucine Aminopeptidases. *Bioorg. Med. Chem.* Vol. 15 (No. 9): 3187 – 3200

[179] Vassiliou, S.; Grabowiecka, A.; Kosikowska, P.; Yiotakis, A.; Kafarski, P. & Belicki, Ł. (2008) Design, Synthesis, and Evaluation of Novel Organophosphorus Inhibitors of Bacterial Ureases. *J. Med. Chem.* Vol. 51 (No. 18): 5736-5744

[180] Vassiliou, S.; Grabowiecka, A.; Kosikowska, P. & Berlicki, L. (2012) Three Component Kabachnik-Fields Condensation Leading to Substituted Aminomethane-P-hydroxy-methylphosphonic Acids as a Tool for Screening of Bacterial Urease Inhibitors. *ARKIVOC* Vol. 2012 (No. 4): 33-43

[181] Weinger, J. S.; Kitchen, D.; Scaringe, S. A.; Strobel, S. A. & Muth, G. W. (2004) Solid Phase Synthesis and Binding Affnity of Peptidyl Transferase Transition State Mimics Containing 2'-OH at P-site Position A76. *Nucl. Acids Res.* Vol. 32 (No. 4):1502-1511

[182] Venkatraman, S.; Wu, W.; Prongay, A.; Girijavallabhan, V. & Njoroge, F. G. (2009) Potent Inhibitors of HCV-NS3 Protease Derived from Boronic Acids. *Bioorg. Med. Chem. Lett.* Vol. 19 (No. 1): 180-183

[183] Verma, R. P. & Hansch, C. (2007) Matrix Metalloproteinases (MMPs): Chemical–Biological Functions and (Q)SARs. *Bioorg. Med. Chem.* Vol. 15 (No. 6): 2223-2268

[184] Wei, D.-Q.; Du, Q.-S.; Sun, H. & Chou, K. H. (2006) Insights from Modeling the 3D Structure of H5N1 Influenza Virus Neuraminidase and its Binding Interactions with Ligands. *Biochem. Biophys. Res. Commun.* Vol. 344 (No. 3): 1048-1055

[185] Wheatley, J. L. & Holyoak, T. (2007) Differential P1 Arginine and Lysine Recognition in the Prototypical Proprotein Convertase Kex2. *Proc. Natl. Acad. Sci. U.S.A.* Vol. 104 (No. 16): 6626-6631

[186] Williams, I. H. (2010) Catalysis: Transition-state Molecular Recognition? *Beilstein J. Org. Chem.* Vol. 6: 1026-1034

[187] Wolfe, M. S. (2012) -Secretase Inhibitors and Modulators for Alzheimer's Disease. *J. Neurochem.* Vol. 120 (Suppl. 1): 89-98

[188] Wolfenden, R. (1972) Analogue Approaches to the Structure of the Transition State in Enzyme Reactions. *Acc. Chem. Res.* Vol. 5: 10-18

[189] Wolfenden, R. (1976) Transition State Analog Inhibitors and Enzyme Catalysis, *Annu. Rev. Biophys. Bioeng.* Vol. 5: 271-306

[190] Wolfenden, R. (1999) Conformational Aspects of Inhibitor Design: Enzyme-Substrate Interactions in the Transition State. *Bioorg. Med. Chem. Lett.* Vol. 7 (No. 5): 647-652

[191] Wolfenden, R. (2003) Thermodynamic and Extrathermodynamic Requirements of Enzyme Catalysis. *Biophys. Chem.* Vol. 105 (No. 2-3): 559-572

[192] Wood, J. M.; Maibaum, J.; Rahuel, J.; Grütter, M. G.; Cohen, N. C.; Rasetti, V.; Rüger, H.; Göschke, R.; Stutz, S.; Fuhrer, W.; Schilling, W.; Rigollier, P.; Yamaguchi, Y.; Cumin, F.; Baum, H.-P.; Schnell, C. R.; Herold, P.; Mah, R.; Jensen, C.; O'Brien, E.; Stanton, A. & Bedigian, M. P. (2003) Structure-based Design of Aliskiren, a Novel Orally Effective Renin Inhibitor. *Biochem. Biophys. Res. Commun.* Vol. 308 (No.4): 698-705

[193] Wu., X.; Öhrngren, P.; Ekegren, J. K.; Unge, J.; Unge, T.; Wallberg, H.; Samuelssom, B.; Hallberg, A. & Larhed, M. (2008) Two-Carbon-Elongated HIV-1 Protease Inhibitors with a Tertiary-Alcohol-Containing Transition-State Mimic. *J. Med. Chem.* Vol. 51 (No.): 1053-1057

[194] Wu, D.; Zhang, L.; Kong, Y.; Du, J.; Chen, S.; Chen, J.; Ding, J.; Jiang, H. & Shen, X. (2008a) Enzymatic Characterization and Crystal Structure Analysis of the D-Alanine-D-alanine Ligase from Helicobacter pylori. *Proteins* Vol. 72, (No. 4): 1148–1160

[195] Xu, W.; Cheng, G.; Liew, O. W.; Zuo, Z.; Jiang, H. & Zhu, W. (2009) Novel Non-peptide -Secretase Inhibitors Derived from Structure-based Virtual Screening and Bioassay. *Bioorg. Med. Chem. Lett.* Vol. 19 (No. 12): 3188-3192

[196] Yiotakis, A.; Georgiadis, D.; Matziari, M. & Dive, V. (2004) Phosphinic Peptides: Synthetic Approaches and Biochemical Evaluation as Zn-Metalloprotease Inhibitors. *Curr. Org. Chem.* Vol. 8 (No. 12): 1135-1158

[197] Zambelli, B.; Musialini, F., Benini, S. & Ciurli, S. (2011) Chemistry of Ni^{2+} in Urease: Sensing, Trafficking, and Catalysis. *Acc. Chem. Res.*Vol. 44 (No. 7): 520-530

[198] Zhang, X.; Schmitt, A. C.; Jiang, W.; Wasserman, Z. & Decicco, C. P. (2003) Design and Synthesis of Potent, Non-peptide Inhibitors of HCV NS3 Protease. *Bioorg. Med. Chem. Lett.* Vol. 13 (No.6): 1157-1160

[199] Zhang, X. & Xu, W. (2008) Aminopeptidase N (APN/CD13) as a Target for Anti-cancer Agent Design. *Curr. Med. Chem.* Vol. 15 (No.27): 2850-2865

[200] Zucker, S. & Cao, J. (2009) Selective Matrix Metalloproteinase (MMP) Inhibitors in Cancer Therapy. *Cancer Bio. Ther.* Vol. 8 (No. 24): 2371-2323

Colon Cancer: Current Treatments and Preclinical Models for the Discovery and Development of New Therapies

Samuel Constant, Song Huang,
Ludovic Wiszniewski and Christophe Mas

Additional information is available at the end of the chapter

1. Introduction

More than 10 years after the first sequencing of the human genome and despite major advances in scientific and technological expertise into drug research and development processes (R&D), the fact remains that we are facing a dearth of new drugs. Indeed, the number of drugs approved by the US Food and Drug Administration (FDA) has roughly fallen to 50% over the last ten years [1]. Unfortunately for pharmaceutical companies, at present this attrition in drug discovery combined with the expiration of major product patents logically lead to the development of generics. Facing both a major medical need and an obvious economical challenge, there is an urgent need to make significant improvements in the research output.

Analyses of the clinical trials landscape reveal that a large number of promising drug leads fail in late stages, mainly in phase II, with an overall failure rate of 67% (Fig. 1a). All studies agree on the reasons by pinpointing either insufficient efficacy (~55%) or safety issues (~20%) as major causes of human trials failure [2, 3]. Remarkably, the therapeutic area showing the largest number of failures is oncology, with only 29% of success rate in Phase II and 34% in Phase III (Fig.1b). Within oncology indications, the status of colorectal cancer (CRC) is the most dramatic with an overall drug approval of only 3% (Fig.1c) over the last 10 years! More surprisingly, more than half of the drugs currently approved to treat CRC work through the general inhibition of DNA synthesis and cellular division, instead of targeting molecular processes specifically involved in CRC progression (Table 1). These observations highlight the necessity to both reduce failure rates in the clinic and shorten the time required for developing innovative therapies.

From this perspective, one of the obvious strategies would be:

1. to directly target the key regulators of CRC cancers

2. to streamline the critical Phase II and Phase III to obtain faster and more reliable responses regarding the drug's efficacy.

This strategy may save years of efforts and millions of dollars, giving that the average usual time for developing a new drug is ten years and with a total cost amount to billions of dollars.

But in contrast, because a new drug has to show a benefit compared to an already approved treatment, the number of patients involved in a pivotal trials is increasing more and more in order to reach significance, and a similar trend is noted for the duration of the trial, that is directly linked to safety. Therefore, regarding the constraints imposed by regulatory authorities nowadays, it seems difficult to save on size and length of clinical trials.

In the mid-1990s, the pharmaceutical community has already attempted to increase R&D productivity by embarking in a technological shift. That was the time of the inevitable high-throughput screening, which combined with the "all-Omics" supposed to reduce costs and blew up success rates [4]. As we have seen, this approach, maybe too reductionist in the sense that it does not allow getting an idea of the full biological properties (ADME, toxicity,etc…) of a compound at an early stage, has favored the quantity instead of quality and has not kept its promises [1].

Today, efforts have to be made to clearly address the early clinical discovery steps, with the goal to better qualify "leads" to increase the signal-to-noise ratio of drugs entering into clinical trials. This point of view is supported by the important failure rate subsisting in Phases III (Fig1b), suggesting an overestimation of the efficacy of candidate molecules during preclinical tests. One of the important reasons may be the use of irrelevant models or models not predictive enough. Therefore, the development of relevant and predictive models is key to increase the quality of preclinical researches and to increase the success rate of new drugs.

Consequently, the foundations of the drug discovery process have to be reconsidered by giving definitively more emphasis to the quality of preclinical validations and by encouraging the design of new pertinent models, including human 3D (three dimensional) *in vitro* cell models and tissue explants.

This article is intended to give an overview of the current knowledge about CRC and the different models commonly used to study CRC, in order to identify the most suitable biosystems for optimal development of new CRC therapies. The first part will describe the pathology and its molecular basis, and the various drugs that are currently in clinical use or under development. Then, in the second part we will review and discuss the use of cancer cell line collections, genetically engineered mouse models (GEM), primary human tumors xenografts (PDX) and *ex vivo* organotypic cultures (EVOC) to identify and validate anticancer colon therapeutics.

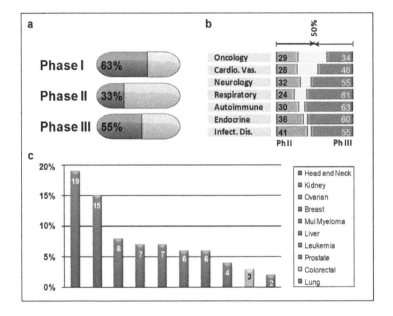

Figure 1. Success rate of drug development. Overall success rate of clinical trials for phases I-III from 2003 to 2010 corresponding to 4275 drugs and 7300 indications (a), success rate for phase II and III divided according to therapeutic areas (b) and overall success rate within specific oncologic areas (c). Source: Hay et al, 13th BIO CEO & Investor Conference, 2011, New-York.

2. Colorectal Cancer

Colorectal cancer is one of the major health concerns in the Western world. CRC is the second most frequently diagnosed cancer in men and women, right after lung cancer. It represents the second leading cause of cancer-related deaths, both in the United States and in Europe, with a significant rate of 9% and 13% of total cancer deaths, respectively (Fig.2). The vast majority (~75%) of colon cancers are sporadic adenocarcinomas, arising from mutations in the epithelial cells lining the wall of the intestine that is in continuous renewal. CRC often begins as an adenomatous polyp, a benign growth on the interior surface of the organ. Most of polyps remain benign, but over the years some of them become progressively more dysplastic, accumulate mutations and progress to carcinoma and ultimately, to metastasis.

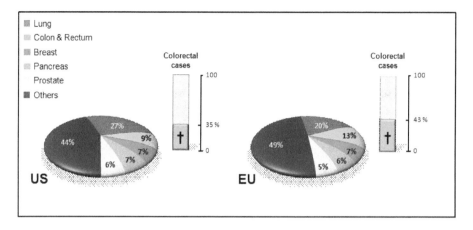

Figure 2. Cancer deaths anticipated in 2011. Estimated leading cancer sites mortality in US and in European Union (EU-27) for the year 2011 expressed as percent of total cancer deaths. Column diagrams highlight the mortality rate within the population specifically affected by colon cancer. Rates are standardized to the World Standard Population. Source: American Cancer Society and Malvezzi et al, Annals of oncology, 2011, 22(4):947-56.

2.1. Molecular mechanisms

Loss of APC function is the initial molecular event that leads to adenoma formation. Indeed, germline mutations in the gene APC have been identified as the cause of familial adenomatous polyposis (FAP), an inheritable intestinal cancer syndrome [5], and APC is mutated in more than 80% of all sporadic cancers [6]. APC belongs to the WNT signaling pathway (Figure 3) where it interacts with other proteins like AXINS and GSK3β to make a complex that down-regulates the cellular levels of β-CATENIN (see [7] for review). Activating mutations in β-CATENIN gene have also been observed in more than 10% of CRC [8]. When activated, β-CATENIN interacts in the nucleus with the transcriptional complex LEF/TCF to induce the expression of growth promoting genes, like MYC and CYCLIN D1. Additional waves of genetic and epigenetic alterations (KRAS, P53, etc...) will follow this early set of molecular changes to sustain the progression of the transformation process until carcinoma and metastasis stages.

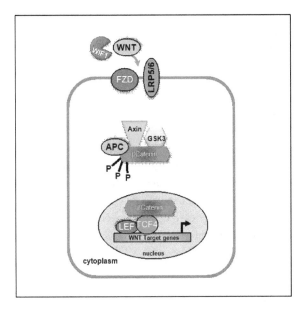

Figure 3. Shematic representation of the WNT signaling pathway. WNT proteins bind to receptors of the Frizzled and LRP families on the cell surface. Through several cytoplasmic components, the signal is transduced to β-CATENIN, which enters the nucleus and forms a complex with LEF and TCF4 to activate transcription of WNT target genes. Mutations in APC, Axin and β-CATENIN genes lead to constitutive activation of WNT signaling and ultimately to cancer development.

2.2. Clinical management

It is commonly accepted that CRC results from complex interactions between inherited and environmental factors, with a large contribution of dietary and life style factors as suggested by wide geographical risk variations. However, the primary risk factor of CRC is age, as 90% of the cases are diagnosed over the age of 50 years [9]. Surgical removal remains the most efficient treatment for early stage colorectal cancer, and may be curative for cancers that have not spread. Patients whose cancer is detected at an early, localized stage present a 5-year survival around 90% [9]. For these reasons, US and European Union have implemented preventive screening programs that have contributed to slightly reduce morbidity and mortality [10].

Unfortunately, as in many other forms of cancer, colon cancer does not display too many symptoms, develops slowly over a period of several years, and only manifests itself when the disease begins to extend. Adjuvant chemotherapy in combination with surgery or radiation is then the usual treatment. However, 5 of the 9 anti-CRC drugs approved by the FDA today are basic cytotoxic chemotherapeutics that attack cancer cells at a very fundamental level (i.e. the cell division machinery) without specific targets, resulting in poor effectiveness and strong side-effects (e.g., oxaliplatin; Table 1)

Moreover, in more advanced cases, when CRC has spread to distant organs in the form of metastasis and escape any surgical therapy, the 5-year survival dramatically drops to 12% [9]. These figures underline the urgent need to expand the standard therapy options by turning to more focused therapeutic strategies. In recent years, combination of basic chemo-therapies with targeted therapies, in the form of humanized monoclonal antibodies directed against the vascular endothelial growth factor VEGF (Bevacizumab) to prevent the growth of blood vessels to the tumor, or directed against the EGF receptor (Cetuximab, Panitumu-mab) to block mitogenic factors that promote cancer growth, have been introduced as possi-ble therapeutic protocol and used routinely to treat standard CRCs, as well as metastatic CRCs (Table 1). During the preparation of this manuscript (August 2012), another recombi-nant protein active against angiogenesis, Aflibercept, has been approved by the FDA for the treatment of metastatic CRC in second-line therapy (Table 1). This new VEGF inhibitor has demonstrated a significant advance over currently available therapy in a Phase III study (improvement in response rate and in overall survival; [11]).

Nonetheless, CRC remains a devastating disease since nearly 35-40% of all patients diag-nosed will die from the disease (Fig.2). Accordingly, the expansion and the development of new path of therapy, like drugs specifically targeting the self-renewal of intestinal can-cer stem cells - a tumor cell population from which CRC is supposed to relapse [12] – remains relevant.

Generic	Trade Name	Type	Class	Target
► Capecitabine	Xeloda	small molecule	antineoplastic prodrug (Fluorouracil)	DNA synthesis
► Fluorouracil	Efudex Adrucil Fluoroplex	small molecule	antineoplastic	DNA synthesis
► Irinotecan	Camptosar	small molecule	antineoplastic prodrug (Camptothecin)	DNA synthesis
► Leucovorin	Wellcovorin	small molecule	antineoplastic adjunct	DNA synthesis
► Oxaliplatin	Eloxatin	small molecule	antineoplastic	DNA synthesis
► Aflibercept	Zaltrap	Recombinant protein	antiangiogenesis	VEGF
► Bevacizumab	Avastin	mAb	antiangiogenesis	VEGF
► Cetuximab	Erbitux	mAb	antineoplastic	EGFr
► Panitumumab	Vectibix	mAb	antineoplastic	EGFr

Table 1. Anti-cancer colorectal drugs approved by the Food and Drug Administration. Drugs are presented sorted by type, i.e. small molecule or biologics (including recombinant protein and monoclonal antibody, noted mAb). Source: National Cancer Institute database, 2012.

2.3. Designing new therapies

A classical approach of drug design in oncology is to identify modulators of specific signal transduction pathways that are important for tumor growth, survival, invasion, and metastasis. Because aberrant WNT signaling has been shown to drive the earliest step of colorectal tumorigenesis (see before), the WNT/β-CATENIN pathway appears critical for CRC and therefore represents a target of choice for the development of CRC therapeutics.

2.3.1. Oncogenic WNT/β-CATENIN pathway as a therapeutic target

Many experiments have demonstrated that disruption of the WNT signaling pathway lead to consistent growth inhibition and apoptosis of CRC cell lines and effective inhibition of tumor growth in CRC animal models. These results can be achieved by modulating the pathway at different levels, from the membrane receptor to the final nuclear transcription factors (Figure 3). A significant number of proof of principle studies have already been published, including targeted inhibition of WNT1-2, FZD or LRP5/6 receptors by antibodies or inhibitory fusion proteins [13-15], inactivation of the pathway by re-expression of WIF1 (WNT-inhibitory factor-1) or through restoration of tumor suppressors APC and Axin expression [16], expression of a dominant-negative mutant to block the transcription factor TCF4 [17], and finally direct inhibition of β-CATENIN using RNA interfering technologies in vitro and in vivo [18, 19]. Taken together, these data provide a strong biological rationale for drugging the WNT/β-CATENIN signaling pathway.

In addition, recent evidence also points to a role for WNT/β-CATENIN signaling in the modulation of cancer stem cells. It is now well documented that a number of critical pathways regulating stem cell maintenance and normal developmental processes (e.g. HEDGEHOG-GLI, NOTCH, TGF) are also involved in the self-renewal and differentiation of cancer stem cells whose tumors are initiated [20]. Consequently, in a way similar to the HEDGEHOG-GLI pathway [21], a large number of high-throughput cell-based screening strategies, mainly designed to disrupt TCF/β-CATENIN interaction, have led to the identification of promising molecules as inhibitors of WNT/β-CATENIN pathway (reviewed by [22]).

However, currently few of these compounds have progressed beyond the preclinical stages. To date, the only compound designed to specifically disrupt β-CATENIN is developed for the treatment of Familial Adenomatous Polyposis (FAP), an inherited form of colon cancer. This new RNAi-based therapeutic known as CEQ508 consists of a modified E.coli bacterium that is able to express and deliver a shRNA to the epithelial cells of the gastrointestinal mucosa after ingestion by the patient [23]. CEQ508, which has shown efficiency in silencing β-CATENIN and preventing polyp formation in the APC^{min} FAP mouse model, is now in a Phase I clinical trial (Table 2).

Alternatively, a possible way of interfering with the WNT/β-CATENIN cascade, even if not direct, may reside in the manipulation of KLF4 levels. KLF4 (Kruppel-like factor 4) is a tumor suppressor factor which is typically deficient in a variety of cancers, including colorectal cancer. In addition to controlling the cell cycle regulator cyclin D1, KLF4 has also been shown to inhibit the expression of β-CATENIN [24]. Therefore, the modulation of KLF4 expression may represent a novel therapeutic approach for β-CATENIN-driven malignancies. LOR-253 [25], a compound that stimulates KLF4 through the inhibition of the human metal-regulatory transcription 1 (MTF1), is currently in a Phase I clinical study (Table 2).

It is noteworthy that despite the significance of this signaling axis for the treatment of sporadic colorectal cancer, none of the therapies engaged to date in CRC clinical trials are directly targeting WNT/β-CATENIN pathway members. Nonetheless, considering the huge effort done at the research level to identify potential antagonists and the few candidate already engaged into preclinical studies, no doubt that innovative therapies will emerge from this promising pathway in a near future.

2.3.2. Acquired tumor resistance and targeted therapies

In the recent years, a cohort of oncogenes, including BRAF, KRAS, NRAS, PI3K, PTEN and SMAD4, have been found mutated in CRC with significant frequencies ranging from 6% (NRAS) to 40% (KRAS) [26]. These observations pinpoint one of the most challenging aspects of anticancer therapy that is intrinsic or acquired drug resistance. Indeed, several studies have shown that these mutations are associated with the lack of response to Cetuximab and Panitumumab (anti-EGFR therapies) observed in a subset of chemorefractory metastatic CRCs, suggesting that the corresponding deregulated signaling pathways are responsible for the occurrence of resistance of the tumor to the clinical treatment [27-28]. As a result, downstream key components (mostly protein kinases) of these constitutively activated growth-related signaling cascades have become targets for drug development. Small molecules inhibitors of BRAF (ARQ 736), MEK (Selumetinib, PD-0325901), PI3K (PX-866, BEZ235, BKM120), and MET (Tivantinib) that were able to reverse resistance to EGFR inhibitor therapy in pre-clinical studies [29-31] are currently in CRC Phase II clinical studies (Table 2). This new class of drugs appears therefore as a promising third-line therapeutic strategy for colon cancer patients, especially after recurrence of tumor resistance. However, a recent publication reporting the apparition of resistance to PI3K and AKT inhibitors mediated by β-CATENIN overactivation, may temper this enthusiasm. Depending on the tumor status, from pro-apoptotic tumor suppressor, PI3K or AKT inhibitors could become metastatic inducers [32]. Similar side effect induction mechanisms have also been reported in CRC for the BRAF(V600E) inhibitor Vemurafenib that triggers paradoxical EGFR activation [33]. All together, the complexity of these results supports the arrival of a personalized medicine, where a careful profiling of tumors will be useful to stratify patient population in order to test drugs sensitivity and combination with the ultimate goal to make treatments safer and more effective.

2.3.3. New anti-angiogenesis therapies

As previously mentioned, until recently the humanized monoclonal antibody Bevacizumab against VEGF was the only anti-angiogenesis agent approved by FDA. It is now completed by Aflibercept, a recombinant protein consisting of the key domains of VEGF receptors 1 and 2. The compound captures and blocks all isoforms of VEGF-A and VEGF-B growth factors, as well as placental growth factors [34]. Due to improvement in the understanding of the critical role of angiogenesis in the maintenance of CRC tumors and the spread of their metastasis, anti-angiogenesis has become an area of active investigation [35]. However, the recent failure in Phase III first-line studies of two promising compounds (Sunitunib in 2009 and Cediranib in 2010) has cast serious doubt on that strategy. Therefore, the approval of Aflibercept provides timely support to the further development of anti-angiogenics as treatment for metastatic CRC. Today, 4 additional therapeutic agents that target VEGF, Ramucirumab [36], Icrucumab [37], Regorafenib [38] and Vatalanib [39-40] are under clinical evaluation (Table 2). This battery of anti-angiogenics is supplemented by AMG386, a recombinant peptide-antibody fusion protein (peptibody) which targets another signaling pathway involved in tumoral angiogenesis, the angiopoietin axis [41]. AMG386, which inhibits the interaction between the ligands ANGIOPOIETIN-1 and ANGIOPOIETIN-2 with their TIE2 receptor, is currently in Phase II. Finally, a phase III trial was also recently initiated (May 2012) to evaluate TAS-102, a combination agent composed of the cytotoxic pyrimidine analog TFT and a thymidine phosphorylase inhibitor (TPI) with antineoplastic activity (Table 2). TAS-102 mechanism of action is based on the inhibition of the thymidine phosphorylase (TYMP) also known as the platelet-derived endothelial cell growth factor, a potent angiogenic factor [42]. In this context, it is important to point out that differences in the efficiency to block angiogenesis and tumor progression have been observed between preclinical models and clinical trials, when comparing antibodies with small molecules [35]. These discrepancies in clinical outcome underline the necessity to validate compounds on relevant models, preferentially based on human tissues, very early during drug development process.

2.3.4. Other cellular mechanisms under target

Modifications in the epigenetic landscape are commonly associated with cancer, but on the contrary to genetic mutations, these changes are potentially reversible and therefore druggable. Most of the epigenetic drugs discovered to date modulate DNA methylation or histone acetylation. Four epigenetic drugs have already been approved by FDA for use in clinic against various cancers. An additional one, the histone deacetylase (HDAC) inhibitor Resminostat [43] is currently being studied in patients with CRC, in a phase I/II trial (Table 2).

Drug	Company	Type	Target	Status
► ARQ 736	ArQule	small molecule	BRAF	Phase I
► Selumetinib	Array BioPharma	"	MEK	Phase II
► PD-0325901	Pfizer	"	MEK	Phase I
► PX-866	Oncothyreon	"	PI3K	Phase II
► BEZ235	Novartis	"	PI3K	Phase I
► BKM120	Novartis	"	PI3K	Phase II
► Tivantinib	ArQule	"	MET	Phase II
► Brivanib	BMS	"	VEGFR2 PDGFRβ	Phase III
► Regorafenib	Bayer	"	VEGFR2-3 PDGFRβ FGFR	Phase III
► Vatalanib	Bayer / Novartis	"	VEGFR1-3	Phase III
► LOR-253	Lorus Therapeutics	"	MTF1 inhibitor	Phase I
► TAS-102	Taiho Pharma	"	TYMS TYMP	Phase III
► Resminostat	4SC	"	HDAC inhibitor	Pasel/II
► CEQ508	Marina Bio	biologics (shRNA)	βCATENIN	Phase I/II
► Icrucumab	ImClone Systems	biologics (humanized mAb)	VEGFR-1	Phase II
► Ramucirumab	ImClone Systems	"	VEGFR-2	Phase II
► AMG 386	Amgen	biologics (peptibody)	Tie-2R	Phase II
► GL-ONC1	Genelux	biologics (oncolytic virus)	Tumoral cells	Phase I/II
► ColoAd1	PsiOxus	"	"	Phase I/II
► NV1020	Medigene	"	"	Phase II
► Reolysin	Oncolytics	"	"	Phase I/II
► JX594	Jennerex	"	"	Phase I/II

Table 2. Anti-cancer drugs in colorectal clinical trials. This table gives an overview of the main colorectal cancer thera-pies being currently evaluated in clinical trials. Drugs are presented sorted by type, i.e. small molecule or biologics. For each compound, the pathway target and clinical status is provided. Source: National Cancer Institute database, 2012 and the clinical database of the *Journal of Gene Medicine* (http://www.wiley.com/legacy/wileychi/genmed/clinical).

2.3.5. Unconventional approaches

Oncolytic viral therapy represents an appealing alternative therapeutic strategy for the treat-ment of CRC, both as single agent or in combination with existing clinical regimens. Onco-lytic viruses, like the vaccinia virus (a virus previously used for worldwide vaccination against smallpox), have the property to selectively infect and destroy tumor cells with limit-ed or no toxicity to normal tissues. These viruses efficiently replicate in tumor tissue, cause tumor lyses and stimulate antitumor immune response. During the last decade, numerous mutants have been engineered to improve their tumor specificity and antitumor efficacy, and to allow tracking of viral delivering by non-invasive imaging [44]. No less than five on-colytic virotherapies are currently evaluated in clinical trials for metastatic CRC indication, including ColoAd1, derived from an adenovirus [45], NV1020, derived from an Herpes simplex virus [46], Reolysin, a reovirus [47], and JX-594 [48] and GL-ONC1 [49] both derived from vaccinia viruses, reflecting the many hopes carried by this emerging treatment modality. However, it is noteworthy to mention that there are still some difficulties to viral infection. Solid tumors have a complex microenvironment that includes disorganized surrounding stroma, poor vascular network as well as high interstitial fluid pressure. All these parameters will limit viral delivery since viral penetration directly depends on cellular packing density and adhesion between cancer cells [50]. Moreover, hypoxia reduces viral replication, and therefore oncolytic efficiency, without affecting tumoral cells viability [51]. These observations highlight how choosing the right experimental validation model, e.g. 3D cell cultures or spheroids *in vitro*, or patient primary-derived xenografts that retain tumoral architecture complexity *in vivo*, will be critical for future clinical success.

This inventory of new drugs for the treatment of colorectal cancer highlights the diversity of approaches being considered to combat the disease. Whether based on small molecules, humanized antibodies or modified viruses, their success in further clinical assessment is largely related to the quality of their preclinical evaluation. This is why both the choice of appropriate existing model systems and the development of more clinically relevant and predictive pre-clinical models appear critical in overcoming the high attrition rates of compounds entering clinical trials.

Current research is also focusing on the development of biomarkers that will be useful for the early detection of CRC, as well as for fine-tuning drug regimen and following efficacy during trials and treatments. To date, only a few markers have been recommended for practical use in clinic [52] but large-scale genomics technology combined with advanced statistical analyses should generate soon new biomarker panels for CRC diagnosis [53]. Then, it will be interesting to see how these biomarkers could be implemented in preclinical stages to improve drug selection.

3. Preclinical models

3.1. Colon cancer cell lines

It is worth mentioning that most of our understanding of the molecular mechanisms involved in CRC come from studies done on mouse or human cell lines that represent only a highly selected fraction of the original tumor and that may have acquired *in vitro* additional genetic abnormalities. Moreover, isolated cells grown on plastic dish flooded with growth factors appear retrospectively as a very poor model system to elucidate human CRC biology, especially with regard to the importance of growth signaling pathways (EGF/FGF) and tumor/stroma interactions in CRC progression. Clearly, the scientific community has taken into account these limitations, as shown by the growing interest for more complex models (e.g. 3D spheroids). However, although imperfect, colon cancer cell lines still represent a unique resource that can be extremely valuable in term of genetic manipulation and high-throughput screening, with cell viability, cell proliferation or promoter specific reporter ac-tivity being the usual endpoints followed. Several initiatives have been launched to maximize their utility in large scale drug discovery programs.

3.1.1. NCI-60 cancer cell lines collection

The NCI60 is a collection of 59 human cancer cell lines derived from diverse tissues, includ-ing colon (HT-29, COLO-205, HCT-15), which was established in the early 1990s by the Sanger institute (http://www.sanger.ac.uk/genetics/CGP/NCI). In an attempt to identify new active molecules, over 100,000 chemical compounds were pharmacologically tested in this cell line set. But disappointingly, most of the selected positive candidates were typical cyto-toxics, affecting cancer cells via general fundamental cellular processes, like cell cycle regu-lation. These cell lines are under further characterization by sequencing for mutations in known human oncogenes. Interestingly, this resource can be screened on demand for any chemical or biological agent. As an example, the NCI60 has been recently used to determine the permissivity of standard cancer cell lines to VACV infection and replication, with the aim to better characterize viral oncolytic therapeutic strategies [54].

3.1.2. The Cancer Genome Project

The emergence of tumor acquired resistance to pharmacological inhibitors linked to muta-tions in driver oncogenes has recently revived the interest for cancer cell lines. Indeed, an extensive characterization of cell lines at the genomic and genetic levels will allow determin-ing a genetic profile predictive of drug sensitivity. Such a signature will help to stratify pa-tient population and identify efficient therapeutics combination, as long as cell lines reflect real tumor biology. In this perspective, the Sanger Cancer Institute has started the genetic characterization of a panel of 800 cancer cell lines (The Cancer Genome Project, http://www.sanger.ac.uk/genetics/CGP). Using current high throughput techniques this program intends to provide information on mutations, copy number variations, single nucleotide polymorphisms (SNPs) and microsatellite instability of usual cancer cell lines.

3.1.3. The Cancer Cell Line Encyclopedia

Similarly, the cancer cell line encyclopedia project is a joint initiative between The Novartis Institutes for Biomedical research and scientists from the Broad Institute (http://www.broad-institute.org/ccle/home) to provide a detailed genetic and pharmacologic characterization of a panel of 1000 human cancer cell lines, including more than 60 CRC cell lines. Again, the ultimate purpose of this project is to establish genetic maps that would predict anticancer drug sensitivity [55].

3.1.4. Biomimetic cell culture models

The derivation of a cancer cell line from the primary tumor is not an obvious process, and for many cancers, few if any cell line can be obtained. A success rate of less than 10% has been reported for the establishment of human colon cancer cell lines grew immediately *in vitro* from fresh tumors [56]. Elasticity of the surrounding microenvironment has been pointed out as a critical parameter of *in vitro* cell growth. Indeed, culture plastic dishes are much more rigid than the epithelial wall of the intestine (10000 kPa vs 40 kPa). More importantly, depending on the stiffness of the substrate, cells can be differentially sensitive to drugs in term of spreading and apoptosis-induction, notably because of the expression and presentation of surface receptors [57]. Therefore, the choice of an appropriate biomimetic substrate that will preserve the *in vivo* phenotype appears decisive not only for cell survival but also for clinical relevance. Soft polymer surface, with different degrees of stiffness reproducing the original tumor environment have been engineered (ExCellness Biotech) and are now available to improve 2D or 3D cultures.

3.1.5. Colon cancer stem cell models

Cancer stem cells (CSCs) are a discrete self-renewing tumor cell subpopulation that can differentiate into multiple lineages, drive tumor growth and metastasis. Moreover, CSCs are thought to be responsible for tumor recurrence after chemotherapy and radiotherapy. One of the characteristic of the CSCs is their ability to form spherical cell colonies when they are cultured in chemically defined serum-free medium at a relative low density [58]. This model, also called colonospheres, constitutes a unique *in vitro* system to elaborate therapeutic strategies that specifically target colon CSCs, like oncolytic adenoviruses developed to target specific CSCs antigens (e.g. CD44 or LGR5). In addition, sorting of CSCs based on specific surface epitopes expression has also been used to enrich culture in tumor initiating cells in order to increase the success rate of cell line establishment and therefore improve cell line representation for CRC.

3.2. Multicellular Spheroid models

Early stage development of novel anti cancer treatment requires *in vitro* methods able to deliver fast, reliable and predictive results. To select the most active molecule lead in a library, pharmaceutical industry has turned its attention to High Throughput Screening (HTS) tests which mimic human tissues. Furthermore, 3-Dimensional (3D) test system has been widely accepted as being more informative and relevant than classical 2D cell systems. Combination of HTS and 3D models such as the multicellular tumor spheroid model has been pointed out having the potential to increase predictability of clinical efficacy from *in vitro* validation therefore contributing savings in both development cost and time [59]. Advantages of spheroids compared to classical 2D cell line culture have been reported [60]. Indeed, proteomic analysis of multicellular spheroids versus monolayers cultures identifies differential protein expression relevant to tumor cell proliferation, survival, and chemoresistance.

Consequently, spheroids strategy has been used for the screening of new anticancer agents, like compounds that modulate apoptosis pathways [61].

Standardized spherical microtissue production in a 96 or 384-well hanging-drop multiwell plate format on robotic platform has been successfully achieved by 3D Biomatrix and In-sphero AG. Formation of standardized spheroids rely on the use of A431.H9, a human epi-thelial carcinoma cells, [62] or the colon cancer cell line HCT116 [63]. Interestingly, loss of cancer drug activity in HCT-116 cells during spheroid formation in a 3D spheroid cell cul-ture system has been reported [64]. Spheroid cell models also enable the study of colon can-cer chemoresistance and metastasis [65].

3.3. Colon cancer animal models

3.3.1. Chemically induced animal models

Colon cancer can be induced in mouse by specific carcinogens like 1,2-dimethylhydrazine (DMH) and azoxymethane (AOM). Exposure of the mouse intestine to these chemicals trig-gers rapid and reproducible tumor induction which recapitulates the adenoma-carcinoma sequence that occurs in human sporadic CRCs, with the notable exception however of the invasive and metastatic stage. The application of colon carcinogenesis treatment to CRC mouse model, like the Apc$^{min/+}$ animals, results in an increased tumor incidence by up to 6 fold. Interestingly, differences in genetic mutations that arise in chemically induced colon tumor models are largely carcinogen specific. K-Ras mutations are predominant in the DMH model, while AOM treated mice exhibit tumors with activating mutations in the β-catenin gene [66]. These models could therefore be useful to assess therapies targeting specific CRC signaling axis.

3.3.2. Apc $^{min/+}$ mice

The multiple intestinal neoplasia (Min) mouse was identified following random mutagene-sis with ethylnitrosourea [67]. A mutation in the Apc gene was identified as the cause of the disease, like in the human Familial Adenomatous Polyposys (FAP). However, Although Apc$^{min/+}$ mice spontaneously form a large number of benign adenomas in the small intestine, colon tumors develop in fewer than half of the animals, in contrast to human FAP patients which routinely develop invasive carcinomas.

3.3.3. Genetically Engineered Mouse models (GEMs)

The main purpose for developing genetically engineered mice is to model the human dis-ease in order to first better understand the biological processes underlying normal and ma-lignant cell physiology, and second to establish a reliable preclinical model mimicking the true biology of human cancer and useful for drug discovery. In an attempt to accurately model the phenotype observed in FAP or sporadic CRC patients, a constellation of Apc ge-netically engineered mice, all based on the loss of the wild-type Apc allele, have been created (see [68] for review). To date, GEMs have been extensively used to demonstrate the function of candidate genes in CRC tumorigenesis, and the fact that tumors occur and develop naturally in the host constitutes undeniably an advantage of transgenic models compare to xenograft models.

The main disadvantage, except the time and the cost required to generate and maintain such animals, lies in the fact that none of these Apc mouse models consistently display metastasis, while treating metastasis is the current challenge.

3.4. Xenograft Models

The development of cancer xenograft models allows *in vivo* testing required for the predictive assessment of the clinical tolerability and efficacy of therapeutic agents. For decades, xenografts have been generated from human tumor cell lines that have been selected by *in vitro* culture.

3.4.1. Subcutaneous xenografts

As standard, tumor cells are implanted subcutaneous in the hindflank region of immunodeficient mice (e.g. Nude, NSG) to prevent rejection. Tumor growth during the treatment period is monitored either by measuring the tumor mass on the animals using Vernier calipers or by recording the activity of specific markers, like luminescent (Luciferase) or fluorescent (GFP) reporters, using non invasive imaging. At the end of the experiment, animals are euthanized and tumors are collected for histological or genetic analyses. Many applications are possible: complex growth competition assays can be performed inside a same tumor by injecting a mix of genetically modified tumor cell population, each expressing a specific reporter (Red/Green assay). These assays allow the identification of new oncogenic targets, revealed by growth advantage, and therefore critical for tumor development [69]. Subcutaneous xenografts are useful for the study of tumor / stroma / vascular network interactions, which is not possible in cell lines. Nonetheless, this heterotypic human/mouse model has its limitations since some murine ligands are not able to activate human receptors (e.g. HGF/MET, [70]). In addition, some CRC cell lines, even if implanted subcutaneous, can produce distant metastasis to the lung or the lymphatic nodes, allowing to study the effect of therapies specifically designed against metastatic dissemination and growth (C. Mas, pers. comm.).

Here it is interesting to note that at the preclinical level, the *in vivo* antiangiogenic activity of Sunitinib (see "New anti-angiogenesis therapies" section before) was evaluated in sub-cutaneous xenograft tumor models derived from HT29 and Colo205 human colon carcinoma cell lines implanted in athymic mice [71-72]. However, thereafter no advantage in anti-tumor efficacy could be shown in Phase III trial. Although the reasons for this failure are not clearly established, the genetic heterogeneity observed in primary CRC patient tumors could explain this lack of efficacy: *in vitro* selected cell lines are not enough representative of CRC patient's tumors. This observation suggests that new models including large tumor panels able to recapitulate the biological heterogeneity of patient's populations appear necessary for an accurate evaluation of molecular targeted agents.

3.4.2. Orthotopic xenografts

A number of observations suggest that the behavior of tumor cells can be significantly different when implanted as a subcutaneous xenograft, compared to their behavior when grown into the tissue of origin. For these reasons, orthotopic models are thought to be better predictors of drug efficacy and are more clinically relevant. To this purpose, intracolonic xenografts have been developed. Technically, a small incision is made in the abdomen of the immunodeficient mouse, directly over the colon, and CRC cells are implanted under the serosa of the colon. Local tumor growth on the colon is then monitored. Although more realistic, the use of orthotopic xenograft models does not guarantee success. The efficacy of Semaxanib, an antiangiogenic molecule, has been tested in preclinical stages using an intracolonic Xenograft [73] but compound development was stopped after negative results from Phase III. Again, representation of patient heterogeneity should be taken into account at the preclinical level.

Finally, if the use of selected tumor lines and the value of the mouse as a host could be questionable in xenograft models, the response end points, survival end points, and tumor cell killing end points that are usually used during *in vivo* efficacy studies remain in line with clinical investigations.

3.4.3. Patient-derived xenograft models (PDXs)

In order to circumvent the difficulties of establishing new cell lines, as well as to establish an *in vivo* model preserving the histopathological characteristics of the original tumor, investigators have developed a new xenograft system based on the direct grafting of human tumor fragment into immunodeficient mice (Figure 4). Several CRC patient-derived xenograft collections (PDX) have been reported, with an average tumor take rate of over 60% [56, 74-75]. They can be cryopreserved and re-established in mice as needed, or maintained as xenografts from mice to mice. Intensive characterization has demonstrated that the architecture of PDX tumors, their gene expression profile and their chromosomal instability remains very similar to the parental tumor, even after successive passages [75-76]. Importantly, high correlation between drug activity in PDX and clinical outcome has been reported, making this model a valuable pharmacological tool for drug development [74-75]. Moreover, because they are derived from tumor fragment, PDX tumors retains the genetic heterogeneity existing in the original human tumor and are therefore useful for studies exploring acquired drug resistance mechanisms [75, 77]. The use of PDX as a model for tumor-stroma interaction is however less obvious since by the fourth passages human tumor stroma is replaced by the murine host [75]. All together, the above considerations highlight the potential of the PDX model to accelerate drug development and predictive biomarker discovery in CRC.

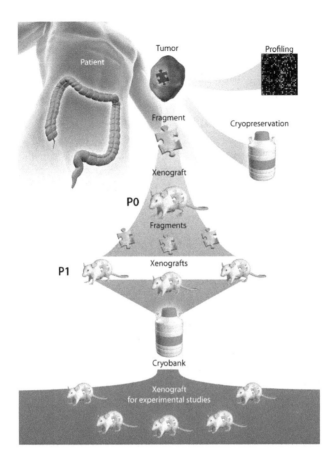

Figure 4. The PDX model. Sequential steps leading to the establishment of a CRC primary Patient-Derived Tumor Xenograft collection. Briefly, a CRC tumor fragment coming from surgical waste is directly xenografted in an immunodeficient mouse (Passage 0). After successful engraftment, new fragments are taken from the mouse hosted human tumor and xenografted again in multiple immunodeficient mice (Passage 1). A collection of fragments from the resulting tumors can then be cryopreserved in a tissue bank for subsequent experiments or directly re-engrafted in mice for expansion (P2, P3, etc…). At any step, tumor fragments can be analyzed and compared to the parental tumor in terms of gene expression, genetic mutations, genomic stability or histopathological features.

3.5. *Ex-Vivo* Organotypic Culture models (EVOCs)

As previously mentionned, current 2D monolayer culture systems are not enough predictive of *in vivo* tumor behavior. Indeed, 3D environement is required to provide essential signaling necessary for establishing and maintaining tumor specific morphogenic programs. Thus, an *ex vivo* methodology which can recapitulate physiological processes and generate multiple experimental replicates from a single tumor, saving at the same time animals involved in *in vivo* experiments will be of great benefit. *Ex vivo* organotypic cultures (EVOCs), by preserving the original cancer microenvironement (e.g. epithelial-stromal interaction) fulfill this requirement. Recently, a number of culture methods have been perfected leading to the development of breast, lung, liver and colon EVOC tumor models [78-81]. EVOCs allow the evaluation of tumor morphology, proliferation, viability and resistance to therapy *in vitro*. Moreover, differential gene-expression profiling across tumor and stroma compartments can be performed, without any contamination coming from a murine host as seen in xenograft models [78]. Recent observations have shown that CRC EVOCs mimic closely the *in vivo* situation, at the immunohistochemical level [81], but also in term of oncogenic pathway fonctionallity and pharmacodynamic properties [78]. Importantly, dose-response experiments with the PIK3 inhibitor LY294002 demonstrate that CRC EVOCs may be used to predit tumor sensitivity to drugs in a patient-specific manner [78]. EVOCs represent therefore a highly promising *in vitro* tumor model, when combined with automated medium-throughput analyses, has the potential to significantly enhance preclinical drug evaluation studies.

4. Conclusion

The development of relevant and predictive models is key to increase the quality of preclinical researches and to increase the success rate of new drugs. Many progresses have been made in this area to get as closer as possible to *in vivo* situations of human CRC cancers. Even though cell lines and animal models are still indispensable, the Xenograft Models, EVOCs as well as the 3D culture of CRC cancer cells hold the promises for the development of new, more efficient and safer drugs.

Author details

Samuel Constant, Song Huang, Ludovic Wiszniewski and Christophe Mas[*]

*Address all correspondence to: christophe.mas@oncotheis.com

OncoTheis, 14 Chemin des aulx, CH-1228 Plan-les-Ouates, Geneva, Switzerland

References

[1] Scannell, J. W., Blanckley, A., Boldon, H., & Warrington, B. (2012). Diagnosing the decline in pharmaceutical R&D efficiency. *Nat Rev Drug Discov*, 11, 191-200.

[2] Arrowsmith, J. (2011a). Trial watch: Phase II failures: 2008-2010. *Nat Rev Drug Discov*, 10, 328-9.

[3] Arrowsmith, J. (2011b). Trial watch: phase III and submission failures: 2007-2010. *Nat Rev Drug Discov*, 10, 87.

[4] Mayr, L. M., & Fuerst, P. (2008). The future of high-throughput screening. J Biomol Screen.; , 13, 443-8.

[5] Groden, J., Thliveris, A., Samowitz, W., Carlson, M., Gelbert, L., Albertsen, H., Joslyn, G., Stevens, J., Spirio, L., Robertson, M., et al. (1991). Identification and characterization of the familial adenomatous polyposis coli gene. *Cell*, 66, 589-600.

[6] Powell, S. M., Zilz, N., Beazer-Barclay, Y., Bryan, T. M., Hamilton, S. R., Thibodeau, S. N., Vogelstein, B., & Kinzler, K. W. (1992). APC mutations occur early during colorectal tumorigenesis. *Nature*, 359, 235-7.

[7] Clevers, H., & Nusse, R. (2012). Wnt/β-catenin signaling and disease. *Cell*, 149, 1192-205.

[8] Morin, P. J., Sparks, A. B., Korinek, V., Barker, N., Clevers, H., Vogelstein, B., & Kinzler, K. W. (1997). Activation of beta-catenin-Tcf signaling in colon cancer by mutations in beta-catenin or APC. *Science*, 275, 1787-90.

[9] Howlader, N., Noone, A. M., Krapcho, M., Neyman, N., Aminou, R., Altekruse, S. F., Kosary, C. L., Ruhl, J., Tatalovich, Z., Cho, H., Mariotto, A., Eisner, M. P., Lewis, D. R., Chen, H. S., Feuer, E. J., & Cronin, K. A. (2012). SEER Cancer Statistics Review, 1975Vintage 2009 Populations). *National Cancer Institute*.

[10] Zavoral, M., Suchanek, S., Zavada, F., Dusek, L., Muzik, J., Seifert, B., & Fric, P. (2009). Colorectal cancer screening in Europe. *World J Gastroenterol*, 15, 5907-5915.

[11] Gaya, A., & Tse, V. (2012). A preclinical and clinical review of aflibercept for the management of cancer. *Cancer Treat Rev*, 38, 484-93.

[12] Merlos, Suárez., et al. (2011). The Intestinal Stem Cell Signature Identifies Colorectal Cancer Stem Cells and Predicts Disease Relapse. *Cell Stem Cell*, 8, 511-24.

[13] He, B., You, L., Uematsu, K., Xu, Z., Lee, A. Y., Matsangou, M., Mc Cormick, F., & Jablons, D. M. (2004). A monoclonal antibody against Wnt-1 induces apoptosis in human cancer cells. *Neoplasia*, 6, 7-14.

[14] You, L., He, B., Xu, Z., Uematsu, K., Mazieres, J., Fujii, N., Mikami, I., Reguart, N., Mc Intosh, J. K., Kashani-Sabet, M., Mc Cormick, F., & Jablons, D. M. An anti-Wnt-2 monoclonal antibody induces apoptosis in malignant melanoma cells and inhibits tumor growth. *Cancer Res*, 64(15), 5385-9.

[15] De Almeida, V. I., Miao, L., Ernst, J. A., Koeppen, H., Polakis, P., & Rubinfeld, B. (2007). The soluble wnt receptor Frizzled8CRD-hFc inhibits the growth of teratocarcinomas in vivo. *Cancer Res*, 67, 5371-9, Taniguchi H, Yamamoto H, Hirata T, Miyamoto N, Oki M, Nosho K, Adachi Y, Endo T, Imai K, Shinomura Y. '05 Frequent epigenetic inactivation of Wnt inhibitory factor-1 in human gastrointestinal cancers. Oncogene.; 24:7946-52.

[16] Morin, P. J., Sparks, A. B., Korinek, V., Barker, N., Clevers, H., Vogelstein, B., & Kinzler, K. W. (1997). Activation of beta-catenin-Tcf signaling in colon cancer by mutations in beta-catenin or APC. *Science*, 275(5307), 1787-90.

[17] Van de Wetering, M., Sancho, E., Verweij, C., de Lau, W., Oving, I., Hurlstone, A., van der Horn, K., Batlle, E., Coudreuse, D., Haramis, A. P., et al. (2002). The β-catenin/TCF-4 complex imposes a crypt progenitor phenotype on colorectal cancer cells. *Cell*, 111, 241-250.

[18] Verma, U. N., Surabhi, R. M., Schmaltieg, A., Becerra, C., & Gaynor, R. B. (2003). Small interfering RNAs directed against beta-catenin inhibit the in vitro and in vivo growth of colon cancer cells. *Clin Cancer Res*, 9, 1291-300.

[19] Scholer-Dahirel, A., Schlabach, M. R., Loo, A., Bagdasarian, L., Meyer, R., Guo, R., Woolfenden, S., Yu, K. K., Markovits, J., Killary, K., Sonkin, D., Yao, Y. M., Warmuth, M., Sellers, W. R., Schlegel, R., Stegmeier, F., Mosher, R. E., & Mc Laughlin, M. E. (2011). Maintenance of adenomatous polyposis coli (APC)-mutant colorectal cancer is dependent on Wnt/beta-catenin signaling. *Proc Natl Acad Sci U S A*, 108, 17135-40.

[20] Van der Flier, L. G., & Clevers, H. (2009). Stem cells self-renewal, and differentiation in the intestinal epithelium. *Annu Rev Physiol*, 71, 241-60.

[21] Mas, C., Ruiz, i., & Altaba, A. Small molecule modulation of HH-GLI signaling: current leads, trials and tribulations. *Biochem Pharmacol*, 80, 712-23.

[22] Takahashi-Yanaga, F., & Kahn, M. Targeting Wnt signaling: can we safely eradicate cancer stem cells? *Clin Cancer Res*, 6(12), 3153-62, 2010 Jun 8.

[23] Vaze, M. B., Wu, T. S., Shaguna, Templin. M., & Polisky, B. Engineering of trans kingdom RNAi (tkRNAi) against gastrointestinal polyps. *Cancer Research*, 72(8, 1).

[24] Zhang, N., Zhang, J., Shuai, L., Zha, L., He, M., Huang, Z., & Wang, Z. Krüppel-like factor 4 negatively regulates β-catenin expression and inhibits the proliferation, invasion and metastasis of gastric cancer. *Int J Oncol*, 40(6), 2038-48.

[25] Cukier, H., Peralta, R. , Hongnan, J. , Huesca, M., Yoon, L., & Aiping, Y. (2012). Preclinical dose scheduling studies of LOR-253, a novel anticancer drug, in combination with chemotherapeutics in lung and colon cancers. *Annual Meeting of the American Association for Cancer Research; Chicago, IL. Philadelphia (PA): AACR; Cancer Res*, 72(8), Abstract nr 3710.

[26] Forber, S. A., et al. (2011). COSMIC: mining complete cancer genomes in the Catalogue of Somatic Mutations in Cancer. *Nucleic Acids Res*, 39, D945-50.

[27] Sartore, Bianchi., et al. (2009). PIK3CA mutations in colorectal cancer are associated with clinical resistance to EGFR-targeted monoclonal antibodies. *Cancer Res*, 69, 1851-7.

[28] De Roock, W., De Vriendt, V., Normanno, N., Ciardiello, F., & Tejpar, S. (2011). KRAS, BRAF, PIK3CA, and PTEN mutations: implications for targeted therapies in metastatic colorectal cancer. *Lancet Oncol*, 12, 594-603.

[29] Mueller, A., Bachmann, E., Linnig, M., Khillimberger, K., Schimanski, C. C., Galle, P. R., & Moehler, M. (2012). Selective PI3K inhibition by BKM120 and BEZ235 alone or in combination with chemotherapy in wild-type and mutated human gastrointestinal cancer cell lines. *Cancer Chemother Pharmacol*, 69, 1601-15.

[30] Misale, , et al. (2012). Emergence of KRAS mutations and acquired resistance to anti-EGFR therapy in colorectal cancer. *Nature*, 486, 532-6.

[31] Munshi, N., Jeay, S., Li, Y., Chen, C. R., France, Ashwell. DS, et al. (2010). ARQ 197, a novel and selective inhibitor of the human c-Met receptor tyrosine kinase with anti-tumor activity. *Mol Cancer Ther*, 9, 1544-53.

[32] Tenbaum, S. P., et al. (2012). β-catenin confers resistance to PI3K and AKT inhibitors and subverts FOXO3a to promote metastasis in colon cancer. *Nat Med*, 18, 892-901.

[33] Prahallad, A., Sun, C., Huang, S., Di Nicolantonio, F., Salazar, R., Zecchin, D., Beijers-bergen, R. L., Bardelli, A., & Bernards, R. (2012). Unresponsiveness of colon cancer to BRAF(V600E) inhibition through feedback activation of EGFR. *Nature*, 483(7387), 100-3.

[34] Holash, J., Davis, S., Papadopoulos, N., Croll, S. D., Ho, L., Russell, M., Boland, P., Leidich, R., Hylton, D., Burova, E., Ioffe, E., Huang, T., Radziejewski, C., Bailey, K., Fandl, J. P., Daly, T., Wiegand, S. J., Yancopoulos, G. D., & Rudge, J. S. (2002). VEGF-Trap: a VEGF blocker with potent antitumor effects. *Proc Natl Acad Sci*, 99, 11393-11398.

[35] Ferrarotto, R., & Hoff, P. M. (2012). Antiangiogenic Drugs for Colorectal Cancer: Exploring New Possibilities. *Clin Colorectal Cancer*, in press.

[36] Spratlin, J. L., Cohen, R. B., Eadens, M., et al. (2010). Phase I pharmacologic and biologic study of ramucirumab (IMC-1121B), a fully human immunoglobulin G1 monoclonal antibody targeting the vascular endothelial growth factor receptor-2. *J Clin Oncol*, 28, 780-7.

[37] Schwartz, J. D., Rowinsky, E. K., Youssoufian, H., Pytowski, B., & Wu, Y. (2010). Vascular endothelial growth factor receptor-1 in human cancer: concise review and rationale for development of IMC-18F1 (Human antibody targeting vascular endothelial growth factor receptor-1). *Cancer*, 116(4), 1027-32.

[38] Grothey, A., Sobrero, A. F., Siena, S., et al. (2012). Results of a phase III randomized, double-blind, placebo-controlled, multicenter trial (CORRECT) of regorafenib plus best supportive care (BSC) versus placebo plus BSC in patients (pts) with metastatic colorectal cancer (mCRC) who have progressed after standard therapies. *J Clin Oncol*, 30(4), abstract LBA385.

[39] Hecht, J. R., Trarbach, T., Hainsworth, J. D., Major, P., Jäger, E., Wolff, R. A., Lloyd-Salvant, K., Bodoky, G., Pendergrass, K., Berg, W., Chen, B. L., Jalava, T., Meinhardt, G., Laurent, D., Lebwohl, D., & Kerr, D. (2011). Randomized, placebo-controlled, phase III study of first-line oxaliplatin-based chemotherapy plus PTK787/ZK 222584, an oral vascular endothelial growth factor receptor inhibitor, in patients with metastatic colorectal adenocarcinoma. *J Clin Oncol*, 29, 1997-2003.

[40] Van Cutsem, E., Bajetta, E., Valle, J., Köhne, C. H., Hecht, J. R., Moore, M., Germond, C., Berg, W., Chen, B. L., Jalava, T., Lebwohl, D., Meinhardt, G., Laurent, D., & Lin, E. (2011). Randomized, placebo-controlled, phase III study of oxaliplatin, fluorouracil, and leucovorin with or without PTK787/ZK 222584 in patients with previously treated metastatic colorectal adenocarcinoma. *J Clin Oncol*, 29, 004-10.

[41] Neal, J., & Wakelee, H. (2010). AMG-386, a selective angiopoietin-1/-2-neutralizing peptibody for the potential treatment of cancer. *Curr Opin Mol Ther*, 12, 487-95.

[42] Temmink, O. H., Emura, T., de Bruin, M., Fukushima, M., & Peters, G. J. (2007). Therapeutic potential of the dual-targeted TAS-102 formulation in the treatment of gastrointestinal malignancies. *Cancer Sci*, 98, 779-89.

[43] Mandl-Weber, S., Meinel, F. G., Jankowsky, R., Oduncu, F., Schmidmaier, R., & Baumann, P. (2010). The novel inhibitor of histone deacetylase resminostat (RAS2410) inhibits proliferation and induces apoptosis in multiple myeloma (MM) cells. *Br J Haematol*, 149, 518-28.

[44] Russell, S. J., Peng, K. W., & Bell, J. C. (2012). Oncolytic virotherapy. *Nat Biotechnol*, 30, 658-670.

[45] Kuhn, I., Harden, P., Bauzon, M., Chartier, C., Nye, J., Thorne, S., Reid, T., Ni, S., Lieber, A., Fisher, K., Seymour, L., Rubanyi, G. M., Harkins, R. N., & Hermiston, T. W. (2008). Directed evolution generates a novel oncolytic virus for the treatment of colon cancer. *PLoS One*, 3, e2409.

[46] Geevarghese, S. K., Geller, D. A., de Haan, H. A., Hörer, M., Knoll, A. E., Mescheder, A., Nemunaitis, J., Reid, T. R., Sze, D. Y., Tanabe, K. K., & Tawfik, H. (2010). Phase I/II study of oncolytic herpes simplex virus NV1020 in patients with extensively pretreated refractory colorectal cancer metastatic to the liver. *Hum Gene Ther*, 21, 1119-28.

[47] Stoeckel, J., & Hay, J. G. (2006). Drug evaluation: Reolysin--wild-type reovirus as a cancer therapeutic. *Curr Opin Mol Ther*, 8, 249-60.

[48] Park, B. H., Hwang, T., Liu, T. C., Sze, D. Y., Kim, J. S., Kwon, H. C., Oh, S. Y., Han, S. Y., Yoon, J. H., Hong, S. H., Moon, A., Speth, K., Park, C., Ahn, Y. J., Daneshmand, M., Rhee, B. G., Pinedo, H. M., Bell, J. C., & Kirn, D. H. (2008). Use of a targeted oncolytic poxvirus, JX-594, in patients with refractory primary or metastatic liver cancer: a phase I trial. *Lancet Oncol*, 9, 533-42.

[49] Pedersen, J. V., Karapanagiotou, E. M., Biondo, A., Tunariu, N., Puglisi, M., Den-
      holm, K. A., Sassi, S., Mansfield, D., Yap, T. A., De Bono, J. S., & Harrington, K. J.
      (2011). A phase I clinical trial of a genetically modified and imageable oncolytic vac-
      cinia virus GL-ONC1 with clinical green fluorescent protein (GFP) imaging. *J Clin
      Oncol*, 29, abstr 2577.

[50] Minchinton, A. I., & Tannock, I. F. (2006). Drug penetration in solid tumours. *Nature
      Rev Cancer*, 6, 583-92.

[51] Pipiya, T., Sauthoff, H., Huang, Y. Q., et al. (2005). Hypoxia reduces adenoviral repli-
      cation in cancer cells by downregulation of viral protein expression. *Gene Ther*, 12,
      911-17.

[52] Cappellani, A., Zanghi, A., Di Vita, M., Zanet, E., Veroux, P., Cacopardo, B., Caval-
      lero, A., Piccolo, G., Lo, Menzo. E., Merabito, P., et al. (2010). Clinical and biological
      markers in gastric cancer: update and perspectives. *Front Biosci*, 2, 403-412.

[53] García-Bilbao, A., Armañanzas, R., Ispizua, Z., Calvo, B., Alonso-Varona, A., Inza, I.,
      Larrañaga, P., López-Vivanco, G., Suárez-Merino, B., & Betanzos, M. Identification of
      a biomarker panel for colorectal cancer diagnosis. *BMC Cancer*, 12, 43.

[54] Ascierto, M. L., Worschech, A., Yu, Z., Adams, S., Reinboth, J., Chen, N. G., Pos, Z.,
      Roychoudhuri, R., Di Pasquale, G., Bedognetti, D., Uccellini, L., Rossano, F., Ascierto,
      P. A., Stroncek, D. F., Restifo, N. P., Wang, E., Szalay, AA, & Marincola, F. M. (2011).
      Permissivity of the NCI-60 cancer cell lines to oncolytic Vaccinia Virus GLV-1h68.
      BMC Cancer, 11, 451.

[55] Barretina, , et al. (2012). The Cancer Cell Line Encyclopedia enables predictive model-
      ling of anticancer drug sensitivity. *Nature*, 483, 603-7.

[56] Dangles-Marie, V., Pocard, M., Richon, S., Weiswald, L. B., Assayag, F., Saulnier, P.,
      Judde, J. G., Janneau, J. L., Auger, N., Validire, P., Dutrillaux, B., Praz, F., Bellet, D., &
      Poupon, M. F. (2007). Establishment of human colon cancer cell lines from fresh tu-
      mors versus xenografts: comparison of success rate and cell line features. *Cancer Res*,
      67, 398-407.

[57] Rehfeldt, F., Engler, A. J., Eckhardt, A., Ahmed, F., & Discher, D. E. (2007). Cell re-
      sponses to the mechanochemical microenvironment--implications for regenerative
      medicine and drug delivery. *Adv Drug Deliv Rev*, 59, 1329-1339.

[58] Kanwar, S. S., Yu, Y., Nautiyal, J., Patel, B. B., & Majumdar, A. P. (2010). The Wnt/
      beta-catenin pathway regulates growth and maintenance of colonospheres. *Mol Can-
      cer*, 9, 212.

[59] Kunz-Schughart, L. A., Freyer, J. P., Hofstaedter, F., & Ebner, R. The use of 3-D cul-
      tures for high-throughput screening: the multicellular spheroid model. *J Biomol
      Screen*, 9(4), 273-85.

[60] Gaedtke, L., Thoenes, L., Culmsee, C., Mayer, B., & Wagner, E. (2007). Proteomic
      Analysis Reveals Differences in Protein Expression in Spheroid versus Monolayer

Cultures of Low-Passage Colon Carcinoma Cells. *Journal of Proteome Research*, 6, 4111-4118.

[61] Herrmann, R., Fayad, W., Schwarz, S., Berndtsson, M., & Linder, S. J Screening for Compounds That Induce Apoptosis of Cancer Cells Grown as Multicellular Spheroids. *Biomol Screen*, 13(1), 1-8.

[62] Tung, , et al. (2011). High-throughput 3D spheroid culture and drug testing using 384 hanging drop array. *Analyst*, 136, 473-478.

[63] Drewitz, M., Helbling, M., Fried, N., Bieri, M., Moritz, W., Lichtenberg, J., & Kelm, J. M. (2011). Towards automated production and drug sensitivity testing using scaffold-free spherical tumor microtissues. *Biotechnol. J*, 6, 1488-1496.

[64] Karlssona, H., Fryknäsa, M., Larssona, R., & Nygren, P. (2012). Loss of cancer drug activity in colon cancer HCT-116 cells during spheroid formation in a new 3-D spheroid cell culture system. *Exp Cell Res*, 318(13), 1577-85.

[65] Fan, X., Ouyang, N., Teng, H., & Yao, H. (2011). Isolation and characterization of spheroid cells from the HT29 colon cancer cell line. *Int J Colorectal Dis*, 26, 1279-1285.

[66] Rosenberg, D. W., Giardina, C., & Tanaka, T. (2009). Mouse models for the study of colon carcinogenesis. *Carcinogenesis*, Feb, 30(2), 183-96.

[67] Moser, A. R., Pitot, H. C., & Dove, W. F. (1990). A dominant mutation that predisposes to multiple intestinal neoplasia in the mouse. *Science*, 247, 322-324.

[68] Mc Cart, A. E., Vickaryous, N. K., & Silver, A. (2008). Apc mice: models, modifiers and mutants. *Pathol Res Pract*, 204(7), 479-90.

[69] Zbinden, M., Duquet, A., Lorente-Trigos, A., Ngwabyt, S. N., Borges, I., Ruiz, i., & Altaba, A. (2010). NANOG regulates glioma stem cells and is essential in vivo acting in a cross-functional network with GLI1 and P53. *EMBO J*, 29, 2659-74.

[70] Rong, S., Bodescot, M., Blair, D., Dunn, J., Nakamura, T., Mizuno, K., Park, M., Chan, A., Aaronson, S., & Vande, Woude. G. F. (1992). Tumorigenicity of the met proto-oncogene and the gene for hepatocyte growth factor. *Mol Cell Biol*, 12, 5152-8.

[71] Mendel, D. B., Laird, A. D., Xin, X., Louie, S. G., Christensen, J. G., Li, G., Schreck, R. E., Abrams, T. J., Ngai, T. J., Lee, L. B., Murray, L. J., Carver, J., Chan, E., Moss, K. G., Haznedar, J. O., Sukbuntherng, J., Blake, R. A., Sun, L., Tang, C., Miller, T., Shirazian, S., Mc Mahon, G., & Cherrington, J. M. (2003). In vivo antitumor activity of SU11248, a novel tyrosine kinase inhibitor targeting vascular endothelial growth factor and platelet-derived growth factor receptors: determination of a pharmacokinetic/pharmacodynamic relationship. *Clin Cancer Res*, 9, 327-37.

[72] Marzola, P., Degrassi, A., Calderan, L., Farace, P., Nicolato, E., Crescimanno, C., Sandri, M., Giusti, A., Pesenti, E., Terron, A., Sbarbati, A., & Osculati, F. (2005). Early antiangiogenic activity of SU11248 evaluated in vivo by dynamic contrast-enhanced

magnetic resonance imaging in an experimental model of colon carcinoma. *Clin Cancer Res*, 11, 5827-32.

[73] Fong, T. A., Shawver, L. K., Sun, L., Tang, C., App, H., Powell, T. J., Kim, Y. H., Schreck, R., Wang, X., Risau, W., Ullrich, A., Hirth, K. P., & Mc Mahon, G. (1999). SU5416 is a potent and selective inhibitor of the vascular endothelial growth factor receptor (Flk-1/KDR) that inhibits tyrosine kinase catalysis, tumor vascularization, and growth of multiple tumor types. *Cancer Res*, 59, 99-106.

[74] Fichtner, I., et al. (2004). Anticancer drug response and expression of molecular markers in early-passage xenotransplanted colon carcinomas. *Eur. J. Cancer*, 40, 298-307.

[75] Julien, S., Merino-Trigo, A., Lacroix, L., Pocard, M., Goere, D., Mariani, P., Landron, S., Bigot, L., Nemati, F., Cuilliere-Dartigues, P., Weiswald, L. B., Lantuas, D., Morgand, L., Pham, E., Gonin, P., Dangles-Marie, V., Job, B., Dessen, P., Bruno, A., Pierre, A., De The, H., Soliman, H., Nunes, M., Lardier, G., Calvet, L., Demers, B., Prevost, G., Vrignaud, P., Roman-Roman, S., Duchamp, O., & Berthet, C. (2012). Characterization of a large panel of patient-derived tumor xenografts representing the clinical heterogeneity of human colorectal cancer. *Clin Cancer Res*, In Press.

[76] Guenot, D., et al. (2006). Primary tumour genetic alterations and intra-tumoral heterogeneity are maintained in xenografts of human colon cancers showing chromosome instability. *J. Pathol*, 208, 643-652.

[77] Krumbach, R., et al. (2011). Primary resistance to cetuximab in a panel of patient-derived tumour xenograft models: activation of MET as one mechanism for drug resistance. *Eur. J. Cancer*, 47, 1231-1243.

[78] Vaira, V., Fedele, G., Pyne, S., Fasoli, E., Zadra, G., Bailey, D., Snyder, E., Faversani, A., Coggi, G., Flavin, R., Bosari, S., & Loda, M. (2010). Preclinical model of organotypic culture for pharmacodynamic profiling of human tumors. *Proc Natl Acad Sci U S A*, 107, 8352-6.

[79] Buchsbaum, D. J., Zhou, T., Grizzle, W. E., Oliver, P. G., Hammond, C. J., Zhang, S., Carpenter, M., & Lo, Buglio. A. F. (2003). Antitumor efficacy of TRA-8 anti-DR5 monoclonal antibody alone or in combination with chemotherapy and/or radiation therapy in a human breast cancer model. *Clin Cancer Res*, 9, 3731-41.

[80] Kern, M. A., Haugg, A. M., Eiteneuer, E., Konze, E., Drebber, U., Dienes, H. P., Breuhahn, K., Schirmacher, P., & Kasper, H. U. (2006). Ex vivo analysis of antineoplastic agents in precision-cut tissue slices of human origin: effects of cyclooxygenase-2 inhibition in hepatocellular carcinoma. *Liver Int*, 26, 604-12.

[81] Dame, M. K., Bhagavathula, N., Mankey, C., Da, Silva. M., Paruchuri, T., Aslam, M. N., & Varani, J. (2010). Human colon tissue in organ culture: preservation of normal and neoplastic characteristics. *In vitro Cell Dev Biol Anim*, 46, 114-22.

Chapter 8

Coupled Enzyme Activity and Thermal Shift Screening of the Maybridge Rule of 3 Fragment Library Against *Trypanosoma brucei* Choline Kinase; A Genetically Validated Drug Target

Louise L. Major, Helen Denton and Terry K. Smith

Additional information is available at the end of the chapter

1. Introduction

Infectious diseases caused by parasitic protozoa affect approximately 15% of the global population, and more than 65% of the population in the Third and developing world, yet current drug therapies for protozoal infections are woefully inadequate. As protozoal infections take their toll predominantly in the developing world, market forces are insufficient to promote the development of novel anti-protozoal drugs. In 2000, only ca. 0.1% of global investment in health research was spent on drug discovery for tropical diseases [1].

One such neglected parasitic disease is Human African Trypanosomiasis (HAT) or African sleeping sickness, which is caused by the protozoan parasite *Trypanosoma brucei* and is transmitted by the bite of the Tsetse fly. The WHO estimates that HAT constitutes a serious health risk to 60 million people in sub-Saharan Africa, 300,000-500,000 of whom become infected each year, with an estimated 10,000 fatalities. The related disease in cattle, Cattle Trypanosomiasis or Nagana, also represents a major health concern due to its devastating economic, social and nutritional impact on African families, estimated by the WHO as an annual economic loss of ~US$ 4 billion. As such, the total burden of Trypanosomiasis translates into 1,598,000 Disability-Adjusted Life Years, this is on a par with big killers such as *Mycobacterium tuberculosis* and Malaria [2, 3].

Treatment of HAT is dependent upon four drugs: suramin, melarsoprol, pentamidine and eflornithine.These therapies are often toxic, difficult to administer and increasingly have an acquired drug resistance [4, 5].Developed before the 1950s suramin and melarsoprol are used for chemotherapy of early stages of the disease, as is pentamidine. The arsenical melar-soprol is extremely toxic, with death for ~1 in 20 of cases and treatment failures as high as 30% in certain areas [4, 6]. Treatment of the second stage of the disease, where the parasites cross the blood-brain barrier and invade the central nervous system, is limited to melarso-prol and eflornithine [7].The WHO as a desperate measure recently introduced nifurtimox-eflornithine combination therapy for the treatment of HAT. This is despite nifurtimox, a drug often used to treat Chagas' disease (caused by the related protozoan the South Ameri-can *Trypanosoma cruzi*), having low efficacy against HAT [8].

Hence there is an urgent need for new, more effective, less toxic, cheap and easy to adminis-ter therapeutic agents to treat African sleeping sickness and other closely related parasitic diseases, e.g. Chagas' disease and Leishmaniasis, whose current treatments suffer from simi-lar limitations.

T. brucei is able to survive and multiply in the harsh environment of a mammalian hosts' bloodstream. This is due to the parasite's dense cell-surface coat of the glycosylphosphatidy-linositol anchored variant surface glycoprotein (5 X 10^6 dimers/cell) [9-11], which protects the parasite in two ways. Firstly by acting as a diffusion barrier, such that complement is unable to reach and attack the plasma membrane of *T. brucei*. Secondly *T. brucei* is able to undergo antigenic variation, where by it is able to express a new variant surface glycopro-tein from a repertoire of more than 1000 different genes, before the hosts' innate immune system is able to catch up [12, 13]. This antigenic variation is why a vaccine against this par-asite is not a viable option as a therapy.

Phospholipids account for ~80% of total lipids in *T. brucei* with a significant proportion of these containing a choline-phosphate headgroup; phosphatidylcholine (PC) (~48%) and sphingomyelin (~15%) [14,15]. Sphingomyelin is made from PC via the sphingomyelin syn-thases transferring the choline-phosphate headgroup from PC to a ceramide lipid moiety [16]. These lipids contribute to the structural integrity of the membrane and in addition de-termine membrane fluidity and cell surface charge. Unsurprisingly, the biosynthesis and utilisation of these choline-containing molecules are implicated in a variety of cellular proc-esses, including signaling, intracellular cellular protein sorting and transport [reviewed in 16]. Phosphocholine has been reported to be a required mitogen for DNA synthesis induced by growth factors [17]. Recently we have shown that the essential *T. brucei* neutral sphingo-myelinase is actively involved in post Golgi sorting of the glycosylphosphatidylinositol anchored variant surface glycoprotein mentioned earlier [18].

Most eukaryotes have three alternative pathways by which PC can be synthesised [19 and reviewed in 20]. The first two pathways both involve three consecutive methylations of PE by S-adenosyl-L-methionemethyltransferases [20]. The PE can be derived from two alterna-tive pathways, either from the concerted actions of the CDP-DAG dependantphosphatidyl-serine synthase and phosphatidylserine decarboxylase, or via the CDP-ethanolamine branch of the Kennedy pathway. This involves phosphorylation of ethanolamine by an ethanola-mine kinase, its activation to CDP-ethanolamine by an ethanolamine-phosphate cytidyl-transferase and its transfer to diacylglycerol by an ethanolamine phosphotransferase. The presence of this branch of the Kennedy pathway was demonstrated in *T. brucei* [22], however only recently have the constituent enzymes been characterized [23].

The trypanosomal genomes have revealed that *T. brucei* does not contain homologues for any methyltransferase(s) required to convert PE to PC [24] (neither does *T. cruzi*, but *Leishmania* do). *Plasmodium falciparum* have an alternative single plant-like S-adenosyl-L-methionemethyltransferase [25-27], responsible for phosphoethanolamine conversion to phosphocholine, however there are no trypanosomatid homologues. This rather surprising absence of PE to PC methylation has been confirmed by *in vivo* labellings by ourselves and others [15, 22, 28].

The third alternative pathway for *de novo* synthesis of PC, and the only pathway by which *T. brucei* can *de novo* synthesise PC, utilises the CDP-choline branch of the Kennedy pathway [19, 29-33]. This involves the phosphorylation of choline by a choline kinase, its activation to CDP-choline by a choline-phosphate cytidyltransferase and its transfer to diacylglycerol by a choline phosphotransferase. Biochemical characterisation of the two choline/ethanolamine kinases involved in the initial steps of the Kennedy pathway show that unusually amongst eukaryotes only one of the kinases is able to phosphorylate choline [23].

Collectively this evidence of an absence of redundancy of *de novo* PC synthesis in *T. brucei*, compared with other organisms (including humans), suggests *T. brucei* has a vulnerability to inhibition of their only way to synthesise PC, i.e. the Kennedy pathway. Recently we have exploited this fact by genetically validating the only *T. brucei* choline kinase (*Tb*CK) as a drug target both in culture and in an animal model [34]. Chemical intervention of the *Tb*CK enzyme activity is likely to interfere with the parasite's biology in multiple ways and *Tb*CK is therefore of interest as a target for novel chemotherapeutics.

In this study we interrogate ~630 compounds of the Maybridge Rule of 3 Fragment Library for compounds that interact with, and inhibit *Tb*CK. The Maybridge Rule of 3 Fragment Library is a small collection of quantifiable diverse [35, 36], pharmacophoric rich, chemical entities that comply with the following criteria; MW ≤ 300, cLogP ≤ 3, H-Bond Acceptors ≤ 3, H-Bond Donors ≤ 3, Rotatable bonds (Flexibility Index) ≤ 3, Polar Surface Area ≤ 60 Å^2 and aqueous solubility ≥ 1 mM using LogS and high purity (≥ 95%). Comparisons between two different screening methods, a coupled enzyme activity assay and differential scanning fluorimetry, has allowed identification of compounds that interact and inhibit the *T. brucei* choline kinase, several of which possess selective trypanocidal activity.

2. Experimental

2.1. Materials

All materials unless stated were purchased either from Sigma/Aldrich or Invitrogen. An in house Maybridge Rule of 3 Fragment Library kept in master plates at 200 mM in DMSO (100%), was transferred into working plates with compounds occupying the central 80 wells of a 96-well plate, at 10 mM in 5% DMSO, allowing the two outside columns for positive and negative controls.

2.2. Recombinant expression and purification of *Tb*CK

Large-scale recombinant expression and purification of *Tb*CK was conducted using the construct pET-15bTEV-*Tb*CK in BL21 Rosetta (DE3) cells as described previously [23], except the cells were grown in tryptone phosphate broth [37], harvested by centrifugation at 3500 g for 20 min at 4°C and affinity purified with either a HisTrap™ FF crude column (enzyme activity assay) or a HisTALON Cartridge (thermal shift analysis).

Briefly, pelleted cells were suspended in buffer A (50 mMTris/HCl, pH 8.0, 300 mMNaCl and 10 mM imidazole) and lysed in the presence of DNase I by sonication. The lysate was cleared by centrifugation at 35000 g for 30 min at 4°C and applied to a 1 ml HisTrap™ FF crude column column (GE Healthcare) pre-loaded with Ni^{2+}. Unbound proteins were removed by washing the column with 15 column volumes of buffer A containing 32.5 mM imidazole and *Tb*CK was eluted with 250 mM imidazole in the same buffer. Using a PD10 column, *Tb*CK was buffer exchanged into 50 mMTris/HCl, pH 8.0, 300 mMNaCl, glycerol (15% w/v) and stored at -80°C.

Alternatively, pelleted cells were suspended in 50 mMTris/HCl, pH 8.0, 300 mMNaCl and 5 mM imidazole and lysed by sonication. The lysate was cleared by centrifugation at 35000 g for 30 min at 4°C and applied to a 1 ml HisTALON Cartridge (Clontech).Unbound proteins were removed by washing the column with 10 column volumes of loading buffer, *Tb*CK was eluted with 15 mM imidazole and a final clearing wash of 250 mM imidazole in the same buffer. Using a PD10 column, *Tb*CK was buffer exchanged into 50 mM HEPES pH 8.0, 300 mMNaCl and 15% glycerol prior to storage at -80°C.

Typical yields were > 10 mg per litre of bacterial culture,*Tb*CK was stable and freeze thawing did not lead to any significant loss of activity.

2.3. *T. brucei* choline kinase activity assay

High throughput screening of the Maybridge Rule of 3 Fragment Library was carried out at a final test concentration of 0.5 mM in 96-well plates (final assay volume 200 µl) using a spectrophotometric assay that has been described previously [23]. The screened library working plates consisted of compounds arrayed in 96 well plates at 10 mM in 5% DMSO; columns 1 and 12 contained 5% DMSO only. For high throughput screening, 10 µl from each well of the working plates was added to 110 µl of buffer containing 50 mM MOPS (pH 7.8), 150 mMKCl and 6 mM MgCl$_2$. 3 µg of purified *Tb*CK was added to each well in 30 µl of the same buffer and the plates were mixed and incubated for 5 min at room temperature. A further 30 µl of buffer containing PEP (1 mM final), ATP (0.5 mM final), NADH (0.5 mM final) and pyruvate kinase and lactate dehydrogenase(PK/LDH) (5 units/ml final) was added, and the reaction was started by addition of 30 µl choline (0.5 mM final) to rows 1-11, 30 µl buffer alone was added to row 12 (negative control) and this was used as an intra-plate control (background rate) in conjunction with row 1 (maximal rate). Following mixing the change in absorbance at 341 nm was monitored for 10 min at room temperature. For testing inhibition of the coupling enzymes (PK/LDH), standard buffer conditions were used but the assay contained 1 mM PEP, 0.1 mM ADP and 0.5 mM NADH. The PK/LDH was titrated to give a change in absorbance of approximately 0.05 absorbance units/min in the absence of inhibitor.

2.4. Differential scanning fluorimetry with TbCK

Differential scanning fluorimetry was set up in 96 well PCR plates using a reaction volume of 100 μL. Samples contained 2.1 μM TbCK, 6 mM MgCl$_2$, 50 mM HEPES pH 8.0, 80 mMNaCl, 5.25% glycerol (v/v) and 1.4 x Sypro Orange (Invitrogen), Maybridge Ro3 compounds were screened at 1 mM concentration with a final DMSO concentration of 0.5% (v/v).Two controls with eight repetitions per plate were used for the thermal shift experiments: 0.5% DMSO; 0.5 mM ATP, 0.5% DMSO.

Differential fluorimetric scans were performed in a realtime PCR machine (Stratagene Mx3005P with software MxPro v 4.01) using a temperature scan from 25°C to 95°C at 0.5°C min^{-1}.Data were then exported to Excel for analysis using "DSF analysis" modified from the template provided by Niesen et al. [38].T$_m$ values were calculated by non-linear regression, fitting the Boltzmann equation to the denaturation curves using GraFit. TbCK T$_m$, in the presence of 6 mM MgCl$_2$ and 0.5% DMSO, 41.21 ± 0.03°C (n > 60), T$_m$ for TbCK and 0.5 mM ATP = 44.46 ± 0.05°C (n > 60).

3. Results and discussion

Screening for inhibitors of the genetically validated drug target TbCK is problematic due to the difficulty in following the reaction either continuously or directly. A direct choline kinase activity assay assessing the production of phosphocholine, utilising a modified method of Kim et. al. [39], using TbCK and radiolabelled choline has been performed previously [23]. However this is not suitable for screening purposes, so choline kinase activity was measured by a spectrophotometric coupled assay (Figure 1). This coupled enzyme assay utilises regeneration of ATP from the ADP by-product of the choline kinase by pyruvate kinase, and subsequent oxidation of NADH as the resulting pyruvate is converted to lactate, by lactate dehydrogenase. This assay using coupled enzymes is also problematic, as a compound could potentially inhibit the coupled enzymes giving rise to a false positive.

An alternative approach for screening is differential scanning fluorimetry (Figure 2), allowing identification of compounds that interact with the TbCK protein, either to stabilise or destabilise it, therefore influencing the protein's T$_m$ (melting point) [38-40].

Initially TbCK was subjected to differential scanning fluorimetry to ascertain if this approach was possible. Known components required for enzyme activity were tested to see if thermal shifts were observed.In the presence of 6 mM MgCl$_2$, a T$_m$ of 41.2°C was obtained (Figure 1C, solid dark line). The addition of 0.5 mM ATP resulted in a > 3°C T$_m$ shift for TbCK(Figure 1C, dashed-line). These encouraging results showed TbCK was amenable to differential scanning fluorimetry and allowed validation of this screening method.It is worth noting the surprising low T_m of TbCK, considering that these parasites live within the bloodstream of a mammalian host, i.e. 37°C, or higher with a fever. However, the presence of physiological

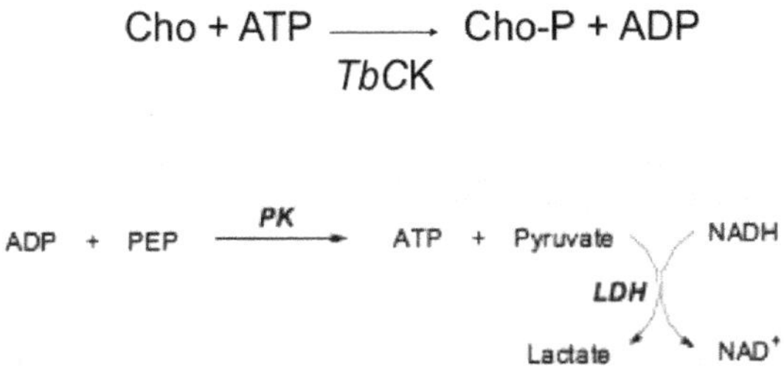

$$Cho + ATP \longrightarrow Cho\text{-}P + ADP$$
$$TbCK$$

$$ADP + PEP \xrightarrow{\ PK\ } ATP + Pyruvate$$

NADH

LDH

Lactate   NAD$^+$

Figure 1. Schematic of the TbCK reaction and coupled assay.

T. brucei choline kinase (TbCK) catalyses the ATP dependent phosphorylation of choline, the ADP is converted back to ATP by pyruvate kinase (PK), which converts phosphoenolpyruvate (PEP) to pyruvate in the process. The resulting pyruvate is reduced to lactate by the NADH dependent lactate dehydrogenase (LDH). The resulting conversion of NADH to NAD$^+$ is monitored, by measuring the reduction in absorbance at 341 nM.

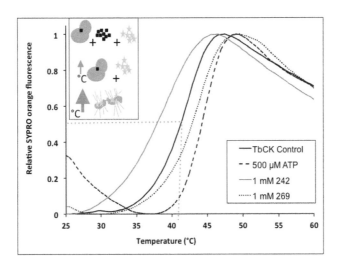

Figure 2. Thermal shift assay; typical differential fluorimetry scans of TbCK.

Differential fluorimetric scans were performed and analysed as described in Experimental. TbCK + DMSO (control) solid dark line, TbCK + 0.5 µM ATP (positive control) dashed line, TbCK + 1 mM compound 242, solid light line, TbCK + 1 mM compound 269, dotted line. T_m of TbCK in the presence of 0.5%DMSO is 41.21 ± 0.03°C (control); T_m of TbCK and 0.5 mM ATP is 44.46 ± 0.05°C (positive control). Insert: schematic representation of the thermal shift assay. A protein will unfold exposing hydrophobic domains as it is denatured due to the increasing temperature. Dyes such as sypro orange (star) are able to bind to these exposed hydrophobic areas giving rise to fluorescence. A plot of this increased fluorescence versus temperature allows determination of T_m (melting point) of the protein. If a compound (squares) is able to interact with the protein it may alter the protein's T_m and thus a library of compounds can be screened to see if they stabilise (increase in T_m) or destabilise (decrease in T_m) the target protein.

An alternative approach for screening is differential scanning fluorimetry (Figure 2), allowing identification of compounds that interact with the TbCK protein, either to stabilise or destabilise it, therefore influencing the protein's T_m (melting point) [38-40].

Initially TbCK was subjected to differential scanning fluorimetry to ascertain if this approach was possible. Known components required for enzyme activity were tested to see if thermal shifts were observed. In the presence of 6 mM $MgCl_2$, a T_m of 41.2°C was obtained (Figure 1C, solid dark line). The addition of 0.5 mM ATP resulted in a > 3°C T_m shift for TbCK(Figure 1C, dashed-line). These encouraging results showed TbCK was amenable to differential scanning fluorimetry and allowed validation of this screening method. It is worth noting the surprising low T_m of TbCK, considering that these parasites live within the bloodstream of a mammalian host, i.e. 37°C, or higher with a fever. However, the presence of physiological relevant levels of ATP does stabilize TbCK by > 3 °C, which may prolong the half-life of the protein in the parasite.

The respective controls in both assay types allowed Z-factors to be determined for all of the plates screened (Figure 3). Both the coupled enzyme activity assay and the thermal shift analysis showed Z-factors to be above 0.5 for all plates, except for plate 5 for the thermal shift assay (but still above 0.45), this is indicative of good reliable assays, with meaningful results [41].

The MayBridge Rule of 3 Fragment Library was distributed over 9 plates (80 compounds per plate) providing space for adequate positive and negative controls, allowing Z-factors to be determined. This was done for each plate for both the choline kinase assay (+) and thermal shift analysis (x). A Z-factor above 0.4 is acceptable and validates the data on that plate as being reliable.

The ~630 compounds from the MayBridge Rule of 3 Fragment Library were assessed for their ability to inhibit the TbCK coupled enzyme activity assay at a single concentration of 0.5 mM (Figure 4A). At this relative high concentration only 9 of the compounds (1.4%) showed > 70% inhibition. These primary hits were retested in triplicate at 0.5 mM (Table 1), 2 of the 9(compounds 320 and 635) were confirmed as being false positives, while the remaining 7 were confirmed to show good inhibition (80-100%) against the TbCK coupled enzyme activity assay. These 7 compounds were then tested against just the coupled enzymes, some inhibition was observed for some of the compounds, but this was insufficient to account for the strong inhibition against the TbCK, thus these 7 compounds were believed to show true TbCK inhibition.

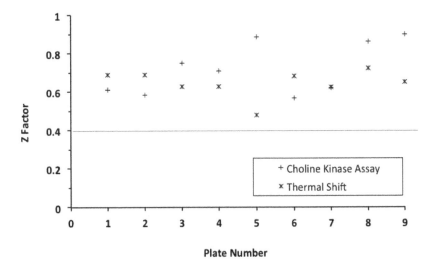

Figure 3. Quality control (Z factors) for the TbCK thermal shift analysis and coupled enzyme activity assay.

It is worth noting the lack of false positives arising from significant inhibition of either of the coupling enzymes, pyruvate kinase and lactate dehydrogenase this is encouraging when screening other ATP utilizing enzymes.

Thermal shift analysis of TbCK with the ~630 compounds from the MayBridge Rule of 3 Fragment Library showed that the vast majority of compounds had little or no affect on the T_m of TbCK (Figure 4B). Relatively few compounds showed an increase in T_m (stabilisation), and only a handful of these showing an increase in $T_m > 1°C$, i.e. compound 269 (Figure 2, dotted line), this was rather surprising given that ATP stabilises TbCK by > 3°C. Significantly more compounds showed a destabilisation affect, with 3 compounds having > 10°C decrease in the Tm, i.e. compound 242 (Figure 2, solid light line). Most of the compounds observed in this screen that show significant destabilisation of TbCK, do not cause similar destabilisation affects with other enzymes that we have screened in a similar manner, the only exceptions are compounds 68 (2-aminothiophene-3-carbonitrile) and 565 (4-(2-amino-1,3-thiazol-4-yl)phenol) (Table 1).

Several drug discovery style studies have shown that an increase in the thermal stability of a protein is proportional to the concentration and affinity of the ligand to the protein in keeping with the equilibrium associated with ligand-protein binding [38, 41-44]. On those occasions where this interaction destabilizes a protein, i.e. lowering T_m, a thermo-dynamic model has been proposed which explains the how the same ligand can stabilise and destabilise different proteins [42]. While the same protein may be stabilized and de-stabilized by very similar ligands, this was exquisitely demonstrated by the changes in thermal stability of Acyl-CoA thioesterase, upon incubation with either CoA (destabilise) or Acyl-CoA (stabilise) [45].

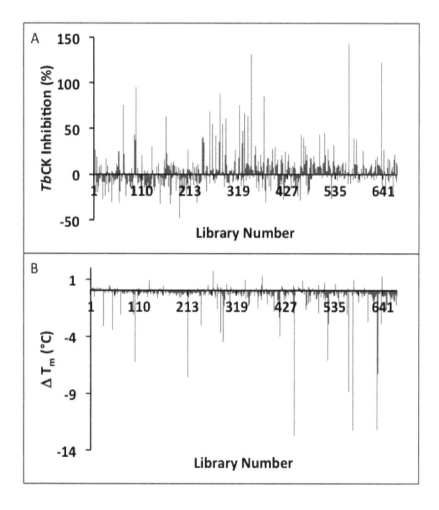

Figure 4. A) Percentage inhibition of *Tb*CK enzyme activity assay for each of the compounds tested. B) Observed thermal shifts of *Tb*CK for each of the compounds tested

Library number[a]	CAS number[b]	Molecular Structure	Compound Name	TbCK activity % inhibition at 500µM Mean ± SD (n=3)	TbCK IC50 (uM)	PK/LDH % inhibition at 500 uM mean (n=2)	TbCK T_mShift[c]	T. brucei % survival[d]
68	4651-82-5		2-aminothiophene-3-carbonitrile	101 ± 3	~758	40	-2.15 ± 0.08	10.3 ± 11
95	933-67-5		7-methyl-1H-indole	84 ± 4	~380	49	-2.16 ± 0.14	4.1 ± 5.2
257	59147-02-3		4-(2-furyl)aniline	80 ± 3	~234	63	0.46 ± 0.08	9.3 ± 8.5
278	199590-00-6		(1-methyl-1H-indol-6-yl)methanol	101 ± 2	25.45 ±1.16	28	0.26 ± 0.09	8.8 ± 10.8
320	39270-39-8		2,3-dihydro-1,4-benzodioxin-6-ylmethanol	6 ± 4	ND	ND	-0.17 ± 0.07	63.1 ± 9.5
346	57976-57-5		3-pyridin-3-ylaniline	100 ± 0	12.35 ± 0.64	68	-1.18 ± 0.06	15.6 ± 9.3
372	143426-51-1		[4-(1H-pyrrol-1-yl)phenyl]methanol	80 ± 1	109.7 ± 10.6	26	1.24 ± 0.04	27 ± 14
565	57634-55-6		4-(2-amino-1,3-thiazol-4-yl)phenol	100 ± 0	~120	85	-8.91 ± 0.49	28.7±19.3
635	64354-50-3		5-methyl-2-phenyl-3-furoic acid	23 ± 4	ND	ND	-2.94 ± 0.16	20.5 ± 7.4

[a] Arbitrary library number

[b] CAS numbers are unique identifiers assigned by the "Chemical Abstracts Service" to describe every chemical described in open access scientific literature.

[c] Tm shift in °C, observed for TbCK in the presence of compound (1mM), value is mean ± SD from the Boltzman curve fitting, see Experimental for details.

[d] Cytotoxicity studies, see Major and Smith 2011 for details, values are percentage of controls in the absence of compound, either mean ± SD (n=3) or mean ± SE (n=2), the latter being in bold.

Table 1. The compounds from the Maybridge Rule of 3 library that show >70% inhibition of TbCK.

All of the compounds in the two data sets (the coupled enzyme activity assay and the thermal shift analysis), were compared to assess any correlation between the two very different methods. In other words looking for compounds that showed a significant change in T_m and a significant inhibition in TbCK enzyme activity (Figure 5A). The vast majority of compounds showed little or no inhibition and little or no shift in T_m. Compounds showing < 40% inhibition of the enzyme activity were removed for clarification (Figure 5B), this highlighted that the majority of compounds that show TbCK enzyme inhibition do not significantly alter the T_m of TbCK. The exceptions are compound 565 with a decrease in T_m~9°C, and compound 68 and 95 with a decrease in T_m~2°C respectively, all show complete inhibition at 0.5 mM (Table 1). Twenty-one compounds showed > 40% enzyme inhibition, 9 of these (43%) displayed > 1°C change in TbCK T_m. This is a substantial enrichment compared to the 7% of compounds with T_m shifts > 1°C observed for the entire library.

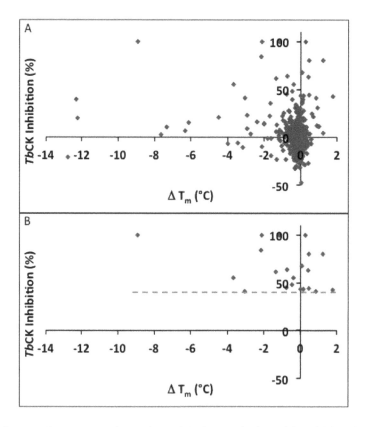

Figure 5. Scatter graph representation showing the correlation between the observed thermal shifts and percentage inhibition of TbCK enzyme activity. A) All of the compounds from the MayBridge Rule of 3 Fragment Library tested. B) For those compounds with > 40% (dotted line) inhibition of TbCK enzyme activity.

Of the compounds identified that alter the T_m of TbCK by > 1°C, ~20% of them inhibit TbCK enzyme activity by > 40%. This suggests that for TbCK thermal shift analysis has allowed significant enrichment, but not total capture of the potential inhibitors of TbCK. However, if a direct assay for a potential drug target was very problematic, prior thermal shift analysis could significantly streamline the number of compounds to be screened, thereby increasing the potential to identify lead compounds. Thermal shift analysis has the disadvantage that good inhibitors could be missed if they do not significantly alter the T_m of the protein.

This raises an interesting question, is it a viable option to target compounds that specifically destabilise an enzyme, causing a decrease in enzyme activity? One could argue this is exactly what pharmaceutical companies are focusing their research efforts upon, but with a slightly different approach. Some of their therapeutic targets rely on finding compounds that disrupt various interactions; hetero- or homo-oligomeric protein-protein, DNA-binding protein and RNA polymerases, many of these are associated with signaling events. Success stories include the identification of HDM2 antagonists associated with P53 activation [46], the identification of anti-cancer agent for the BCL-X_L protein-protein complex and several others, reviewed by Wells and McClendon [47] and more recently by Coyne and colleagues [48].

The techniques utilized to study the formation / disruption of protein-protein complexes are driven by high throughput drug discovery, including fragment based approaches, these include X-ray crystallography, NMR, dynamic light scattering, differential static light scattering, differential scanning fluorimetry [42-50].

In summary, destabilisation by a ligand could affect the oligomeric state of a protein, or in the case of a monomer disrupt intra-molecular interactions, i.e. between stacking α-helixes or β-sheets, causing partial unfolding and thus destabilisation.In the case of TbCK, which we know exists as a dimer, one of several potential mechanisms of destabilisation could be disruption of the dimer interface, whereby a ligand is able to bind to freshly exposed hydrophobic surfaces on the protein, and this interaction allows further destabilisation of the monomer structure.

As it was clear that compounds that inhibit TbCK enzyme activity do not necessarily show a significant increase or decrease in T_m, it was decided to compare inhibition of TbCK enzyme activity with previously determined trypanocidal activities for the compounds [51]. From this comparison (Figure 6) a group of compounds above a threshold of > 70% inhibition of TbCK showed significant trypanocidal activity (circled), suggesting a direct correlation.

Compounds from the May Bridge Rule of 3 Fragment Library with greater than 70% inhibition (dotted line) of the TbCK enzyme activity are circled and numbered. Numbers correspond to arbitrary compound library numbers; see Table 1 for chemical structures and extra data. T. brucei survival data was previously determined [51].

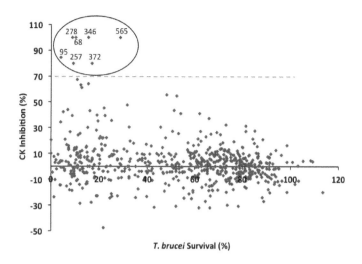

Figure 6. Correlation of the percentage inhibition of *Tb*CK enzyme activity assay and *T. brucei* survival.

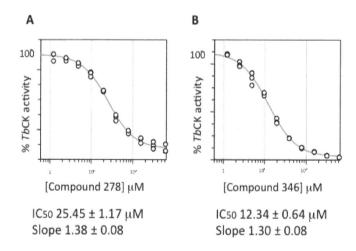

Figure 7. IC50 curves of the promising compounds (278 and 346) that show significant TbCK inhibition.

IC50 values were determined for these compounds (Table 1, Figure 7) ranging from 100s of μM to low μM. For example, compound 278 (1-methyl-(1H-indol-6-yl)methanol) has an IC50 value of 25.45 ± 1.16 μM however the selectivity index is not very good, while compound 346 (3-pyridin-3-ylaniline) has an IC50 value of 12.35 ± 0.64 μM with a high selectivity index.

One of the strengths of the Maybridge Rule of 3 Fragment Library is the chemical diversity, additionally a range of analogous structures can normally be found within it allowing initial structure activity relationships to be formulated. There are several close analogues of compound 278 (1-methyl-(1H-indol-6-yl)methanol), which highlight that the N-methyl indole moiety seems necessary to have any TbCK inhibition and the methanol portion of the molecule can not be replaced by a carboxylic acid. Investigation of the CHEMBL database for similar compounds identified 1-Methyl-1H-pyrrolo[2,3-c]pyridine (CHEMBL594467) which was screened as one of a library of tricyclic and bicyclic analogues of indoloquinoline alkaloids against a variety of protozoan parasites. The analogue mentioned here showed weak trypanocidal activity (624 μM) against *Trypanosoma brucei rhodesiense*, but significantly better (37 μM) against *Plasmodium falciparum* [52].

Another analogue, 1-Methyl-1H-indole (CHEMBL19912) has been shown to interact with human intracellular adhesion molecules and highlights the importance of selectivity [53]. 1H-indol-5-yl-methanol (CHEMBL1650258) has previously been screened against *Leishmania* as a potential PTR1 inhibitor but was shown to be inactive at 500 μM [54]

For the relatively simple compound 346 (3-pyridin-3-ylaniline), there are several analogous structures in the library, including compound 262 (2-(1H-imidazo-1-yl)aniline) which shows ~55% TbCK enzyme inhibition and is trypanocidal. Compound 347 (4-pyridin-3-ylaniline) is a structural isomer of 346 but shows no TbCK enzyme inhibition and is not trypanocidal. The only related structure in the CHEMBL database was 3-(pyridin-3-yl)benzenaminium (CHEMBL1778131) which was shown to be a weakinhibitor of metallo-β−lactamase IMP-1 [55].

4. Conclusions

In this study, screening of a comparatively small fragment library by two different screening methods has allowed identification of several compounds that interact with and inhibit TbCK, a genetically validated drug target against African sleeping sickness. Some of the inhibitory fragments were also selectively trypanocidal, considering these are relatively simple molecules with no optimization, finding low μM inhibitors is very encouraging. Moreover some of the morphological phenotypes of these trypanocidal compounds include cell-cycle arrests similar to those observed for the TbCK conditional knockout grown under permissive conditions.

This study highlights that if faced with a drug target that is problematic to screen, prior thermal shift analysis could significantly triage the number of compounds to be screened, thereby significantly increasing the potential to identify lead compounds. This approach obviously has the limitation that potential inhibitors could be missed if they do not significantly alter the T_m of the protein.

Future follow up work with TbCK will include expanding the structure activity relationship of our most promising hits identified by this study. Their trypanocidal mode of action will be investigated by undertaking various *in vivo* biochemical phenotyping experiments to ascertain if they are inhibiting *Tb*CK, thus causing a lack of *de novo* PC synthesis, known to be essential for the parasite.

The ultimate goal is to identify new easy to make, affordable, easy to administer, drugs in the fight against African sleeping sickness and other closely related protozoan transmitted Third World diseases.

Acknowledgements

This work was supported in part by a Wellcome Trust Senior Research Fellowship (067441) and Wellcome Trust project grants 086658 and 093228. We thank the late and sorely missed Dr Rupert Russell (St Andrews), supported by SUSLA, for access to the May Bridge Rule of 3 Fragment Library.

Author details

Louise L. Major, Helen Denton and Terry K. Smith

Biomedical Sciences Research Centre, The North Haugh, The University, St. Andrews, Fife, Scotland, U.K.

References

[1] WHO web site: http://www.who.int/topics/trypanosomiasis_african/en/

[2] Steverding, D. Parasites & vectors 2010, 3, 15.

[3] Priotto, G.; Kasparian, S.; Mutombo, W.; Ngouama, D.; Ghorashian, S.; Arnold, U.; Ghabri, S.; Baudin, E.; Buard, V.; Kazadi-Kyanza, S.; Ilunga, M.; Mutangala, W.; Pohlig, G.; Schmid, C.; Karunakara, U.; Torreele, E.; Kande, V. Lancet 2009, 374, 56.

[4] Delespaux, V.; de Koning, H. P. Drug resistance updates : reviews and commentaries in antimicrobial and anticancer chemotherapy 2007, 10, 30.

[5] Baker, N.; Alsford, S.; Horn, D. MolBiochemParasit 2011, 176, 55.

[6] Bouteille, B., O. Oukem, S. Bisser, and M. Dumas. 2003. Treatment perspectives for human African trypanosomiasis. Fundam. Clin. Pharmacol. 17:171

[7] Priotto, G., C. Fogg, M. Balasegaram, O. Erphas, A. Louga, F. Checchi, S. Ghabri, and P. Piola. 2006. Three drug combinations for late-stage *Trypanosoma brucei gambiense* sleeping sickness: a randomized clinical trial in Uganda. PLoSClin. Trials 1:e39

[8] Priotto, G., S. Kasparian, W. Mutombo, D. Ngouama, S. Ghorashian, U. Arnold, S. Ghabri, E. Baudin, V. Buard, S. Kazadi-Kyanza, M. Ilunga, W. Mutangala, G. Pohlig, C. Schmid, U. Karunakara, E. Torreele, and V. Kande. 2009. Nifurtimox-eflornithine combination therapy for second-stage African *Trypanosoma brucei gambiense* trypano-somiasis: a multicentre, randomised, phase III, non-inferiority trial. Lancet 374:56-64

[9] M. A. Ferguson; G. A. Cross Myristylation of the membrane form of a *Trypanosoma brucei* variant surface glycoprotein. J. Biol. Chem. 1984, 259, 3011-3015.

[10] M. A. Ferguson; M. G. Low; G.A. Cross Glycosyl-sn-1,2-dimyristylphosphatidylinosi-tol is covalently linked to *Trypanosoma brucei* variant surface glycoprotein. J. Biol. Chem. 1985, 260, 14547-14555.

[11] Ferguson, M.A.J., Brimacombe, J.S., Brown, J.R., Crossman, A., Dix, A., Field, R.A., Guther, M.L.S., Milne, K.G., Sharma, D.K. and Smith, T.K., (1999). The GPI biosyn-thetic pathway as a therapeutic target for African sleeping sickness. Biochim. Bio-phys. Acta 1455, 327-340.

[12] G. A. M. Cross Antigenic variation in trypanosomes: Secrets surface slowly. BioEs-says 1996, 18, 283-287.

[13] N. Aitcheson; S. Talbot; J. Shapiro; K. Hughes; C. Adkin; T. Butt; K. Sheader; G. Ru-denko VSG switching in *Trypanosoma brucei*: antigenic variation analysed using RNAi in the absence of immune selection. MolMicrobiol. 2005, 57, 1608-1622.

[14] Smith, T.K, &Bütikofer, P. (2010) Phospholipid biosynthesis in Trypansomabrucei. Mol Bio Para 172:66-79.

[15] Richmond, G.S,Gibellini, F., Young, S.A., Major, L., Denton, H. Lilley, A. and Smith T.K (2010) Lipidomic Analysis of bloodstream and procyclic form *Trypanosoma brucei* Parasitology 137 (9) I : 1357-1392.

[16] Young SA, Mina JG, Denny PW, Smith TK.(2012) Sphingolipid and ceramide homeo-stasis, potential therapeutic targets Biochem Res Int. 2012;2012:248135.

[17] Li, Z. and Vance, D.E. (2008) Phosphatidylcholine and choline homeostatis J Lipid Res. 49: 1187-1194.

[18] Young, S.A & Smith, T.K, (2010) The essential neutral sphingomyelinase is involved in the trafficking of the variant surface glycoprotein in the bloodstream form of *Try-panosoma brucei*. Molecular Microbiology 76(6): 1461-1482.

[19] Kennedy E.P., and Weiss, S.B. (1956) The function of cytidine coenzymes in the bio-synthesis of phospholipids. J. Biol. Chem. 222:193-214

[20] Gibellini, F & Smith T.K (2010) Critical Review on the Kennedy Pathway for IUBMB Life 62: 414-428.

[21] Kanipes, M.I. and S.A. Henry, 1997 The phospholipid methyltransferases in yeast. Bi-ochimBiophysActa. 1348(1-2): p. 134-41.

[22] Rifkin, M.R., C.A. Strobos, and A.H. Fairlamb, 1995 Specificity of ethanolamine transport and its further metabolism in *Trypanosoma brucei*. J Biol Chem. 270(27): p. 16160-6.

[23] Gibellini. F., Hunter W. N. & Smith, T.K, (2008) Biochemical characterisation of the initial steps of the Kennedy pathway in *Trypanosoma brucei*- the ethanolamine and choline kinases BJ 415 135-144.

[24] Choi, J.Y., W.E. Martin, R.C. Murphy, and D.R. Voelker, 2004 Phosphatidylcholine and N-methylated phospholipids are nonessential in Saccharomyces cerevisiae. J Biol Chem. 279(40): p. 42321-30.

[25] Pessi, G., J.Y. Choi, J.M. Reynolds, D.R. Voelker, and C.B. Mamoun, 2005 In vivo evidence for the specificity of Plasmodium falciparum phosphoethanolamine methyltransferase and its coupling to the Kennedy pathway. J Biol Chem. 280(13): p. 12461-6.

[26] Pessi, G., G. Kociubinski, and C.B. Mamoun, 2004 A pathway for phosphatidylcholine biosynthesis in Plasmodium falciparum involving phosphoethanolamine methylation. ProcNatlAcadSci U S A. 101(16): p. 6206-11.

[27] Witola, W.H., G. Pessi, K. El Bissati, J.M. Reynolds, and C.B. Mamoun, 2006 Localization of the phosphoethanolaminemethyltransferase of the human malaria parasite Plasmodium falciparum to the Golgi apparatus. J Biol Chem. 281(30): p. 21305-11.

[28] Cornell, RB and Northwood, I.C. (2000) Regulation of CTP:phosphocholinecytidyltransferase by amphitropism and relocalization. TIBS 25 441-447

[29] Jackowski, S. and P. Fagone, 2005 CTP: Phosphocholine cytidylyltransferase: paving the way from gene to membrane. J Biol Chem. 280(2): p. 853-6.

[30] Kent, C., 1997 CTP:phosphocholinecytidylyltransferase. BiochimBiophysActa. 1348(1-2): p. 79-90.

[31] Weinhold, P.A. and D.A. Feldman, 1992 Choline-phosphate cytidylyltransferase. Methods Enzymol. 209: p. 248-58.

[32] McMaster, C.R. and R.M. Bell, 1997 CDP-choline:1,2-diacylglycerol cholinephosphotransferase. BiochimBiophysActa. 1348(1-2): p. 100-10.

[33] Carman, G.M.andZeimetz, G.M (1996) Regulation of phospholipid biosynthesis in the yeast Saccharomyces cerevisiae. J. Biol. Chem. 271, 13293-13296.

[34] Simon Young, Federica Gibellini, Keith R. Mathews, William N. Hunter & Terry K. Smith (2012) In the mammalian bloodstream, *Trypanosoma brucei* is totally dependent upon its only choline kinase for survival. Pending submission.

[35] R. A. E. Carr, M. Congreve, C. W. Murray, and D. C. Rees, "Fragment-based lead discovery: leads by design," DrugDiscovery Today, vol. 10, no. 14, pp. 987–992, 2005.

[36] www.maybridge.com/images/pdfs/ro3frag.pdf

[37] J.T. Moore, A. Uppal, F. Maley, G.F. Maley (1993) Overcoming Inclusion Body Formation in a High-Level Expression System. Protein Expression and Purification, 4: 160-163

[38] Niesen, F. H., Berglund, H. and Vedadi, M. (2007) The use of differential scanning fluorimetry to detect ligand interactions that promote protein stability. Nature Protocols, 2, 2212-2221.

[39] Kim, K., Kim, K.H., Storey, M.K., Voelker, D.R. and Carman, G.M. (1999) Isolation and characterization of the *Saccharomyces cerevisiae* EKI1 gene encoding ethanolamine kinase. *JBiolChem* 274: 14857-14866

[40] M. C. Lo, A. Aulabaugh, G. Jin et al., "Evaluation of fluorescence-based thermal shift assays for hit identification in drug discovery," Analytical Biochemistry, vol. 332, no. 1, pp. 153–159, 2004.

[41] Zhang, J,H., Chang, T.D. and Oldenberg, K.R. A simple statistical parameters for use in evaluation and validation of high throughput screening assays 1999 J Biomol Screen 4: 67-73.

[42] Kopen, J. And Schneider, G. Comparison of fluorescence and light scattering based methods to assess formation and stability of protein-protein complexes 2011 J Structural Biology 175: 211-223.

[43] Pantoliano MW, Petrella EC, Kwasnoski JD, Lobanov VS, Myslik J, Graf E, Carver T, Asel E, Springer BA, Lane P, Salemme FR. High-density miniaturized thermal shift assays as a general strategy for drug discovery. J Biomol Screen. 2001 Dec;6(6):429-40.

[44] PiotrasCimmperman, LinaBaranauskienė, SimonaJachimovičiūtė, JelenaJachno, JolantaTorresan, VilmaMichailovienė, JurgitaMatulienė, JolantaSereikaitė, VladasBumelis, DaumantasMatulis

A Quantitative Model of Thermal Stabilization and Destabilization of Proteins by Ligands Biophysical Journal 2008 (Vol. 95, Issue 7, pp. 3222-3231)

[45] Marfori M, Kobe B, Forwood JK. Ligand-induced conformational changes within a hexameric Acyl-CoA thioesterase. J Biol Chem. 2011 Oct 14 ;286(41):35643-9

[46] Grasberger BL, Lu T, Schubert C, Parks DJ, Carver TE, Koblish HK, Cummings MD, LaFrance LV, Milkiewicz KL, Calvo RR, Maguire D, Lattanze J, Franks CF, Zhao S, Ramachandren K, Bylebyl GR, Zhang M, Manthey CL, Petrella EC, Pantoliano MW, Deckman IC, Spurlino JC, Maroney AC, Tomczuk BE, Molloy CJ, Bone RF Discovery and cocrystal structure of benzodiazepinedione HDM2 antagonists that activate p53 in cells.J Med Chem. 2005;48(4):909-12.

[47] Wells, J.A. and McClendon, C.L. Reaching for high-hanging fruit in drug discovery at protein-protein interfaces 2007 450: pp1001-1009

[48] Coyne A.G, Scott, D.E and Abell, C. Drugging challenging targets using fragment-based approaches 2010 Current opinions in Chemical Biology 14:299-307.

[49] Murray C.W. and Rees D.C. The rise of fragment-based drug discovery Nature Chemistry 2009 1:1187-192

[50] Shuker S.B., Hajduk P.J., Meadows R.P. and Fesik, S.W. Discovering high-affinity ligands for proteins SAR by NMR 1996 Science 274: 5292, pp 1531-1534.

[51] Louise L. Major & Terry K. Smith (2011) Screening of the MayBridge Rule of 3 Fragment Library for trypanocidal compounds that interact with the myo-inositol-3-phosphate synthase from *Trypanosoma brucei* Molecular Biology International Vol 2011, Article ID 389364,doi:10.4061/2011/389364).

[52] Van Baelen G, Hostyn S, Dhooghe L, Tapolcsanyi P, Matyus P, Lemiere G, Dommisse R, Kaiser M, Brun R, Cos P, Maes L, Hajos G, Riedl Z, Nagy I, Maes BU, Pieters LStructure-activity relationship of antiparasitic and cytotoxic indoloquinoline alkaloids, and their tricyclic and bicyclic analogues.Bioorg. Med. Chem. (2009) 17:7209-7217

[53] Liu G, Huth JR, Olejniczak ET, Mendoza R, DeVries P, Leitza S, Reilly EB, Okasinski GF, Fesik SW, von Geldern TW Novel p-arylthiocinnamides as antagonists of leukocyte function-associated antigen-1/intracellular adhesion molecule-1 interaction. 2. Mechanism of inhibition and structure-based improvement of pharmaceutical properties.J. Med. Chem. (2001) 44:1202-1210

[54] Stefania Ferrari, Federica Morandi, DomantasMotiejunas, Erika Nerini, Stefan Henrich, Rosaria Luciani, Alberto Venturelli, Sandra Lazzari, SamueleCalò, Shreedhara Gupta, Veronique Hannaert, Paul A. M. Michels, Rebecca C. Wade, and M. Paola Costi Journal of Medicinal Chemistry 201154 (1), 211-221

[55] Vella P, Hussein WM, Leung EW, Clayton D, Ollis DL, Mitic N, Schenk G, McGeary RP The identification of new metallo-BETA-lactamase inhibitor leads from fragment-based screening. Bioorg. Med. Chem. Lett. (2011) 21:3282-3285

Applications of Snake Venom Proline-Rich Oligopeptides (Bj-PROs) in Disease Conditions Resulting from Deficient Nitric Oxide Production

Claudiana Lameu and Henning Ulrich

Additional information is available at the end of the chapter

1. Introduction

Snake venoms contain a complex mixture of proteins and biologically active peptides [1, 2]. Some of these bioactive peptides are derived from precursor proteins that through proteo-lytic processing generate mature active polypeptides [3]. As an example, the protein precursor of natriuretic peptide type-C (CNP) from the Brazilian pit viper *Bothrops jararaca* venom and brain originates CNP, a hormone present in several animal species as well as various isoforms of proline-rich oligopeptides (*Bj*-PROs) [4, 5]. *Bj*-PROs were the first natural inhibitors of angiotensin I-converting enzyme (ACE) described [6]. The metalloproteinase ACE, the key enzyme of the renin-angiotensin system, displays two homologous active sites, one at the C-terminal and the other at the N-terminal of the protein [7]. While both active sites convert angiotensin I into angiotensin II and cleave bradykinin (BK) into BK1-5 and BK1-7, the C-terminal is more effective in hydrolysis of these vasoactive peptides [8].

Bj-PROs are molecules of 5 to 14 amino acids residues with a pyroglutamyl residue (<E) at the N-terminus and a proline residue at the C-terminus. *Bj*-PROs longer than seven amino acids share similar features, including a high content of proline residues and a C-terminal tripeptide sequence Ile–Pro–Pro [13]. Since *Bj*-PROs are ACE inhibitors, they potentiate some pharmacological activities of BK, such as induction of contractile action of smooth muscles of guinea-pig ileum *in vitro* as well as *in vivo* BK-induced effects on central nervous, cardiovascular and anti-nociceptive systems [6, 9, 10]. For this reason, these peptides were initially named bradykinin-potentiating peptides (BPPs). The ability of some *Bj*-PROs inhibiting ACE turned them in structural models to develop the first non-peptide site directed inhibitor of this enzyme. The development of Captopril in the early 1980s became a paradigm

for "rational drug design", a concept much heralded today and made possible by computer imaging and genome science [11].

Many studies on structure–activity of *Bj*-PROs showed that a simple analogous structure to Ala–Pro was optimal for binding to the active site of ACE. Replacement of the carboxyl by a sulfhydryl group enhanced the inhibitory activity of the analogue by 1,000-fold. This compound proved to be one of the most potent competitive inhibitors of ACE and, therefore, turned into a useful drug to treat human hypertension (reviewed by [12]). Captopril was a blockbuster drug and inspired the creation of several generations of similar antihypertensive compounds.

However, due to structural diversity of *Bj*-PROs [13] other mechanisms besides inhibiting ACE were proposed. In fact, some of these peptides augmenting argininosuccinate synthase (AS) activity *in vitro* and *in vivo*, can also induce rises in free intracellular calcium concentration ($[Ca^{2+}]_i$) by acting on muscarinic acetylcholine, BK or yet unidentified receptors [15-18] or reversal inhibition of nicotinic acetylcholine receptor [19]. These novel mechanisms of action, recently identified for *Bj*-PROs explain their anti-hypertensive effects [14-17, 20, 21]. Therefore, investigation of *Bj*-PRO-induced effects through acting on different targets opens possibilities of applications for these peptides in the treatment of several pathologies lacking efficient treatment options.

Here, we describe the targets of various *Bj*-PROs and their potential use to treat different target-related pathologies, as well as discuss chemical properties of these peptides for obtaining an oral pharmaceutical formulation.

2. Targets of proline-rich oligopeptides from Bothrops jararaca

Recently, argininosuccinate synthase (AS) was identified as another target for the *Bj*-PROs, which both *in vitro* and *in vivo* positively modulates the activity of this enzyme [14] which leads to L-arginine synthesis [22]. L-arginine is a nonessential amino acid under normal conditions as it is obtained from the breakdown of proteins or synthesized de novo from citrulline in the kidneys by AS (EC 6.3.4.5) and argininosuccinate lyase (ASL, EC 4.3.2.1). AS catalyses the reversible condensation of citrulline with aspartate with consumption of ATP to form argininosuccinate; ASL catalyzes the conversion of the argininosuccinate to fumarate and L-arginine, which is released into the circulation [22].

In the liver, enzymes involved in the anabolism of L-arginine, AS and ASL are present; however, there is not a net production of L-arginine due to arginase activity (EC 3.5.3.1) as part of the urea cycle, catalyzes the hydrolysis of L-arginine into L-ornithine and urea. The urea is then excreted in the urine and L-ornithine is recycled back into the cycle [23]. Furthermore, AS is the rate-limiting enzyme of the citrulline-nitric oxide (NO) cycle for the supply of L-arginine which is then metabolized by NO synthase (NOS) to form NO and citrulline [24-26]. Citrulline, through the reactions catalyzed by AS and ASL may cycle back to arginine, constituting the citrulline-NO cycle [27, 28]. In summary, AS activity contributes to three major different functions in the adult organism depending on the cell/tissue considered: (i) ammonia detoxification in the liver, (ii) L-arginine production for the whole organism by kidney and (iii) L-arginine synthesis for NO production in many other cells [22].

Three isoforms of NOS catalyze the reaction: the endothelial constitutive NOS (eNOS), the neuronal constitutive NOS (nNOS) and the inducible NOS (iNOS), reviewed in [29, 30]. NO is a gaseous molecule capable of interacting with many intracellular targets for triggering a series of signal transduction pathways, resulting in a stimulatory and inhibitory signals. NO plays roles in cardiovascular, immune and neuronal control. It is directly involved in arterial tension control since it regulates the local and systemic resistance of vascular walls, as well as the sodium balance [31]. The NO produced by endothelial cells reaches neighboring smooth muscle cells where it activates two types of K^+ channels, ATP-sensitive and Ca^{2+}-dependent [32, 33], and thereby induces the relaxation of blood vessels and brings about vascular dilation leading direct consequences in processes like erection, arterial pressure systemic or organ-specific [34].

Due to the great physiological importance of the NO, compounds revealing properties aspotential NO donors have been protected by patents. They are based on the fact that there are many pathological states related to NO deficiency (reviewed by [35]). However, a major problem of NO donors is to achieve a therapeutic dose without reaching a threshold of toxicity. Mostly, if NO is produced in excess around of cells in a pro-oxidant state, NO could react with reactive oxygen species (ROS) such as superoxide and hydrogen peroxide forming peroxynitrite and nitrogen oxide III, which has been linked to pathogenesis of neurodegenerative disorders [35].

The superoxide anion is produced by uncoupling of NOS due to the lack of its natural substrate L-arginine or tetrahydrobiopterin (BH_4) [36], an important cofactor for NOS. Excessive production of superoxide is explained by increased activity and expression of the enzyme arginase, which competes with eNOS for its substrate L-arginine [37]. Other possible sources for elevated concentrations of ROS include increased expression and activity of NADPH and reduced superoxide dismutase activity [38, 39].

In order to compensate for the deficiency of NO production without induction of toxicity, addition of exogenous L-arginine in the maintenance of NO production has been investigated. The inefficiency of swallowed L-arginine in promoting increase of NO can be explained by its low availability, due to the first pass effect, since the viability of L-arginine as substrate for NOS is reduced by the activity of arginase in the liver. Several studies have shown that induction or activation of arginase may lead to impaired NO production and endothelial dysfunction (reviewed by [35]).

Thus, NO presents challenges and opportunities to intervene and promote human health. The study of regulation of NO production becomes important for understanding the mechanisms which maintain NO levels in a safe range and not injurious to the body.

An important mechanism for control and maintenance of NO levels is achieved by its recycling via the NO-citrulline cycle. The obtained L-arginine provided by the citrulline-NO cycle is then directed to sustain NO production, sparing bulk intracellular L-arginine for other metabolic roles [24]. In view of that, compounds that increase AS activity and sustain tightly NO production avoiding an excess production will ensure adequate bioavailability for proper physiological functioning. Guerreiro and colleagues demonstrated that a *Bj*-PRO promotes activation of AS, assayed in the presence of the substrates ATP, citrulline, and aspartate, thus leading to NO production by endothelial cells [14]. More recently, we have demonstrated that other *Bj*-PROs induce NO production by activation of AS or kinin-B2 receptors as well as by M1 muscarinic acetylcholine activation, thereby inducing vasodilatation *in vivo* [16, 17].

The patent entitled "Proline-Rich Peptides, Pharmaceutical Composition, use of one or more peptides and method of treatment" was deposited to protect the use and application of *Bj*-PROs and analogous molecules [patent: BR2007/ 000003]. All applications contemplated by patent BR2007/ 000003 are consistent with the use of PROs as prototype molecules for the development of new drugs aiming to treat a range of pathological states related to deficiency in NO production and AS activity, e.g. lung hypertension, preeclampsia, essential hypertension, coagulopathies and citrullinemia. Some of these applications will be discussed below.

3. Pulmonary hypertension

Pulmonary hypertension (PH) is an increase in blood pressure in the pulmonary artery, vein or capillaries, together known as the lung vasculature. In fetus life, PH is a normal state essential for survival. Since the placenta, not the lung, serves as the organ of gas exchange during embryonic development, most of the right ventricular output crosses from the ductus arteriosus to the aorta, and only 5–10% of the combined ventricular output is directed to the pulmonary vascular bed. Pulmonary vascular constriction plays a key role in maintaining high pulmonary vascular tone during fetal life. At the same time, the fetal lung and pulmonary vasculature must prepare for the dramatic adaptation to air breathing at the time of birth [40].

However, PH can continue even after the birth, called persistent pulmonary hypertension that develops when pulmonary vascular resistance remains elevated, resulting in right-to-left shunting of blood through fetal circulatory pathways. The pulmonary vascular resistance may remain elevated due to pulmonary hypoplasia and cause disease states, like congenital diaphragmatic hernia, as well as impaired development of the pulmonary arteries, resulting in the meconium aspiration syndrome, or failing adaption of the pulmonary vascular bed as occurs with perinatal asphyxia [41]. Moreover, PH has more than one etiological factor, thus it can be classified as idiopathic PH when there is no identifiable cause of this disease; familial PH with a previous disease history; and associated PH when an underlying cause of PH such as connective tissue disease is present [42].

PH has been reported in patients with chronic hemolytic anemias, including sickle cell disease, thalassemia, paroxysmal nocturnal hemoglobinuria, hereditary spherocytosis, malaria, among other disease states [43, 44]. The exact mechanism(s) involved in the development of

PH in these patients is unclear. Hemolysis may result in a nitric oxide deficient state through free hemoglobin scavenging of nitric oxide and release of erythrocyte arginase, which limits L-arginine, a substrate for nitric oxide synthesis [45].

Nitric oxide is synthesized from terminal nitrogen of L-arginine by NOS. All three NOS isoforms are expressed in the lung and are distinguished by regulation of their activities, as well as by specific sites and developmental patterns of expression [46]. The isoform eNOS is expressed in vascular endothelial cells and is believed to be the predominant source of NO production in pulmonary circulation [40]. This hypothesis is corroborated by the fact that NO inhalation in premature newborns with severe respiratory failure due to PH provides improvement of symptoms, accompanied by marked increase in oxygenation [34].

Although large well-designed studies paved the way to Food and Drug Administration (FDA) approval of therapeutic NO inhalation, it is equally important to note that inhaled NO did not reduce the mortality, length of hospitalization, or the risk of significant neurodevelopmental impairment associated with persistent PH in newborn children [40]. It is known that at excessive levels NO can react with reactive oxygen species (ROS) such as superoxide and hydrogen peroxide. Such increase in ROS was observed in the smooth muscle and adventitia of pulmonary arteries from lambs with chronic intrauterine PH [47, 48], forming peroxynitrite, an anion with deleterious tissue-oxidant effects [49].

Inhaled NO is usually delivered with high concentrations of oxygen. Whereas hyperoxic ventilation continues to be a mainstay in the treatment of PH, little is known about the side effects of oxygen supply together with NO. The extreme hyperoxia routinely used in PH management may in fact be toxic to the developing lung due to ROS formation [39, 50, 51]. Superoxide may react with arachidonic acid to increase concentrations of isoprostanes and may also combine with NO to form peroxynitrite [52] with possible induction of vasoconstriction, cytotoxicity, and damage to surfactant proteins and lipids. Moreover, peroxynitrite has been shown to directly induce NOS uncoupling. New data indicate that even brief (30 min) periods of exposure to 100% O_2 are sufficient to increase reactivity of pulmonary vessels in healthy lambs [53, 54], to diminish the response of the pulmonary vasculature to endogenous and exogenous nitric oxide [54], and to increase the activity of cGMP-specific phosphodiesterases [51]. Inhaled NO would theoretically benefit patients with chronic primary or secondary pulmonary hypertension, but its therapeutic application in this setting has been limited by the risk of causing rebound pulmonary hypertension, if it is inadvertently discontinued, and the lack of practical home-based continuous delivery devices.

Therefore, we have proposed an alternative approach for controlled induction of NO production. We believe that cytosolic L-arginine provides a major NO donor. Arginine concentrations subject to metabolic fine-tuning controls will assure that the amino acid is kept in a homeostatic concentration range. These effects could be achieved by the action of Bj-PRO on AS, a target unexplored by the pharmaceutical industry. Compounds inducing an increase in AS expression and activity are promising for the treatment of diseases related with deficient NO production.

4. Preeclampsia

Preeclampsia, a pregnancy-specific syndrome characterized by hypertension, proteinuria and edema, causes fetal and maternal morbidity and mortality with high incidence in developing countries [55]. Symptoms of preeclampsia are currently combated by sodium restriction, rest and medication for blood pressure control to avoid complications for the mother and prolong the pregnancy for fetal maturation [56-58]. However, this attempt is rather unspecific with possible side effects for the developing fetus [59, 60]. Currently, the only therapy of preeclamsia involves placenta removal resulting in pre-term birth [61]. Therefore, novel drug development for pregnancy-specific conditions remains a challenge [59].

The pathology of preeclampsia involves systemic inflammation, oxidative stress, alterations in the levels of angiogenic factors, and vascular reactivity leading to hypertension of the mother and metabolic alterations in the fetus [61, 62]. A number of evidence suggests that clinical manifestations are caused by endothelial malfunction including insufficient production of NO [63, 64]. Levels of eNOS, the enzyme responsible for NO synthesis in the endothelium from L-arginine, are decreased in human umbilical vein endothelial cells from pregnant women suffering from preeclampsia [62] together with impaired AS expression [65]. The low availability of L-arginine uncouples eNOS activity, decreases NO production and increases eNOS-dependent superoxide generation [62, 66], consequently resulting in reduced vasodilatation or in inflammatory processes observed in preeclampsia [66, 67]. Therefore, it is expected that the sustained concentration of L-arginine in endothelial cells is likely to play a critical role not only in the control of systemic blood pressure, but also in inhibition of inflammatory processes [68].

Recently, we have reported that a *Bj*-PRO containing ten amino acid residues (*Bj*-PRO-10c), activating AS, is able to correct dysfunction of human umbilical vein endothelial cells from pregnant women suffering from preeclampsia [65] (Figure 1).

Bj-PRO-10c, besides augmenting the activity of AS both *in vitro* and *in vivo* [14] increases significantly eNOS expression of human umbilical vein endothelial cells obtained from pregnant women suffering from preeclampsia [65]. It was observed that the increase in NO levels induced by *Bj*-PRO-10c diminished the oxidative stress of the endothelial cells of preeclamptic women, shown as a 50% reduction in superoxide levels [65] (Figure 1).

Most importantly, *Bj*-PRO-10c promoted NO production only in endothelial cells from patients suffering from the disorder and not in normotensive pregnant women. In agreement, *Bj*-PRO-10c is a molecule endowed with antihypertensive activity that reduced blood pressure in hypertensive but not in normotensive rats [69]. These observations led to suggest that *Bj*-PRO-10c promotes its anti-hypertensive effect in mothers with preeclampsia without any effect on the blood pressure of the fetus, a problem with drugs currently used for minimizing health problems arising from preeclampsia. Taken together, *Bj*-PRO-10c becomes a potential tool for the development of an efficient drug for preeclampsia treatment.

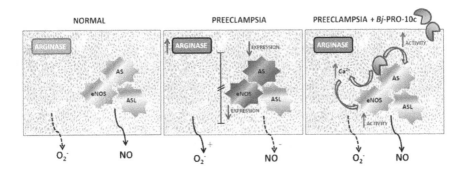

Figure 1. *Bj*-PRO-10c-induced effects on endothelial cell from healthy and pregnant women suffering from preeclampsia. In endothelial cells from normotensive pregnant women (NORMAL), NO production is adequate to maintain normal gestation. In cells from patients with the disease (PREECLAMPSIA) both decreased NO production and increased superoxide (O₂) production are observed together with enhanced activity of the enzyme arginase, reduced expression of eNOS and AS and uncoupled eNOS. When endothelial cells from pregnant women suffering from preeclampsia are exposed to *Bj*-PRO-10c (PREECLAMPSIA + *Bj*-PRO-10c), production of NO and superoxide return to normal ranges, since *Bj*-PRO-10c initiates a signaling cascade including increases of cytosolic calcium concentration activating eNOS and augmenting AS activity.

5. Citrullinemia

Citrullinemia, a disorder causing serious episodes of neurological symptoms associated with hyperammonemia involving disorientation, abnormal behaviors (aggression, irritability, and hyperactivity), seizures, coma, and potentially death from brain edema [70], occurs in two variants: CTLN1 (MIM#215700) or classical neonatal onset, and CTLN2 (MIM#603471) or adult-onset [71-74]. Classical citrullinemia in children is associated with a mutation in the AS gene [75]. However, in CTLN2 the enzyme reveals normal kinetic properties and is quantitatively deficient only in the liver of adult-onset citrullinemia patients [71-74]. The most successful therapy of CTLN2 has been liver transplantation [76, 77] because this treatment prevents hyperammonemic crises and corrects consequent metabolic disturbances [70].

It has been reported that administration of L-arginine to CTLN2 patients is effective in decreasing blood ammonia concentration [78, 79]. For ammonia detoxification, arginine needs to enter the liver via the portal vein where is metabolized by mitochondrial arginase to provide ornithine for citrulline and aspartate synthesis and for the priming of the urea cycle [80]. However, care must be taken when administering L-arginine, as fatal cases caused by L-arginine hydrochloride overdose have been reported [81]. In general, the dose of L-arginine supplementation used in the treatment of hyperammoaemia is in the high range between 100 and 700 mg/kg body weight per day [82-85]. In animal models the effects of hyperargininaemia can be observed, reflecting toxic effects of high L-arginine concentration and making it possible to predict side effects of L-arginine supplementation including cognitive deficits, epilepsy and a progressive spastic diplegia [86]. Therefore, drugs augmenting AS activity, the step-limiting enzyme of urea cycle, may be a promising strategy for CTLN2 therapy, since AS is the step-limiting enzyme of the urea cycle. A consequence of increased AS activity, a final common pathway is triggered resulting in the excretion of waste nitrogen as urea [87].

As previously mentioned, CTLN2 is not associated with genetic mutation of the AS gene; however, Saheki et al. identified the SLC25A13 gene as being defective in CTLN2 patients. This gene encodes for a Ca^{2+}-dependent mitochondrial solute carrier, designated citrin [88]. According to Saheki et al., it is difficult to predict disease-causing effects of citrin deficiency in CTLN2, since children carrying citrin gene mutations may suffer from CTLN2 after more than 10 years or several decades of being asymptomatic [70]. In view of that, an option to prevent CLTN2 in infants with mutation of the citrin gen is being sought, having in mind that the nutritional management with appropriate intake of proteins only avoids accumulation of nitrogen [70].

Based on information discussed here, the strategy to increase AS activity in the liver could be an effective treatment for CTLN2 as well to prevent that children diagnosed as carrying SLC25A13 mutations from developing CTLN2 in the future [89]. We believed that direct pharmacological and clinical studies with *Bj*-PROs for these proposals, could turn them into a powerful therapeutic tool. The efficiency of *Bj*-PRO action can yet be improved by the rational design of a compound which in the liver accelerates the urea cycle for eliminating ammonia or even preventing its accumulation.

6. Conclusion

AS as molecular target for drug development will be important for the treatment of a wide variety of diseases associated with deficiency of NO production, and also could transform *Bj*-PROs or their synthetic analogous into blockbuster medicine, as happened in the 80s with Captopril [90, 91]. The properties of *Bj*-PROs enhancing AS activity [14, 17], provides a precise pharmacological tool for controlling pathophysiological mechanisms with advantages of uncontrolled application of exogenous L-arginine or NO donors [92]. For instance, the effect of exogenous NO donors is not subject to physiological control, thus being more susceptible of generating undesired ROS [93, 94]. For all these reasons, keeping NO production in a safe level, so that a deleterious threshold would not be reached, is of particular interest. In this way, *Bj*-PROs should serve as structural models for the development of therapeutic agents for the treatment of various diseases related to NO deficiency, as cause or effect, as well AS deficiency.

Chemical properties of *Bj*-PROs make these peptides even more attractive potential lead compounds for drug development. For instance, *Bj*-PRO-10c is able to penetrate cells, where it remains as an intact molecule for hours [14]. Moreover, *Bj*-PROs contain a notable high proline content [13], which gives them some resistance to hydrolysis by aminopeptidases, carboxypeptidases and endopeptidases [95]. Nevertheless, cyclodextrins or nanocompounds could provide carriers for *Bj*-PROs, since drug release could be controlled in accordance with therapeutic propose [96, 97].

Acknowlegments

H.U. acknowledges grant support from Fundação de Amparo à Pesquisa do Estado de São Paulo (FAPESP) and (Conselho Nacional de Desenvolvimento Científico e Tecnológico (CNPq), Brazil. C.L. is grateful for a postdoctoral fellowship awarded by FAPESP.

Author details

Claudiana Lameu and Henning Ulrich

Department of Biochemistry, Institute of Chemistry, University of São Paulo, São Paulo, Brazil

References

[1] Tanen DA, Ruha AM, Graeme KA, Curry SC, Fischione MA. Rattlesnake envenoma-tions: unusual case presentations. Arch Intern Med. 2001 Feb 12;161(3):474-9.

[2] Walter FG, Bilden EF, Gibly RL. Envenomations. Crit Care Clin. 1999 Apr;15(2): 353-86, ix.

[3] Kini RM. Molecular moulds with multiple missions: functional sites in three-finger toxins. Clinical and experimental pharmacology & physiology. 2002 Sep;29(9):815-22.

[4] Hayashi MA, Murbach AF, Ianzer D, Portaro FC, Prezoto BC, Fernandes BL, et al. The C-type natriuretic peptide precursor of snake brain contains highly specific in-hibitors of the angiotensin-converting enzyme. J Neurochem. 2003 May;85(4):969-77.

[5] Murayama N, Hayashi MA, Ohi H, Ferreira LA, Hermann VV, Saito H, et al. Cloning and sequence analysis of a Bothrops jararaca cDNA encoding a precursor of seven bradykinin-potentiating peptides and a C-type natriuretic peptide. Proceedings of the National Academy of Sciences of the United States of America. 1997 Feb 18;94(4): 1189-93.

[6] Ferreira SH. A Bradykinin-Potentiating Factor (Bpf) Present in the Venom of Bo-throps jararca. Br J Pharmacol Chemother. 1965 Feb;24:163-9.

[7] Wei L, Alhenc-Gelas F, Corvol P, Clauser E. The two homologous domains of human angiotensin I-converting enzyme are both catalytically active. The Journal of biologi-cal chemistry. 1991 May 15;266(14):9002-8.

[8] Jaspard E, Wei L, Alhenc-Gelas F. Differences in the properties and enzymatic specif-
     icities of the two active sites of angiotensin I-converting enzyme (kininase II). Studies
     with bradykinin and other natural peptides. The Journal of biological chemistry. 1993
     May 5;268(13):9496-503.

[9] Camargo AC, Graeff FG. Subcellular distribution and properties of the bradykinin
     inactivation system in rabbit brain homogenates. Biochemical pharmacology. 1969
     Feb;18(2):548-9.

[10] Ribeiro SA, Corrado AP, Graeff FG. Antinociceptive action of intraventricular brady-
     kinin. Neuropharmacology. 1971 Nov;10(6):725-31.

[11] van Dongen M, Weigelt J, Uppenberg J, Schultz J, Wikstrom M. Structure-based
     screening and design in drug discovery. Drug discovery today. 2002 Apr 15;7(8):
     471-8.

[12] Camargo AC, Ianzer D, Guerreiro JR, Serrano SM. Bradykinin-potentiating peptides:
     beyond captopril. Toxicon. 2012 Mar 15;59(4):516-23.

[13] Ianzer D, Konno K, Marques-Porto R, Vieira Portaro FC, Stocklin R, Martins de Ca-
     margo AC, et al. Identification of five new bradykinin potentiating peptides (BPPs)
     from Bothrops jararaca crude venom by using electrospray ionization tandem mass
     spectrometry after a two-step liquid chromatography. Peptides. 2004 Jul;25(7):
     1085-92.

[14] Guerreiro JR, Lameu C, Oliveira EF, Klitzke CF, Melo RL, Linares E, et al. Arginino-
     succinate synthetase is a functional target for a snake venom anti-hypertensive pep-
     tide: role in arginine and nitric oxide production. The Journal of biological chemistry.
     2009 Jul 24;284(30):20022-33.

[15] Lameu C, Hayashi MA, Guerreiro JR, Oliveira EF, Lebrun I, Pontieri V, et al. The cen-
     tral nervous system as target for antihypertensive actions of a proline-rich peptide
     from Bothrops jararaca venom. Cytometry A. 2010 Mar;77(3):220-30.

[16] Morais KL, Hayashi MA, Bruni FM, Lopes-Ferreira M, Camargo AC, Ulrich H, et al.
     Bj-PRO-5a, a natural angiotensin-converting enzyme inhibitor, promotes vasodilata-
     tion mediated by both bradykinin B(2)and M1 muscarinic acetylcholine receptors. Bi-
     ochemical pharmacology. 2011 Mar 15;81(6):736-42.

[17] Morais KLP, Ianzer D, Santos RAS, Miranda JRR, Melo RL, Guerreiro JR, et al. The
     structural diversity of proline-rich oligopeptides from Bothrops jararaca (Bj-PROs)
     provides synergistic cardiovascular actions Submitted.

[18] Negraes PD, Lameu C, Hayashi MA, Melo RL, Camargo AC, Ulrich H. The snake
     venom peptide Bj-PRO-7a is a M1 muscarinic acetylcholine receptor agonist. Cytom-
     etry A. 2011 Jan;79(1):77-83.

[19] Nery AA, Trujillo CA, Lameu C, Konno K, Oliveira V, Camargo AC, et al. A novel
     physiological property of snake bradykinin-potentiating peptides-reversion of

MK-801 inhibition of nicotinic acetylcholine receptors. Peptides. 2008 Oct;29(10): 1708-15.

[20] Ianzer D, Xavier CH, Fraga FC, Lautner RQ, Guerreiro JR, Machado LT, et al. BPP-5a produces a potent and long-lasting NO-dependent antihypertensive effect. Therapeutic advances in cardiovascular disease. 2011 Dec;5(6):281-95.

[21] Lameu C, Pontieri V, Guerreiro JR, Oliveira EF, da Silva CA, Giglio JM, et al. Brain nitric oxide production by a proline-rich decapeptide from Bothrops jararaca venom improves baroreflex sensitivity of spontaneously hypertensive rats. Hypertens Res. 2010 Dec;33(12):1283-8.

[22] Husson A, Brasse-Lagnel C, Fairand A, Renouf S, Lavoinne A. Argininosuccinate synthetase from the urea cycle to the citrulline-NO cycle. European journal of biochemistry / FEBS. 2003 May;270(9):1887-99.

[23] Aminlari M, Shahbazkia HR, Esfandiari A. Distribution of arginase in tissues of cat (Felis catus). Journal of feline medicine and surgery. 2007 Apr;9(2):133-9.

[24] Flam BR, Eichler DC, Solomonson LP. Endothelial nitric oxide production is tightly coupled to the citrulline-NO cycle. Nitric Oxide. 2007 Nov-Dec;17(3-4):115-21.

[25] Shen LJ, Beloussow K, Shen WC. Accessibility of endothelial and inducible nitric oxide synthase to the intracellular citrulline-arginine regeneration pathway. Biochemical pharmacology. 2005 Jan 1;69(1):97-104.

[26] Xie L, Gross SS. Argininosuccinate synthetase overexpression in vascular smooth muscle cells potentiates immunostimulant-induced NO production. The Journal of biological chemistry. 1997 Jun 27;272(26):16624-30.

[27] Hattori Y, Campbell EB, Gross SS. Argininosuccinate synthetase mRNA and activity are induced by immunostimulants in vascular smooth muscle. Role in the regeneration or arginine for nitric oxide synthesis. The Journal of biological chemistry. 1994 Apr 1;269(13):9405-8.

[28] Hecker M, Sessa WC, Harris HJ, Anggard EE, Vane JR. The metabolism of L-arginine and its significance for the biosynthesis of endothelium-derived relaxing factor: cultured endothelial cells recycle L-citrulline to L-arginine. Proceedings of the National Academy of Sciences of the United States of America. 1990 Nov;87(21):8612-6.

[29] Alderton WK, Cooper CE, Knowles RG. Nitric oxide synthases: structure, function and inhibition. The Biochemical journal. 2001 Aug 1;357(Pt 3):593-615.

[30] Knowles RG, Moncada S. Nitric oxide synthases in mammals. The Biochemical journal. 1994 Mar 1;298 (Pt 2):249-58.

[31] Umans JG, Levi R. Nitric oxide in the regulation of blood flow and arterial pressure. Annual review of physiology. 1995;57:771-90.

[32] Bolotina VM, Najibi S, Palacino JJ, Pagano PJ, Cohen RA. Nitric oxide directly activates calcium-dependent potassium channels in vascular smooth muscle. Nature. 1994 Apr 28;368(6474):850-3.

[33] Murphy ME, Brayden JE. Nitric oxide hyperpolarizes rabbit mesenteric arteries via ATP-sensitive potassium channels. J Physiol. 1995 Jul 1;486 (Pt 1):47-58.

[34] McCurnin DC, Pierce RA, Chang LY, Gibson LL, Osborne-Lawrence S, Yoder BA, et al. Inhaled NO improves early pulmonary function and modifies lung growth and elastin deposition in a baboon model of neonatal chronic lung disease. American journal of physiology. 2005 Mar;288(3):L450-9.

[35] Lameu C, de Camargo AC, Faria M. L-arginine signalling potential in the brain: the peripheral gets central. Recent patents on CNS drug discovery. 2009 Jun;4(2):137-42.

[36] Mata-Greenwood E, Jenkins C, Farrow KN, Konduri GG, Russell JA, Lakshminrusimha S, et al. eNOS function is developmentally regulated: uncoupling of eNOS occurs postnatally. American journal of physiology. 2006 Feb;290(2):L232-41.

[37] Sankaralingam S, Xu H, Davidge ST. Arginase contributes to endothelial cell oxidative stress in response to plasma from women with preeclampsia. Cardiovascular research. 2010 Jan 1;85(1):194-203.

[38] Brennan LA, Steinhorn RH, Wedgwood S, Mata-Greenwood E, Roark EA, Russell JA, et al. Increased superoxide generation is associated with pulmonary hypertension in fetal lambs: a role for NADPH oxidase. Circulation research. 2003 Apr 4;92(6):683-91.

[39] Wedgwood S, Lakshminrusimha S, Fukai T, Russell JA, Schumacker PT, Steinhorn RH. Hydrogen peroxide regulates extracellular superoxide dismutase activity and expression in neonatal pulmonary hypertension. Antioxidants & redox signaling. 2011 Sep 15;15(6):1497-506.

[40] Steinhorn RH. Therapeutic approaches using nitric oxide in infants and children. Free radical biology & medicine. 2011 Sep 1;51(5):1027-34.

[41] Stayer SA, Liu Y. Pulmonary hypertension of the newborn. Best practice & research. 2010 Sep;24(3):375-86.

[42] Simonneau G, Galie N, Rubin LJ, Langleben D, Seeger W, Domenighetti G, et al. Clinical classification of pulmonary hypertension. Journal of the American College of Cardiology. 2004 Jun 16;43(12 Suppl S):5S-12S.

[43] Barnett CF, Hsue PY, Machado RF. Pulmonary hypertension: an increasingly recognized complication of hereditary hemolytic anemias and HIV infection. Jama. 2008 Jan 23;299(3):324-31.

[44] Machado RF, Gladwin MT. Pulmonary hypertension in hemolytic disorders: pulmonary vascular disease: the global perspective. Chest. 2010 Jun;137(6 Suppl):30S-8S.

[45] Morris CR, Kuypers FA, Kato GJ, Lavrisha L, Larkin S, Singer T, et al. Hemolysis-associated pulmonary hypertension in thalassemia. Annals of the New York Academy of Sciences. 2005;1054:481-5.

[46] Shaul PW. Regulation of endothelial nitric oxide synthase: location, location, location. Annual review of physiology. 2002;64:749-74.

[47] Barr FE, Tirona RG, Taylor MB, Rice G, Arnold J, Cunningham G, et al. Pharmacokinetics and safety of intravenously administered citrulline in children undergoing congenital heart surgery: potential therapy for postoperative pulmonary hypertension. The Journal of thoracic and cardiovascular surgery. 2007 Aug;134(2):319-26.

[48] Smith HA, Canter JA, Christian KG, Drinkwater DC, Scholl FG, Christman BW, et al. Nitric oxide precursors and congenital heart surgery: a randomized controlled trial of oral citrulline. The Journal of thoracic and cardiovascular surgery. 2006 Jul;132(1): 58-65.

[49] Lopez BL, Liu GL, Christopher TA, Ma XL. Peroxynitrite, the product of nitric oxide and superoxide, causes myocardial injury in the isolated perfused rat heart. Coronary artery disease. 1997 Mar-Apr;8(3-4):149-53.

[50] Farrow KN, Lakshminrusimha S, Reda WJ, Wedgwood S, Czech L, Gugino SF, et al. Superoxide dismutase restores eNOS expression and function in resistance pulmonary arteries from neonatal lambs with persistent pulmonary hypertension. American journal of physiology. 2008 Dec;295(6):L979-87.

[51] Farrow KN, Groh BS, Schumacker PT, Lakshminrusimha S, Czech L, Gugino SF, et al. Hyperoxia increases phosphodiesterase 5 expression and activity in ovine fetal pulmonary artery smooth muscle cells. Circulation research. 2008 Feb 1;102(2):226-33.

[52] Lakshminrusimha S, Russell JA, Wedgwood S, Gugino SF, Kazzaz JA, Davis JM, et al. Superoxide dismutase improves oxygenation and reduces oxidation in neonatal pulmonary hypertension. American journal of respiratory and critical care medicine. 2006 Dec 15;174(12):1370-7.

[53] Lakshminrusimha S, Russell JA, Steinhorn RH, Ryan RM, Gugino SF, Morin FC, 3rd, et al. Pulmonary arterial contractility in neonatal lambs increases with 100% oxygen resuscitation. Pediatric research. 2006 Jan;59(1):137-41.

[54] Lakshminrusimha S, Russell JA, Steinhorn RH, Swartz DD, Ryan RM, Gugino SF, et al. Pulmonary hemodynamics in neonatal lambs resuscitated with 21%, 50%, and 100% oxygen. Pediatric research. 2007 Sep;62(3):313-8.

[55] Sibai B, Dekker G, Kupferminc M. Pre-eclampsia. Lancet. 2005 Feb 26-Mar 4;365(9461):785-99.

[56] Khalil A, Muttukrishna S, Harrington K, Jauniaux E. Effect of antihypertensive therapy with alpha methyldopa on levels of angiogenic factors in pregnancies with hypertensive disorders. PloS one. 2008;3(7):e2766.

[57]   Podymow T, August P. Update on the use of antihypertensive drugs in pregnancy. Hypertension. 2008 Apr;51(4):960-9.

[58]   Lindheimer MD, Taler SJ, Cunningham FG. Hypertension in pregnancy. J Am Soc Hypertens. 2010 Mar-Apr;4(2):68-78.

[59]   Thadhani R. Inching towards a targeted therapy for preeclampsia. Hypertension. 2010 Feb;55(2):238-40.

[60]   Sachdeva P, Patel BG, Patel BK. Drug use in pregnancy; a point to ponder! Indian journal of pharmaceutical sciences. 2009 Jan;71(1):1-7.

[61]   Myatt L, Webster RP. Vascular biology of preeclampsia. J Thromb Haemost. 2009 Mar;7(3):375-84.

[62]   Escudero C, Sobrevia L. A hypothesis for preeclampsia: adenosine and inducible nitric oxide synthase in human placental microvascular endothelium. Placenta. 2008 Jun;29(6):469-83.

[63]   Lopez-Jaramillo P, Arenas WD, Garcia RG, Rincon MY, Lopez M. The role of the L-arginine-nitric oxide pathway in preeclampsia. Therapeutic advances in cardiovascular disease. 2008 Aug;2(4):261-75.

[64]   Rytlewski K, Olszanecki R, Korbut R, Zdebski Z. Effects of prolonged oral supplementation with l-arginine on blood pressure and nitric oxide synthesis in preeclampsia. European journal of clinical investigation. 2005 Jan;35(1):32-7.

[65]   Benedetti G, Morais KL, Guerreiro JR, de Oliveira EF, Hoshida MS, Oliveira L, et al. Bothrops jararaca peptide with anti-hypertensive action normalizes endothelium dysfunction involved in physiopathology of preeclampsia. PloS one. 2011;6(8):e23680.

[66]   Lowe DT. Nitric oxide dysfunction in the pathophysiology of preeclampsia. Nitric Oxide. 2000 Aug;4(4):441-58.

[67]   Schulz E, Jansen T, Wenzel P, Daiber A, Munzel T. Nitric oxide, tetrahydrobiopterin, oxidative stress, and endothelial dysfunction in hypertension. Antioxidants & redox signaling. 2008 Jun;10(6):1115-26.

[68]   Noris M, Todeschini M, Cassis P, Pasta F, Cappellini A, Bonazzola S, et al. L-arginine depletion in preeclampsia orients nitric oxide synthase toward oxidant species. Hypertension. 2004 Mar;43(3):614-22.

[69]   Ianzer D, Santos RA, Etelvino GM, Xavier CH, de Almeida Santos J, Mendes EP, et al. Do the cardiovascular effects of angiotensin-converting enzyme (ACE) I involve ACE-independent mechanisms? new insights from proline-rich peptides of Bothrops jararaca. J Pharmacol Exp Ther. 2007 Aug;322(2):795-805.

[70]   Saheki T, Kobayashi K, Iijima M, Horiuchi M, Begum L, Jalil MA, et al. Adult-onset type II citrullinemia and idiopathic neonatal hepatitis caused by citrin deficiency: in-

volvement of the aspartate glutamate carrier for urea synthesis and maintenance of the urea cycle. Molecular genetics and metabolism. 2004 Apr;81 Suppl 1:S20-6.

[71] Saheki T, Nakano K, Kobayashi K, Imamura Y, Itakura Y, Sase M, et al. Analysis of the enzyme abnormality in eight cases of neonatal and infantile citrullinaemia in Japan. Journal of inherited metabolic disease. 1985;8(3):155-6.

[72] Saheki T, Ueda A, Hosoya M, Kusumi K, Takada S, Tsuda M, et al. Qualitative and quantitative abnormalities of argininosuccinate synthetase in citrullinemia. Clinica chimica acta; international journal of clinical chemistry. 1981 Feb 5;109(3):325-35.

[73] Saheki T, Ueda A, Iizima K, Yamada N, Kobayashi K, Takahashi K, et al. Argininosuccinate synthetase activity in cultured skin fibroblasts of citrullinemic patients. Clinica chimica acta; international journal of clinical chemistry. 1982 Jan 5;118(1):93-7.

[74] Saheki T, Kobayashi K, Inoue I. Hereditary disorders of the urea cycle in man: biochemical and molecular approaches. Reviews of physiology, biochemistry and pharmacology. 1987;108:21-68.

[75] Gao HZ, Kobayashi K, Tabata A, Tsuge H, Iijima M, Yasuda T, et al. Identification of 16 novel mutations in the argininosuccinate synthetase gene and genotype-phenotype correlation in 38 classical citrullinemia patients. Human mutation. 2003 Jul; 22(1):24-34.

[76] Kawamoto S, Strong RW, Kerlin P, Lynch SV, Steadman C, Kobayashi K, et al. Orthotopic liver transplantation for adult-onset type II citrullinaemia. Clinical transplantation. 1997 Oct;11(5 Pt 1):453-8.

[77] Todo S, Starzl TE, Tzakis A, Benkov KJ, Kalousek F, Saheki T, et al. Orthotopic liver transplantation for urea cycle enzyme deficiency. Hepatology (Baltimore, Md. 1992 Mar;15(3):419-22.

[78] Hoshi N, Mukai S, Oishi M, Takano M, Shinzawa J, Watanabe S, et al. A case of hepatic angiosarcoma supplied by both hepatic artery and portal vein. Fukushima journal of medical science. 2006 Jun;52(1):13-9.

[79] Imamura Y, Kobayashi K, Shibatou T, Aburada S, Tahara K, Kubozono O, et al. Effectiveness of carbohydrate-restricted diet and arginine granules therapy for adult-onset type II citrullinemia: a case report of siblings showing homozygous SLC25A13 mutation with and without the disease. Hepatol Res. 2003 May;26(1):68-72.

[80] Nissim I, Luhovyy B, Horyn O, Daikhin Y, Nissim I, Yudkoff M. The role of mitochondrially bound arginase in the regulation of urea synthesis: studies with [U-15N4]arginine, isolated mitochondria, and perfused rat liver. The Journal of biological chemistry. 2005 May 6;280(18):17715-24.

[81] Gerard JM, Luisiri A. A fatal overdose of arginine hydrochloride. Journal of toxicology. 1997;35(6):621-5.

[82] Batshaw ML, Wachtel RC, Thomas GH, Starrett A, Brusilow SW. Arginine-responsive asymptomatic hyperammonemia in the premature infant. The Journal of pediatrics. 1984 Jul;105(1):86-91.

[83] Walser M, Batshaw M, Sherwood G, Robinson B, Brusilow S. Nitrogen metabolism in neonatal citrullinaemia. Clinical science and molecular medicine. 1977 Aug;53(2): 173-81.

[84] Brusilow SW, Valle DL, Batshaw M. New pathways of nitrogen excretion in inborn errors of urea synthesis. Lancet. 1979 Sep 1;2(8140):452-4.

[85] Summar M. Current strategies for the management of neonatal urea cycle disorders. The Journal of pediatrics. 2001 Jan;138(1 Suppl):S30-9.

[86] Iyer R, Jenkinson CP, Vockley JG, Kern RM, Grody WW, Cederbaum S. The human arginases and arginase deficiency. Journal of inherited metabolic disease. 1998;21 Suppl 1:86-100.

[87] Coman D, Yaplito-Lee J, Boneh A. New indications and controversies in arginine therapy. Clinical nutrition (Edinburgh, Scotland). 2008 Aug;27(4):489-96.

[88] Kobayashi K, Sinasac DS, Iijima M, Boright AP, Begum L, Lee JR, et al. The gene mutated in adult-onset type II citrullinaemia encodes a putative mitochondrial carrier protein. Nature genetics. 1999 Jun;22(2):159-63.

[89] Closs EI. Expression, regulation and function of carrier proteins for cationic amino acids. Current opinion in nephrology and hypertension. 2002 Jan;11(1):99-107.

[90] Smith CG, Vane JR. The discovery of captopril. Faseb J. 2003 May;17(8):788-9.

[91] Smith CG, Vane JR. The discovery of captopril: a reply. Faseb J. 2004 Jun;18(9):935.

[92] Angus DC, Linde-Zwirble WT, Tam SW, Ghali JK, Sabolinski ML, Villagra VG, et al. Cost-effectiveness of fixed-dose combination of isosorbide dinitrate and hydralazine therapy for blacks with heart failure. Circulation. 2005 Dec 13;112(24):3745-53.

[93] Beckman JS. Ischaemic injury mediator. Nature. 1990 May 3;345(6270):27-8.

[94] Lipton SA, Choi YB, Pan ZH, Lei SZ, Chen HS, Sucher NJ, et al. A redox-based mechanism for the neuroprotective and neurodestructive effects of nitric oxide and related nitroso-compounds. Nature. 1993 Aug 12;364(6438):626-32.

[95] Cheung HS, Cushman DW. Inhibition of homogeneous angiotensin-converting enzyme of rabbit lung by synthetic venom peptides of Bothrops jararaca. Biochim Biophys Acta. 1973 Feb 15;293(2):451-63.

[96] Shen TT, Bogdanov A, Jr., Bogdanova A, Poss K, Brady TJ, Weissleder R. Magnetically labeled secretin retains receptor affinity to pancreas acinar cells. Bioconjugate chemistry. 1996 May-Jun;7(3):311-6.

[97] Uekama K, Hirayama F, Irie T. Cyclodextrin Drug Carrier Systems. Chemical reviews. 1998 Jul 30;98(5):2045-76.

Permissions

The contributors of this book come from diverse backgrounds, making this book a truly international effort. This book will bring forth new frontiers with its revolutionizing research information and detailed analysis of the nascent developments around the world.

We would like to thank Hany El-Shemy, for lending his expertise to make the book truly unique. He has played a crucial role in the development of this book. Without his invaluable contribution this book wouldn't have been possible. He has made vital efforts to compile up to date information on the varied aspects of this subject to make this book a valuable addition to the collection of many professionals and students.

This book was conceptualized with the vision of imparting up-to-date information and advanced data in this field. To ensure the same, a matchless editorial board was set up. Every individual on the board went through rigorous rounds of assessment to prove their worth. After which they invested a large part of their time researching and compiling the most relevant data for our readers. Conferences and sessions were held from time to time between the editorial board and the contributing authors to present the data in the most comprehensible form. The editorial team has worked tirelessly to provide valuable and valid information to help people across the globe.

Every chapter published in this book has been scrutinized by our experts. Their significance has been extensively debated. The topics covered herein carry significant findings which will fuel the growth of the discipline. They may even be implemented as practical applications or may be referred to as a beginning point for another development. Chapters in this book were first published by InTech; hereby published with permission under the Creative Commons Attribution License or equivalent.

The editorial board has been involved in producing this book since its inception. They have spent rigorous hours researching and exploring the diverse topics which have resulted in the successful publishing of this book. They have passed on their knowledge of decades through this book. To expedite this challenging task, the publisher supported the team at every step. A small team of assistant editors was also appointed to further simplify the editing procedure and attain best results for the readers.

Our editorial team has been hand-picked from every corner of the world. Their multi-ethnicity adds dynamic inputs to the discussions which result in innovative outcomes. These outcomes are then further discussed with the researchers and contributors who give their valuable feedback and opinion regarding the same. The feedback is then collaborated with the researches and they are edited in a comprehensive manner to aid the understanding of the subject.

Apart from the editorial board, the designing team has also invested a significant amount of their time in understanding the subject and creating the most relevant covers. They scrutinized every image to scout for the most suitable representation of the subject and create an appropriate cover for the book.

The publishing team has been involved in this book since its early stages. They were actively engaged in every process, be it collecting the data, connecting with the contributors or procuring relevant information. The team has been an ardent support to the editorial, designing and production team. Their endless efforts to recruit the best for this project, has resulted in the accomplishment of this book. They are a veteran in the field of academics and their pool of knowledge is as vast as their experience in printing. Their expertise and guidance has proved useful at every step. Their uncompromising quality standards have made this book an exceptional effort. Their encouragement from time to time has been an inspiration for everyone.

The publisher and the editorial board hope that this book will prove to be a valuable piece of knowledge for researchers, students, practitioners and scholars across the globe.

List of Contributors

Asli N. Goktug, Sergio C. Chai and Taosheng Chen
High Throughput Screening Center, Department of Chemical Biology and Therapeutics, St. Jude Children's Research Hospital, USA

Sonia Lobo Planey
The Commonwealth Medical College, Scranton, PA, USA

Luis Jesús Villarreal-Gómez
Center of Engineering and Technology, University Autonomous of Baja California, Tijuana, BC., México

Irma Esthela Soria-Mercado
Marine Science Faculty, University Autonomous of Baja California, Ensenada, BC., México

Ana Leticia Iglesias and Graciela Lizeth Perez-Gonzalez
Center of Engineering and Technology, University Autonomous of Baja California, Tijuana, BC., México

Charles J. Malemud
Arthritis Research Laboratory, Division of Rheumatic Diseases, Case Western Reserve University School of Medicine, Cleveland, Ohio, USA

Jie Yanling, Liang Xin and Li Zhiyuan
Guangzhou Institutes of Biomedicine and Health, Chinese Academy of Sciences, China

Karolina Gluza and Pawel Kafarski
Department of Bioorganic Chemistry, Faculty of Chemistry, Wroclaw University of Technology, Wybrzeze Wyspianskiego, Wroclaw, Poland

Samuel Constant, Song Huang, Ludovic Wiszniewski and Christophe Mas
OncoTheis, 14 Chemin des aulx, CH-1228 Plan-les-Ouates, Geneva, Switzerland

Louise L. Major, Helen Denton and Terry K. Smith
Biomedical Sciences Research Centre, The North Haugh, The University, St. Andrews, Fife, Scotland, U.K.

Claudiana Lameu and Henning Ulrich
Department of Biochemistry, Institute of Chemistry, University of São Paulo, São Paulo, Brazil

Printed in the USA
CPSIA information can be obtained
at www.ICGtesting.com
JSHW011436221024
72173JS00004B/820